Contents

Clinical contributors and consultants

Deborah B. Benvenuto, RN, CRNI
Nurse Educator, Intravenous Therapy
Intravenous Nurses Society
Cambridge, Mass.

Kay Coulter, RN, CRNI
Nurse Consultant
Coulter Consulting
Clearwater, Flor.

Noreen Coyne, RN, MSN, CRNI, OCN
National Director of Infusion
Therapy
Staff Builders Homehealth Care
Lake Success, N.Y.

Brenda Dugger, RN, MS, CRNI, CNA
Director Infusion Therapy,
Psychological Services and
Consultation
Saint Joseph's Hospital of Atlanta

Judith O. Fesz, RN, BSN, MN
Advanced Practice Nurse
Community In Home Services of
University of Pittsburgh Medical
Center

Anne Marie Frey, RN, BSN, CRNI
Clinical Nurse—Level Four: I.V.
Team
The Children's Hospital of
Philadelphia

Sandra L. Gilmore, RN, BSN, MS
Advanced Practice Nurse
Community In Home Service of
University of Pittsburgh Medical
Center

Gloria Gotaskie, RN, MSN, OCN
Oncology Clinical Nurse Specialist
University of Pittsburgh Cancer
Institute

Barbara G. Grimes, RN, BSN, JD
Attorney-at-Law
Medlaw Consulting Services
Gulfport, Miss.

Peggi Guenter, RN, PhD, CNSN
Editor-in-Chief
Nutrition in Clinical Practice
Silver Spring, Md.

Lynn C. Hadaway, MEd, RNC, CRNI
Principal
Hadaway & Associates
Milner, Ga.

Sandra J. Hamilton, RN, BSN, MEd,
CRNI
Infusion Specialist and Regional
Coordinator of Pharmacy Nursing
Services
Vencare Pharmacy Services
Boise, Idaho

Virginia Higgins, RN, BSN, MBA
Director, Clinical Application Services
Pall Medical
East Hills, N.Y.

Edward J. Hoey, RN, BSN
Care Team Leader
Thomas Jefferson Home Infusion
Service
Bryn Mawr, Pa.

Debra A. Jarck, RN, MSN, CNS, ACNP,
CCRN
Berkshire Medical Center
Pittsfield, Mass.

Diane S. Komon, RN, CRNI
Manager IV Therapy Team
University of Michigan Health
System
Ann Arbor

Thomas T. Lawson, PhD
Director, Clinical Affairs
RadioTherapeutics Corporation
Mountain View, Calif.

Kathleen A. McGrory, RN
Clinical Support Liaison
Thomas Jefferson University Hospital
Bryn Mawr, Pa.

Doris A. Millam, RN, BSN, MS, CRNI
IV Therapy Consultant and Educator
IV Therapy Resources
Glenview, Ill.

Lynne M. Murphy, RN, MSN, CNSN
Nutrition Support Nurse
Veterans Affairs Medical Center
Washington, DC

Barbara Ross Nolet, RN, MA
President
Northwest Management Associates
Tacoma, Wash.

Darla Pistella-Annonio, RN, BSN, MS
Advanced Practice Nurse
Community In Home Health
Services
McKeesport, Pa.

Carol M. Renner, RN, BSN, CRNI
Manager, Clinical Education Services
Cardio Thoracic Systems, Inc.
Cupertino, Calif.

Deborah Richardson, RN, MS, CNS
Clinical Nurse Specialist
Infusion Therapy Team
M.D. Anderson Cancer Center
Houston

Mary Jo Sikora, RN, BSN, MBA, CRNI
Quality Improvement Manager
MVI Home Care
Girard, Ohio;
President
V.A.L.O.R. Consulting
Poland, Ohio

Cynthia C. Small, RN, BSN, MSN
Medical-Surgical Nursing Instructor
Lake Michigan College
Benton Harbor, Mich.

Donna Ayers Snelson, RN, MSN
Associate Professor
College Misericordia
Dallas, Pa.

Jacquelyn A. Spangler, RN, MSN, CRNI
Director
University of Pittsburgh Medical
Center Home Health
Cheswick, Pa.

Catherine Ultrino, RN, MSN, OCN
Nurse Manager
Boston Regional Medical Center
Stoneham, Mass.

Stacy A. Weigman, MS, PharmD, RPh
Project Manager
Adis International
Langhorne, Pa.

Foreword

The use of the intravenous (IV) route to deliver all types of infusion agents continues to be a mainstay in patient care. Each year, millions of people receive IV medications in a variety of settings, from hospitals to clinics to the patient's home. Tens of thousands of patients have vascular access devices inserted to deliver fluids, medications, blood or blood products, chemotherapy, or parenteral nutrition solutions.

Infusion therapists and other health care providers use approximately 5 million central venous catheters and 200 million peripheral IV catheters each year. Infusion therapy as a specialty becomes increasingly more complex as new infusion devices are created, new facts about IV solutions and medications are released, and new responsibilities emerge for those of us caring for patients who receive one of the many forms of infusion therapy.

Each time you care for such a patient, you need precise information on indications, dosage, preparation and storage, incompatibilities, administration techniques, contraindications and cautions, and the nursing interventions for each IV drug or solution you give. You also need to fully understand the many facets of infusion therapy, such as how to clear an occluded catheter, which blood products are safe for which patients, and why some patients would benefit more from a peripherally inserted central catheter than a tunneled central venous catheter. The *Handbook of Infusion Therapy* provides all that information and more.

The book gives you fast access to crucial details and helps you more safely and effectively administer IV drugs and solutions. It also provides all the background information you need to really understand infusion therapy. Detailing everything from butterfly needles to implanted vascular access devices to transfusions of leukocyte-poor RBCs, and from abciximab to Zovirax, the *Handbook of Infusion Therapy* examines all facets of infusion therapy, and it does it all clearly and simply.

I think you'll find, as I have, that the *Handbook of Infusion Therapy* is a remarkably useful tool for all health care professionals. Whether you're a student, a new graduate, or an experienced nurse, I'm convinced this book will become one of your most treasured resources and your absolute best reference for infusion therapy.

Deborah Richardson, RN, MS, CNS
Clinical Nurse Specialist
Infusion Therapy Team
M. D. Anderson Cancer Center
Houston

How to use *Handbook of Infusion Therapy*

The *Handbook of Infusion Therapy* is divided into four units. The first unit, consisting of four chapters, introduces infusion therapy. Chapter 1 looks at the past, present, and future of infusion therapy. Chapter 2 examines safety issues, such as how to prevent infection and needle-stick injuries as well as how to recognize, prevent, and treat allergic reactions to latex. Chapter 3 probes the legal issues inherent in infusion therapy, such as risk management, standards of competency, the role of unlicensed assistive personnel in infusion therapy, and documentation guidelines. Chapter 4 examines the latest infusion therapy equipment, including administration sets, filters, and infusion delivery devices, from elastomeric pumps to patient-controlled analgesia pumps to implantable infusion pumps.

The second unit covers peripheral and central infusion therapy, with separate chapters on managing therapy using peripheral catheters, midline catheters, PICCs, central venous catheters, vascular access ports, and four main alternative access routes—epidural, intraperitoneal, intraosseous, and subcutaneous. Each chapter covers advantages and disadvantages of that particular type of therapy; how to select a patient, vein, and device for the therapy; how to insert the device; how to maintain and care for the device; complications that might occur and how to handle them; what to teach the patient about the device; how the device is removed; and what documentation guidelines to follow.

The third unit deals with special infusions and includes separate chapters on administering blood and blood products, parenteral nutrition, and chemotherapy. In these chapters, for instance, you'll learn what filters you need to administer leukocyte-poor blood, how to calculate a patient's caloric intake when he's receiving parenteral nutrition, and how to prevent or alleviate the most common complications of chemotherapy.

Throughout the book, you'll find of particular help special sections highlighting the use of infusion therapy equipment. These "Equipment Expertise" sections offer helpful tips for making the most of available infusion therapy devices. You'll also appreciate the "Staying Safe" sections, which outline preventive measures you can take to avoid some of the hazards associated with infusion therapy procedures. And the "Clinical Pearls" sections offer tips gathered from infusion therapy experts around the nation.

The fourth unit is an alphabetical compendium of monographs for virtually all the IV drugs and solutions in use today. The information in each drug entry is organized under standard headings. *Indications & Dosages* gives the indications for IV use of the drug, with dosages for adults and children. It lets you know which drug dosages need to be adjusted for conditions such as renal failure. *Preparation & Storage* tells how the drug is supplied, how to store it, what its shelf life is, and how to reconstitute or dilute it, as appropriate. *Incompatibility* tells what medications shouldn't be mixed with the drug in direct combination. *Administration* gives specific instructions for delivering the drug by the appropriate method: direct injection, intermittent infusion, or continuous infusion. Rates are provided when available. *Contraindications & Cautions* tells what conditions contraindicate use of the drug and when to be especially careful in administering the drug. *Special Considerations,* the final heading, covers key nursing concerns not included elsewhere. Wherever appropriate, this section contains information on the treatment of an overdose. It may also provide tips on drug administration, patient monitoring, therapy modifications for special patients, and patient teaching.

Special symbols denote the availability of trade names in Canada. A solid diamond indicates that the trade name is available in Canada as well as the United States. An open diamond indicates that the trade name is available only in Canada.

You'll also find a pregnancy risk rating with each entry and, where appropriate, the controlled substance schedule. The pregnancy risk category identifies a drug's potential for causing birth defects. It's based on Food and Drug Administration (FDA) ratings, package inserts, and highly respected drug references. Five categories (A, B, C, D, and X) distinguish different levels of risk. Drugs in category A are generally considered safe to use in pregnancy; drugs in category X are generally contraindicated. Drugs with the designation NR are not rated.

The controlled substance schedule is an FDA classification for drugs with a high potential for abuse. Schedule I drugs, such as heroin and LSD, have high abuse potential and no accepted medical use in the United States. Schedule II, III, IV, and V drugs have progressively declining potentials for abuse.

In the book's appendices, you'll find a guide to electrolyte components of IV solutions, nomograms for estimating body surface area in children and adults, a chart highlighting selected infusion therapy products, and a list of postal addresses, Web site addresses, and phone numbers for major infusion therapy organizations. A guide to selected references points you toward other reliable sources of infusion therapy information.

The index lists equipment and procedures discussed throughout the early chapters and the generic and trade names of the IV drugs and solutions.

ABBREVIATIONS

abbreviation	meaning	abbreviation	meaning
ACE	angiotensin-converting enzyme	IND	investigational new drug
ADH	antidiuretic hormone	INR	international normalized ratio
AIDS	acquired immunodeficiency syndrome	IU	International Unit
ALT	serum alanine aminotransferase	IV	intravenous
APTT	activated partial thromboplastin time	kg	kilogram
AST	serum aspartate aminotransferase	L	liter
AV	atrioventricular	LD	lactate dehydrogenase
b.i.d.	twice daily	M	molar
BUN	blood urea nitrogen	m^2	square meter
cAMP	cyclic 3', 5' adenosine monophosphate	MAO	monoamine oxidase
CBC	complete blood count	mcg	microgram
CDC	Centers for Disease Control and Prevention	mEq	milliequivalent
CK	creatine kinase	mg	milligram
CMV	cytomegalovirus	MI	myocardial infarction
CNS	central nervous system	ml	milliliter
COPD	chronic obstructive pulmonary disease	mm^3	cubic millimeter
CPR	cardiopulmonary resuscitation	NaCl	sodium chloride
CSF	cerebrospinal fluid	ng	nanogram (millimicrogram)
CV	cardiovascular	NSAID	nonsteroidal anti-inflammatory drug
CVA	cerebrovascular accident	OSHA	Occupational Safety and Health Administration
D_5W	dextrose 5% in water	OTC	over-the-counter
DIC	disseminated intravascular coagulation	PCA	patient-controlled analgesia
DNA	deoxyribonucleic acid	PO	by mouth
ECG	electrocardiogram	p.r.n.	as needed
EEG	electroencephalogram	PT	prothrombin time
EENT	eyes, ears, nose, throat	PTT	partial thromboplastin time
FDA	Food and Drug Administration	PVC	premature ventricular contraction
g	gram	q	every
G	gauge	q.i.d.	four times daily
GI	gastrointestinal	RBC	red blood cell
G6PD	glucose-6-phosphate dehydrogenase	RDA	recommended daily allowance
GU	genitourinary	RNA	ribonucleic acid
HIV	human immunodeficiency virus	RSV	respiratory syncytial virus
h.s.	at bedtime	SA	sinoatrial
IM	intramuscular	SC	subcutaneous
		SIADH	syndrome of inappropriate antidiuretic hormone
		SL	sublingual
		t.i.d.	three times daily
		U	units
		USP	United States Pharmacopeia
		WBC	white blood cell

I

UNDERSTANDING
INFUSION THERAPY

1

Introduction to infusion therapy

At one time, infusion therapy was essentially synonymous with intravenous therapy, the administration of fluids—from saline solutions to blood to chemotherapeutic agents—through veins. Over the past several decades, though, the term has come to mean much more.

Infusion therapy has grown from nurses using simple butterfly needles and being severely restricted in their scope of practice in this field to the development of long-term IV access and needleless systems, common use of advanced technologies, and a significantly broader scope of practice for nurses in all areas of health care. With the advent of managed care, infusion therapy is being used more and more often in clinics, long-term care facilities, nurse-operated infusion centers, doctor's offices, and even patients' homes.

Regardless of the setting, the nurse is a key figure in the team of professionals devoted to providing improved standards of care and better management of complications. This chapter explores the history of infusion therapy, what infusion therapy means today, and what infusion therapy organizations are doing to help maintain the quality of care provided by infusion specialists throughout the nation.

Definition

Today, the term infusion therapy refers to the therapeutic administration of fluids or drugs to diagnose or treat an illness or to help maintain homeostasis. Of the total number of patients admitted to hospitals throughout the United States, peripheral IV lines are inserted in 80% to 95% of them. Many home care agencies and extended care facilities are noting a surge in the use of infusion therapy as increasingly ill patients are discharged from the hospital to the home or to less acute health care settings.

An understanding of the history of this dynamic and vital specialty can help define the role of infusion therapy nurses in today's health care system.

History

Infusion therapy has gone through many changes in the last century. (See *Highlights of infusion therapy,* page 4.) In 1940, Massachusetts General Hospital became the first hospital in the nation to implement an IV therapy program for its nurses. The period that followed marked the beginning of IV therapy as a specialty.

The duties of the IV nurse specialist at that time included administering IV solutions and transfusions, cleaning administration sets, and sharpening needles. Nurses inserted IV lines, but few IV teams existed anywhere.

The first plastic catheter was invented in 1945 and was later modified by the medical supply firm Becton Dickinson. The catheter, called Intracath, was a through-the-needle device that could remain in place longer than steel needles alone, was more comfortable for the patient, and caused fewer infections. The development of this catheter led to the development of similar catheters during the 1950s and early 1960s. Intracath consisted of a metal needle with a catheter threaded through it, the opposite of today's over-the-needle catheters. A soft plastic sleeve enveloped the catheter. After the needle pierced the lumen of the vein, the catheter was threaded through the needle and into the vein.

Several years after the Intracath was developed, peripherally inserted central catheters (PICCs) were introduced. Inserted in a peripheral vein, then threaded into a central vein, PICCs met the increasing demand for more advanced long-term peripheral venous access devices.

Highlights of infusion therapy

1492	Blood infused from three youths into ailing Pope. All four died.
1638	Heart and circulatory system described by physiologist William Harvey.
1658	Using a quill and a pig's bladder, wine and opium infused into dogs by Christopher Wren.
1664	First infusion of unpurified compounds into humans performed by J.D. Moore.
1667	First successful transfusions made from one animal to another.
1818	First successful transfusion performed by James Blundell.
1830	Gold-plated steel 14G needle developed.
1832	Saline injected by Thomas Latta into 25 victims of cholera as a way of treating the disease.
1855	Hollow needle and syringe invented.
1900	IV saline used as a parenteral fluid in critically ill patients.
1913	Blood transfusions first performed by direct infusion.
1923	Pyrogens discovered in distilled water.
1925	Dextrose given by IV infusion to provide calories.
1933	First IV solutions produced.
1939	Essential amino acids discovered; led to development of protein hydrolysate infusion.
1940	First IV nurse in the United States worked at Massachusetts General Hospital. First intraosseous infusion performed.
1945	First plastic catheter introduced; later became Intracath.
1950	Rochester plastic needle developed by anesthesiology resident at Mayo Clinic. Plastic IV tubing replaces rubber tubing.
1952	Vacuum bottles replaced by plastic bags.
1960	Central line cannulization first described.
1965	Peripherally inserted central catheters first used.
1967	IV hyperalimentation (developed by Stanley Dudrick) first used.
1970	IV teams emerged. Electronic rate controllers and central lines developed.
1971	Recommendations for safe IV therapy made by CDC as a result of an epidemic of infections caused by contaminated IV fluids.
1973	National Intravenous Therapy Association (NITA) formed. Tunneled silicone catheter first inserted by Broviac.
1975	First fat emulsion (Intralipid) approved for use.
1980	Double-lumen Hickman catheter developed. *National Standards of Intravenous Practice* issued by NITA.
1982	Implanted ports introduced.
1985	First credentialing examination offered by NITA.
1986	Patient-controlled analgesia used for first time. Total parenteral alimentation developed.
1987	NITA name changed to Intravenous Nurses Society (INS).
1995	CDC recommendations for preventing intravascular infections revised.
1996	Credentialing examination for LPN/LVN offered by INS.
1998	Revised *Intravenous Nursing Standards of Practice* of the INS published.

Adapted from *Journal of Intravenous Nursing,* courtesy of Lippincott Williams & Wilkins.

Then in 1973, Dr. John W. Broviac created a catheter for long-term use in a central vein. Eventually, Dr. Robert O. Hickman would take Broviac's concept and modify it into what is known today as the Hickman catheter, a popular catheter for long-term use.

During the 1980s, catheter manufacturers developed polyurethane and silicone catheters, which allowed the use of larger central veins, a plus for patients receiving large volumes of fluid and for those who needed monitoring of pressures within a central vein. Implantable ports were developed in the early 1980s. These ports allow long-term use for patients requiring infusion therapy outside the hospital.

Other advances include in-line filters, popular for their ability to remove foreign particles and organisms during an infusion. Portable pumps and controllers fostered the development of such concepts as patient-controlled analgesia, which gives the patient more control over his medication therapy.

Infusion therapy organizations

Numerous infusion therapy organizations currently exist to educate, certify, and recognize the importance of infusion therapy in today's health care environment. Here's a sampling of the more prominent of those organizations.

Intravenous Nurses Society
The National Intravenous Therapy Association was formed in 1973 to provide education and networking opportunities for IV therapy nurses. The association's name was changed to the Intravenous Nurses Society (INS) in 1987, to incorporate "nurses" into the title.

The INS developed the *Intravenous Nursing Standards of Practice,* an authoritative document that outlines standards related to the nurse's scope of practice, educational requirements, clinical management, and the use of access devices for delivering infusion therapy. These standards guide orientation and training programs, define performance criteria, and protect and preserve the patient's right to safe, quality care. The INS began offering certification examinations for IV nurses in 1985.

League of Intravenous Therapy Education
The League of Intravenous Therapy Education (LITE) creates standards of patient care, educates practitioners of infusion therapy, and

identifies guidelines for competence and excellence in the field. LITE believes that all practitioners of infusion therapy should be adequately educated and possess skills beyond those required for state licensure. The group maintains that the establishment of those requirements is the responsibility of the health care provider.

LITE also believes that only practitioners who have successfully met those requirements should be permitted to practice infusion therapy. They contend that all practitioners of infusion therapy have a responsibility to maintain and improve their knowledge, competence, and excellence in practice.

National Association of Vascular Access Networks

The National Association of Vascular Access Networks (NAVAN) is a multidisciplinary association designed to improve patient care as it relates to infusion therapy. NAVAN believes improvement of care occurs through education, research, and the standardization of infusion therapy. NAVAN members include nurses, pharmacists, and physicians as well as account managers, dietitians, technicians, technologists, and sales and industry representatives.

National Home Infusion Association

The National Home Infusion Association (NHIA) was founded to provide information to and representation of professionals participating in infusion therapy. One of the major goals of NHIA is to implement cost-effective methods of providing infusion therapy. Membership in the group consists of nurses, physicians, pharmacists, managers, executives, dietitians, consultants, and reimbursement staff.

Infusion therapy: Today and tomorrow

Infusion therapy is increasingly being used in the home as a means of continuing therapies started in the hospital. Nurse-operated infusion centers are becoming more numerous to handle the growing need for infusion therapy throughout the nation. In addition, regulations passed recently by the Health Care Financing Administration require hospitals to implement outpatient ambulatory infusion centers, a response by the federal government to help contain health care costs.

In the future, infusion specialists will most likely continue to be in high demand. IV teams, still common in many hospitals today, will probably no longer exist as we know them. Instead, infusion specialists will focus on the more technical aspects of infusion therapy and will be increasingly known as vascular access specialists. With so many different types of devices, medications, and supplies available, the vascular access specialist will determine precisely which approach works best for each patient.

Just as they are today, infusion therapy nurses will be required to pursue continuing education in their specialty. The nurse's knowledge and expertise will become more and more imperative for the success of infusion therapy. Nurse educators will be increasingly challenged to teach the hands-on skills and technical knowledge needed to deliver infusion therapy safely.

As insurance companies and regulatory agencies become more involved with monitoring the costs of infusion therapy, so too will the need increase for certification of infusion specialists and more stringent standardizations of practice.

Safety in infusion therapy

Safety is a major concern in infusion therapy, both for the patients receiving the therapy and for the nurses administering it. For patients, principal safety concerns for infusion therapy include the potential for infection, trauma, and errors made by health care workers. For nurses, primary safety risks include injury and disease transmission due to needle puncture. Spills and splashes also pose a threat to nurses, and because standard precautions require the use of gloves when dealing with blood, latex allergies may pose a safety concern for both nurses and patients. This chapter covers each of these potential hazards and what steps nurses can take to minimize risks for themselves and their patients, including how to select safe products.

Risks for patients

Patients stand a direct risk of infection and trauma during infusion therapy and may be exposed to the results of errors in administration, both of medications and infusion fluids. These risks are outlined here.

Infection

Infection related to venipuncture devices is one of the most serious threats to patients receiving infusion therapy, especially immuno-compromised patients. Patients are at risk for sepsis, hepatitis, and HIV infection.

Sepsis

Sepsis can be life-threatening for any patient and is frequently caused by skin contamination or contamination of the hub of an in-fusion device. Skin contamination from short catheters is the most common cause of infection. With long-term vascular access devices (VADs), hub contamination is the most likely source of infection.

Other sources of contamination include extension tubing or T-connectors, glass ampules, injectable medications and medication additives, injection ports on IV tubing, IV fluids, and locking de-vices used as saline or heparin locks.

Besides fungi, the most common organisms associated with catheter-related sepsis are *Escherichia coli, Staphylococcus aureus,* and *Enterobacter.* Because contamination at the entry or exit site is com-mon, facilities that provide infusion therapy should maintain stan-dard treatments for catheter, or line, infections. For example, the protocol when a catheter infection is suspected may involve remov-ing the catheter, culturing its tip, and obtaining blood cultures from both the original and another site. Sometimes the catheter is left in place and the infection treated according to blood culture results.

Nonseptic infections may be treated with IV antibiotics or with urokinase, a drug used to dissolve a catheter thrombus. Septic infec-tions are treated aggressively with IV antibiotics and other support-ive measures, as indicated.

Hepatitis and HIV

The transmission of blood-borne diseases, such as hepatitis B, hep-atitis C, or HIV infection, presents a relatively low risk for patients receiving infusion therapy. Transmission of these diseases from health care workers to patients requires blood-to-blood contact, and documented cases are rare. The risk of transmission of patho-genic organisms through blood transfusions has been slight since stringent screening of blood and blood products began in 1985.

Preventing infection

Hand washing by health care workers is the single most important factor in preventing infection and the transmission of diseases as a result of infusion therapy. Standard precautions, as outlined by OSHA and the CDC, are extremely important for the safety of the patient as well as the nurse. OSHA guidelines for the prevention of transmission of blood-borne pathogens should be followed closely. Infusion therapists should wear gloves when performing venipuncture and using VADs as well as when changing VAD dressings. Gloves should always be changed and hands thoroughly washed between patients and procedures.

Caring for IV sites

The preparation and maintenance of catheter entry sites are critical for preventing infection. Current standards recommend that hair around the venipuncture site should be clipped rather than shaved to prevent skin abrasions that foster the growth of microorganisms. Other recommendations for site preparation include the use of tincture of iodine 1% to 2%, iodophors, 70% isopropyl alcohol, and chlorhexidine.

Site care recommendations vary by catheter, and actual practice varies widely across health care facilities. Standards developed by the Intravenous Nurses Society (INS) suggest changing the site of a peripheral catheter every 48 to 72 hours, depending on the presence of phlebitis and the overall IV infection rate for that facility. Most nurses use 72 hours as the standard frequency for site changes.

Central venous catheters as well as midline, midclavicular, and peripherally inserted central catheters are intended to provide intermediate to long-term vascular access and can be left in place for weeks to months, depending on the type of catheter. Manufacturer recommendations and current literature should serve as guidelines when establishing policies and protocols for dwell time, the frequency of dressing changes, and other care.

Changing solutions and administration sets

To prevent the possible infusion of bacteria that may grow in an IV solution, the IV bag or bottle should be changed every 24 hours. The CDC recommends replacing the bag or bottle and the administration set every 72 hours. The administration set should be changed every 48 hours if a facility has a high incidence of patient phlebitis and infection.

If lipids are mixed in total parenteral nutrition, the tubing should be changed every 24 hours. For a closed system for drug administration, such as an ambulatory infusion pump with a cassette or reservoir, manufacturer's recommendations should be followed.

Trauma

Trauma to the patient's vein or extremity can be caused by a number of factors, many of which are related to insertion error or lack of proper assessment of the site.

Insertion trauma

Repeated attempts at venipuncture may cause bruising, vein trauma, or skin tears, all of which can lead to infection. If the selected vein is too small for adequate blood flow around the catheter, blood flow to the distal extremity may be decreased or cut off entirely. Placing a catheter in an area of flexion may decrease the length of time the catheter remains patent and cause mechanical phlebitis that may result in infection or the formation of a thrombus. This outcome is of particular concern in an outpatient setting, where patients are more active and more likely to use the extremity in which a catheter has been inserted.

When catheters are not anchored securely, mechanical phlebitis or infection may occur from the to-and-fro motion of the catheter inside the vein, which can also introduce pathogens. In addition, the catheter itself can migrate further into the vein, a particularly dangerous consequence of the use of a longer catheter, whose tip lies close to the heart, thus increasing the risk of systemic or cardiac infection or cardiac irritation.

Infusion trauma

Trauma to the vein can also occur during rapid infusion of fluid volumes too large for the vein, from hyperosmolar drugs and solutions, or from solutions with a high or low pH. Tissue damage and loss of an entire extremity can result when vesicants are infused through a line that has slipped out of a vein, allowing the drug to infiltrate the surrounding tissue. Infusion trauma must be considered with all therapy but is of greatest concern with chemotherapeutic agents, which are known vesicants.

Bleeding from either a venous access site or a severed catheter is a potential threat, particularly if the patient is being treated with anticoagulants or has thrombocytopenia or a clotting disorder.

Preventing trauma

Catheters must be chosen wisely to minimize the risk of trauma. (Proper catheter and site selection are enhanced by the experience and education of the nurse.) In addition, selections of the pH and osmolality of the solution to be infused, the delivery device, and the infusion rate should all be carefully considered. Proper selection of these elements can help to prevent trauma to patients, including ambulatory patients who are receiving infusion therapy in outpatient or home settings.

Patient education also plays a role in preventing traumatic injuries related to infusion therapy. Infusion specialists should understand the importance of teaching patients about, among other things, proper site care, avoiding the use of scissors near the line, and keeping site dressings clean and dry.

Errors in medication administration

Most medication administration errors occur when a nurse or pharmacist fails to follow one of the Five Rights: right patient, right drug, right route, right dose, and right time. Errors related to infusion therapy can have devastating consequences for the patient.

Nurses need to take responsibility for more than just venipuncture when managing infusion therapy. Knowledge about the appropriateness of therapy, the patient's condition and allergies, desired rate of administration, drug actions, adverse effects, incompatibilities, contraindications, and potential localized skin reactions from caustic drugs can help protect the patient.

Monitoring IV sites is also crucial in preventing severe infiltrations, phlebitis, and interruptions of the infusion. Constant vigilance by the nurse can help ensure the patient's safety.

Risks for nurses

Injuries from sharp devices pose the greatest safety threat to infusion therapy nurses. A simple miscalculation by the nurse can cause a needle or other sharp object to puncture the nurse's skin. Blood-borne pathogens can then pass from the needle to the nurse's bloodstream, a potentially disastrous consequence of a needle stick.

Needle-stick injuries

Although needle-stick injuries may occur when inserting a needle or catheter, most occur after the puncture has been completed. Needle-stick injuries can happen when placing a used needle into a container that holds sharp implements, or "sharps." Needles that haven't been properly disposed of, such as those left on a chair or bed, under a piece of equipment, or sticking out of an already full disposal unit, may also pose a threat. Needle sticks can occur when removing a needle-containing device, injecting medication, removing a needle from an implanted port, flushing a catheter, or handling blood samples.

Large-gauge, hollow-bore needles used as stylets for catheter insertion, butterfly needles, solid-core suture needles, and noncoring needles used for implanted port access all pose significant risks to the nurse. Needles that involve less risk but that still warrant cautious use include connection needles and needles attached to syringes used to flush catheters or administer medications.

Major risks

The greatest risk of needle sticks involves the transmission of bacteria, viruses, or fungi from an infected patient to the health care worker. Exposure to blood through spills or splashes during vascular access procedures also poses a high risk to nurses.

Diseases most often transmitted to the nurse through exposure to the blood of an infected patient include viral hepatitis, particularly hepatitis B and hepatitis C, and HIV infection. Cases of HIV transmission through needle sticks are less common than they were several years ago because of the precautions instituted to prevent such injuries.

The risk of all infections increases if a needle stick involves deep penetration with a blood-filled, hollow-bore needle such as those used in establishing venous access.

Preventing needle-stick injuries

Preventing needle-stick injuries and injuries from other sharps should be part of the overall safety plan and standards of practice in any setting where infusion therapy is provided. All personnel should follow OSHA standards and CDC guidelines for infusion therapy for preventing the transmission of blood-borne pathogens.

Staff education and routine testing on safety standards are mandatory in most facilities and should be provided at least once a year. Employers are required by OSHA to offer a hepatitis B vaccine, free of charge, to all employees at risk for blood exposure. Direct preventive measures, including standard precautions, proper disposal of sharps, and the use of needleless systems, can be taken as well to minimize the risk of needle-stick injuries.

Standard precautions

Standard precautions involves handling all blood and known or potentially infectious materials as if the materials are in fact infected.

STAYING SAFE

Standard precautions

The CDC has issued standard precautions for preventing undue exposure to contaminants. This list summarizes these standard precautions.

- Handle all body fluids and potentially bloody substances as if they were infectious, regardless of the patient's diagnosis.
- Wash your hands immediately if they become contaminated with blood or bodily fluids. Wash your hands before and after caring for the patient and after removing gloves.
- Wear gloves if you could come into contact with blood, bodily fluids, or contaminated surfaces or objects.
- Handle used needles carefully. Do not bend, break, or reinsert them into their original sheaths or handle them unnecessarily. Discard the needles intact into an impervious disposal box immediately after use.
- Immediately notify your employee health provider of all needle-stick accidents or contamination of open wounds with blood or bodily fluids.
- Promptly clean all blood and bodily fluid spills with a 1:10 dilution of bleach to water (mixed daily) or with an approved disinfectant effective against hepatitis B virus and HIV.

(See *Standard precautions.*) Gloves, goggles, and barrier gowns (which protect against spills and splashes) that meet OSHA standards should be available at all times and consistently used as required when managing patients receiving infusion therapy.

In addition, puncture-resistant, well-designed disposal units should be conveniently placed in all areas where venipuncture is performed. These units should be discarded when full and locked to prevent access by patients and other non-health care personnel.

Disposal of sharps

To prevent accidental injuries, always dispose of used needles immediately. Needles left in a bed or on a chair after a venipuncture or other infusion procedure may expose patients, visitors, and other health care workers to significant risk. Nurses should *never* recap used needles and should teach the same precaution to patients and family members who administer drugs at home.

Although recapping devices are available to make recapping a needle safer, the most prudent policy remains to dispose of uncapped needles in a puncture-resistant container, avoiding risk completely. Bending or breaking needles is *never* safe.

EQUIPMENT EXPERTISE

Components of a needleless system

The risk of needle-stick injuries can be reduced by using a needleless system. One type consists of a blunt-tipped plastic insertion device and a rubber injection port (below, left). The port contains a slit that can open and then reseal immediately. Another type does not require any adaptors (below, right). A needleless system can be used to give piggyback infusions with a heparin or saline lock.

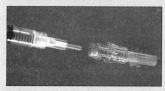 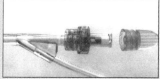

Photos courtesy of Becton Dickinson (left) and Abbott Laboratories (right).

Needleless systems to reduce risk

The emergence of HIV infections has significantly increased awareness of the risk of disease transmission from needle-stick injuries. Numerous safety devices and systems are now available to minimize this risk, including the popular needleless system. OSHA guidelines dictate that safety devices such as needleless systems be made available to all health care workers at risk. The use of these devices is not mandated, however, which leaves the decision for which devices to use up to individual health care facilitys.

Many needleless devices are available, including those that can be used to connect infusion tubing to a catheter or other VAD, draw blood from a vascular access port, transfer a blood sample from a syringe to a specimen tube, transfer medication and diluent from a vial, and connect tubing to an extension. A needleless system typically consists of a blunt-tipped insertion device and a corresponding rubber injection port with a slit that opens and reseals immediately. (See *Components of a needleless system.*)

These products are often used together as an integrated system, but many parts of a system can be adapted to fit other pieces of equipment, such as medication vials and IV tubing. Catheters designed with a shield to house the stylet after venipuncture are also available to limit exposure to blood-borne pathogens. Blood collection products that offer a closed collection system, from the steel needle to the specimen tube, are also available.

Some of the challenges associated with the widespread adoption of needleless systems include safely integrating the many different methods of stylet removal as well as the cost of these systems and the concern expressed by the CDC that use of the devices is associated with an increase in catheter infections.

Despite these concerns, many organizations have adopted needleless systems to minimize risk for their staff, patients, and personnel involved in infectious waste disposal. Hospitals and other health care facilities should initiate blood exposure protocol prior to adopting needleless systems and ensure that the staff is informed about procedures to follow when exposure occurs.

Caring for a needle-stick injury

After exposure from a needle stick or blood splash, clinical risk must be evaluated and the exposed health care worker properly treated. (See *OSHA guidelines for exposure.*) Decisions regarding treatment of exposed health care workers and patients should be made between the exposed individual and an informed, experienced doctor. Evaluation and treatment are personal and sensitive processes that require discretion and complete confidentiality.

Initial treatment

If the needle involved isn't contaminated, basic cleaning of the wound and tetanus prophylaxis, if indicated, will most likely prove adequate. However, if the person was directly exposed to a patient's blood or other bodily fluids, further action is required.

For those cases, the wound or area of exposure should be cleaned thoroughly. Tetanus prophylaxis should be given, if indicated. The employee should also be tested for hepatitis B surface antigen, hepatitis B core antibodies, hepatitis C, and HIV to determine baseline values. The employee has the right to refuse such tests.

Follow-up care

The employer is required to offer confidential medical evaluation and follow-up care at no charge. The exposed individual should be counseled by a knowledgeable doctor regarding the risk of transmission of hepatitis B and C viruses and HIV, depending on the circumstances.

The history and status of the patient at the source of the contamination should be evaluated by a doctor to determine if additional testing and precautions are necessary. (See *Treating exposure to*

STAYING SAFE

OSHA guidelines for exposure

OSHA has issued instructions for employers when an employee has been exposed to blood or bodily fluids. These instructions should be taken into account, along with individual state or insurance requirements, when treating an exposed individual. This chart lists the special instructions according to the individuals and facilities involved. Note that all actions taken by the health care professional should remain confidential, except for sending a written opinion to the employer.

EMPLOYEE	EMPLOYER	HEALTH CARE PROFESSIONAL (HCP)
• Reports incident to employer. • Receives copy of written opinion of HCP.	• **Directs employee to HCP.** • Sends these reports to HCP: – Copy of standard – Job description of employee – Incident report (route, circumstance, etc.) – Source individual's HBV/HIV status (if known) – Employee's HBV vaccine status and other relevant medical information. • Documents events on OSHA 200 and 101 forms, if applicable. • Receives written opinion from HCP. • Provides copy of HCP's written opinion to employee within 15 days of completed evaluation.	• Evaluates exposure incident. • Arranges for testing of employee and source individual (if appropriate). • Notifies employee of results of all testing. • Provides counseling as needed. • Provides postexposure prophylaxis. • Evaluates reported illness. • Sends to employer written opinion and confirmation only: – That employee was informed of evaluation results and the need for further follow-up, if appropriate – Whether HBV vaccine is indicated, and if so, whether vaccine was received.

blood-borne pathogens, page 18.) Appropriate prophylactic treatment following exposure should be offered as needed. Treatment for HIV, including antiviral medications, should be instituted in accordance with the latest CDC guidelines.

The event should be fully documented in accordance with federal and state OSHA regulations as well as existing facility and employer liability guidelines. Injured individuals should immediately file a record of the needle-stick exposure, including results of baseline tests and counseling and treatment they've received, however slight the exposure. By reporting the incident, the nurse helps to protect her potential ability to collect worker's compensation and other forms of insurance if problems occur later.

STAYING SAFE

Treating exposure to blood-borne pathogens

Treating someone exposed to blood-borne pathogens can be complex, depending on the type of exposure and the pathogen involved. The algorithm below offers general guidelines for handling blood-borne exposures.

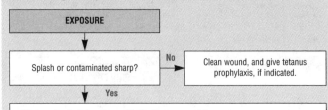

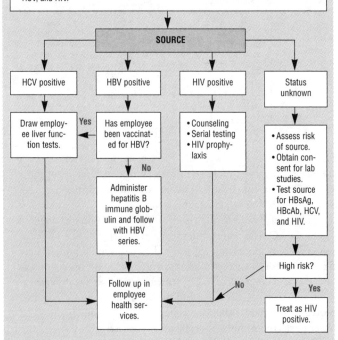

From *Infection Control*, Skidmore-Roth Publishing, Inc., 1996. Adapted with permission.

Latex allergies

Latex allergies have become a serious problem among health care workers at all levels as well as among the lay public. A large number of products contain latex, each of which presents a potential hazard for people with latex allergies no matter where they work. (See *Products containing latex,* page 20.)

Risks and reactions

Individuals at risk include children with spina bifida, patients with congenital urologic abnormalities, and those allergic to bananas, avocados, tropical fruits, and chestnuts. Health care professionals who use gloves frequently or for long periods—particularly people who work in operating rooms, phlebotomists, and emergency department and infusion therapy personnel—face an especially high risk from latex products. All health care workers should understand the potential risk of latex allergies and be able to identify signs and symptoms of typical allergic reactions.

Latex reactions can occur within minutes of an exposure up to 36 to 48 hours afterward. Reactions range from mild, localized urticaria, pruritis, and erythema to generalized urticaria or pruritis, tachycardia, angioedema, dyspnea, bronchospasm, hypotension, and shock.

Preventing latex allergies

All health care facilities should develop policies and procedures that determine measures to protect staff and patients from latex exposure and outline a treatment plan for latex reactions. Protective measures include having latex-free products available and teaching staff members how to identify a latex allergy, what alternative equipment may be used, and what allergy treatments are available. Each patient care unit should stock a tray or box containing latex-free items to use when a patient or staff member is allergic to latex.

Many facilities no longer use latex products for *any* patient, regardless of whether the patient is allergic to latex. Rubber caps, rubber injection ports on tubing, and rubber tourniquets are now available for use. Institutions are required to make these products available to latex-sensitive health care workers. Many manufacturers are now working to eliminate latex entirely from their product lines.

Products containing latex

A wide assortment of patient care products contain latex. Many of those products are used frequently in infusion therapy. Here's a partial list of commonly used products that contain latex:

- absorbent bed pads
- adapters and needleless systems
- adhesive strips
- adhesive tape
- airways
- anesthesia bags and circuits
- blood pressure cuffs
- bulb syringes
- Buretrols
- condom catheters
- dental bite blocks
- dental dams
- disposable hats, shoe covers, and masks used in surgery
- disposable syringes
- drains (rubber and Penrose)
- dressings
- elastic bandages
- electrocardiographic electrode pads
- endotracheal tubes
- enema tips
- face masks
- finger cots
- gastrostomy tubes
- gloves
- handheld resuscitation bags
- heparin or saline lock adapters
- indwelling urinary catheters
- IV bags, latex injection ports
- IV pumps (cassettes)
- IV tubing, latex injection ports
- medication pumps
- multidose medication vials
- nonsterile examination gloves
- orthodontic elastics
- rectal pressure catheters
- rubber suction catheters
- rubber stoppers for medication vials
- sterile surgical gloves
- stethoscope tubing
- straight catheters
- syringes
- tape
- tooth protectors
- tourniquets
- urodynamic catheters
- ventilator bellows
- wheelchair wheels and cushions.

Selecting safe products

Infusion nurses are frequently asked to review a range of products for potential use in their health care facility. Those products may include tape, solutions, catheters, insertion kits, dressings, flush devices, blood drawing implements, safety systems, and delivery devices, such as tubings and pumps.

The selection of each infusion product should be based on the thoughtful evaluation of the product's quality, the safety needs of the facility, and the safety needs of a particular patient population. The setting in which patient care takes place, the cost of the devices, and the personal choice of the practitioner should also be considered.

New products may offer significant improvements in patient care and staff efficiency, but they may also need significant staff education to prevent complications resulting from misuse. Those disadvantages may or may not be enough to reject some products for use.

When evaluating a new product, determine whether a similar product that meets the needs of patients and staff is already being used, and if so, what compelling reasons there might be to make a change. Evaluators should ensure that each product meets all patient and employee safety criteria and is compatible with other products already in use.

Proper research can help identify potential user-related problems and safety hazards. Sales representatives and other clinical liaisons for manufacturers can provide literature reviews, contacts with experienced users, educational materials about the product, and product samples. Clinical trials within the organization as well as interviews with other users can be critical when purchase decisions are being made. Reviewers can also investigate journals, newsletters, and Internet sites of such professional organizations as the INS, the National Home Infusion Association, Oncology Nursing Society, and the National Association of Vascular Access Networks.

Legal issues

Nurses today are assuming greater roles and responsibilities for patient care than ever before. Some of the procedures they're performing include administering vesicant drugs, inserting midline catheters and peripherally inserted central catheters (PICCs), and removing certain types of central lines—procedures previously considered to fall within the role of the doctor only. As a result of these expanded nursing responsibilities, nurses are increasingly becoming targets for litigation when things go wrong.

The legal basis for nursing practice in infusion therapy is determined by the state nurse practice acts, joint policy statements, and institutional policy, which protect you legally as long as you practice within the limitations set up. Nurses practicing infusion therapy may expose themselves to malpractice litigation stemming from improper documentation, failure to follow informed consent procedures, or participating in substandard IV site care.

This chapter focuses on the legal issues involved in risk management, standards of competency, use of unlicensed assistive personnel, documentation, informed consent, and patient education.

Risk management

Risk management for health care facilities is designed to prevent or minimize liability through the use of highly developed risk-reduction strategies. Here's a brief look at fundamental strategies.

Identifying risks

The first step in risk management is to identify those high-risk activities likely to be the subject of litigation or the loss of property, income, or personnel. Identifying these activities can be complicated and may require input from personnel throughout the facility.

Individuals charged with managing risks should estimate potential losses from high-risk activities and determine the steps needed to prevent or minimize loss from those activities. For example, the risk manager should assess the losses that could occur if a nurse sticks herself while putting a used needle in an overfilled needle box.

For such cases, courts often use risk-versus-utility tests to determine whether a risk could have been avoided by alleviating the problem and whether the manufacturer's recommendations were adhered to and the facility's policies maintained. Nurses involved in managing risks from infusion therapy need to identify such potential problems and introduce steps to avoid them.

Preventing and reducing loss

Loss prevention and loss reduction techniques focus on lessening the extent of a loss or preventing the likelihood that the loss will occur. For example, risk managers must ask questions about each high-risk activity. Were safe products in place? Were caregivers taught how to use them? Was patient teaching evaluated properly for its effectiveness?

The patient's rights are of utmost importance in creating strategies for reducing loss. For instance, denying a patient's right to refuse treatment or to grant an informed consent is frequently a basis for litigation. Infusion therapy nurses should always consider the patient's rights as they relate to infusion therapy and make clinical decisions in light of those rights.

Understanding malpractice claims

Many nurses assume that any deviation from normal standards of care can form a basis for negligence, but in fact, deviations need to meet certain criteria before they can reasonably form a basis for negligence. Minimal deviations in practice occur on a regular basis. For example, standing hospital procedures might dictate that skin should be cleaned for 30 seconds prior to inserting an infusion catheter. During a cardiac arrest, however, the skin may be cleaned—appropriately so—for only 2 or 3 seconds. In such cases, no harm occurs.

Deviations that cause harm, however, can form a basis for a claim of negligence. If a malpractice or professional liability claim is filed based on negligence, the person filing the claim (the plaintiff) needs to prove:
• that there was a duty owed by the defendant to the plaintiff
• that the defendant breached a duty by deviating from an accepted standard of care
• that the breach of that duty was the direct, or proximate, cause of damages to the plaintiff
• that damage actually resulted from the breach.

Assault and battery, false imprisonment, and breach of confidentiality can also be cause for patients to bring suit against infusion therapy nurses or the facilities that employ them. For example, if a nurse inserts an infusion device against the wishes of the patient, the nurse could be held liable for assault and battery. If the patient is critically ill and confused, however, it may be necessary to administer emergency medications through an IV line. In such cases, the nurse or the health care facility may need to prove that the greater good at that point was to establish an IV line to deliver lifesaving medications.

Standards of competency

Standards of competency form the foundation for proving a breach of duty in negligence actions. Competency standards—a set of minimum requirements for safe nursing practice—are determined by experts and are based on what any other reasonable, prudent nurse of the same educational level and background would do under the same or similar circumstances.

For example, if a licensed practical nurse (LPN) qualified to deliver infusion therapy is sued, her conduct would be measured against what another equally qualified LPN would reasonably have been expected to do under the same or similar set of circumstances. Likewise, if a registered nurse (RN) is sued, she would be judged by the standards of care pertaining to an RN, not to an LPN. Standards of reasonable conduct may be derived from hospital policy, organizational standards of practice or guidelines, federal and state laws, nursing textbooks or professional journals, and that particular state's Nurse Practice Act.

Nurses obtain and maintain competency through adequate training, successful completion of continuing education programs, and membership in professional organizations that promote ongoing training and provide updated legal, technical, and professional information.

Both RNs and LPNs may legally provide infusion therapy in conjunction with their state's Nurse Practice Act. Individual states may supply broad job responsibilities for these nurses, leaving specific standards to organizations whose mission it is to advance optimal standards for patient care. For instance, the *Intravenous Nursing Standards of Practice,* created by the Intravenous Nurses Society, designates special educational requirements for nurses who provide infusion therapy.

Use of unlicensed assistive personnel

The issue of using unlicensed assistive personnel (UAP) to deliver infusion therapy is becoming increasingly important. Regulation of UAPs and determinations of their roles in infusion therapy are still being debated.

Regulating UAPs

State governments have the authority to regulate UAPs, but many neither license nor certify these individuals. State nursing boards might be allowed to exert little or no disciplinary authority over UAPs.

Some attempts have been made to control the use of UAPs through regulations of individual health care facilities. In addition, certain standards have been established to help define which duties RNs may legally delegate to UAPs. Right now, standards exist for nursing assistants who work in nursing homes that receive Medicaid funding, but the standards don't cover UAPs.

UAP responsibilities in infusion therapy

Infusion therapy organizations agree that the use of UAPs in delivering infusion therapy should be strongly discouraged because of the high risks inherent in infusion therapy. In some instances, nursing assistants may appropriately prepare equipment (such as setting up IV trays), record statistics (such as intake and output), monitor IV sites, and discontinue IV lines.

The current consensus, however, is that UAPs should not be allowed to practice infusion therapy because they lack the education necessary to carry out core competencies safely. Specifically, UAPs should not:

• administer medications
• convert infusions to heparin locks
• hang piggybacks and solutions
• insert a catheter
• manage central lines
• regulate IV rates.

To avoid legal problems inherent in the use of UAPs in infusion therapy, policies and procedures regarding all aspects of infusion therapy should be clearly defined by each health care facility and accompanied by appropriate education.

Documentation

The importance of documenting precisely, accurately, and completely, and of creating a record that assists with the recollection of events and substantiates the care provided cannot be overemphasized. Information contained in the chart serves as the nurse's most important legal protection and often the *only* protection in malpractice cases.

This section discusses documenting procedures, how to avoid common legal pitfalls, and methods of charting.

Documenting procedures

The infusion therapy nurse should always document all procedures performed, including the initiation, monitoring, and discontinuation of an infusion. (See *Documenting an infusion therapy procedure.*) Without adequate documentation, even the brightest, most skilled nurse may not remember what she did for a patient 2 or 3 years after a treatment was administered. At trial, the patient's medical record may be the nurse's best and *only* defense.

Many other aspects of nursing care—from complications to assessment to adherence to facility policies—must be documented accurately and completely.

Documentation for any infusion therapy procedure should include certain basic information about the procedure and its conse-

Documenting an infusion therapy procedure

Precise, accurate documentation about infusion therapy is critical for avoiding legal problems and for more effective communication among staff members caring for the patient. This list summarizes the information that should be contained in each notation related to initiating, monitoring, and discontinuing an infusion.

INITIATING	MONITORING	DISCONTINUING
• Site chosen • Condition of the insertion site before and after insertion (bruising, burns, and other observations) • Type of cannula used • Length and gauge of the cannula • Time and date of insertion • Number of attempts at cannulation • Name and title of the individual responsible for the insertion • Type of medication administered • Flow rate	• Condition of the insertion site and surrounding area • Flow rate • Type of medication being administered • Intake and output • Description of any complications as well as what was done about the complications • Name and title of the individual making the assessment	• Condition of the site and surrounding area • Condition of the cannula upon removal (documented only if a problem occurred) • Reason for discontinuation • Date and time of discontinuation • Name and title of the individual removing the infusion device

quences, if any. Each time you document an infusion therapy procedure, keep in mind times of procedures, changes in the patient's condition, complications, and verification of orders.

Times of procedures

Always try to chart exact times of procedures performed. Nurses tend to record notations on the hour or half hour rather than at the precise time of the procedure. Regimented times of notations appear strange to medical records reviewers and plaintiff attorneys. For instance, a nurse might be asked in court, "Tell me, nurse, did you really go into the patient's room at 8:00, 8:15, 8:30, and again at 8:45 to check the IV site?"

When documenting an assessment, review previous assessments and keep these in mind when documenting the latest assessment. An assessment that varies greatly from previous assessments should alert the nurse to a change in the patient's condition. For example, at 8 a.m., the nurse charts, "Slight discomfort at right-hand IV site." At 11 a.m., the nurse inspects the site and notes redness. She suspects the site is becoming phlebitic and removes the IV. Because of the previous notation, the nurse looked for other complications, which helped make her assessment more accurate and the patient's care safer and more effective.

Changes in the patient's condition

Document all changes in the patient's condition and report them promptly and accurately to the primary health care provider. Conversations with the doctor regarding the patient's condition should also be documented in detail. It is never enough to chart that the doctor was notified. If a nurse contacts a patient's doctor, her documentation should include the date and time of the conversation, exactly what was said and done about the situation, and the patient's response to the treatment.

Complications

Always chart complications of infusion therapy. For instance, if you note erythema and edema at an IV site, document the amount of redness and swelling at the site, your nursing interventions, to whom the incident was reported, and what treatment, if any, was ordered.

Verification of orders

When taking a telephone order or charting a verbal order, repeat the order to the doctor or other prescriber to verify accuracy. When faced with a questionable order, consult other health care providers to clarify issues and help determine the most appropriate plan of action. If the treatment is being questioned, verify the order with the nurse manager. If the order seems obviously wrong or potentially harmful, contact senior medical staff. Do *not* carry out the order. You may be held liable for following questionable orders.

Adhering to policies

Always document according to your facility's policies and procedures. For example, always use abbreviations accepted in writing by the facility. Accepted abbreviations may play a significant role in subsequent litigation.

In the discovery phase of the litigation process, an attorney may request a copy of the standard abbreviations accepted by the facility. If the nurse uses other abbreviations, she may be considered to have deviated from the standard of care the employer has established.

Furthermore, if the deviation leads to confusion and ultimately contributes to the injury of a patient, the nurse may be held liable. The nurse risks similar liabilities for not following other policies and procedures of her particular facility.

Documenting patient education

Always chart patient teaching you've done and the patient's response to that teaching. Even though a health care facility may not require a separate signed consent form for infusion therapy, nurses should be aware that patients have a right to know about the procedures being performed on them.

Avoiding common charting errors

Lawsuits can be won by being accurate and complete in every way in your charting and by avoiding common charting errors, from documenting after the fact to charting ahead of time to obliterating entries.

Documenting after the fact

The period of time after a legal problem has arisen is clearly *not* the proper time for nurses or doctors to add statements to a chart. If documentation prior to that time had been scant, an abundance of writing after the fact may serve as a red flag to an investigator and open the staff to charges of a cover-up.

Charting ahead of time

Never chart ahead of time, and always avoid routine charting. Doing either opens the door to accusations of inaccurate charting and the inherent liabilities that may result.

Charting for someone else

Charting for someone else may make the nurse liable for the other person's inappropriate actions or failure to act. Charting for someone else might be permissible if, for example, a nurse actually sees someone else give a medication and knows positively what was given, the exact amount administered, and the time it was given. Even then, though, the practice is risky and should be avoided.

Using unfamiliar terms

Use only familiar terminology. (See *Sample documentation*, page 30.) Charting terms that the nurse doesn't understand or that are used incorrectly implies incompetence.

Sample documentation

Effective charting for infusion therapy covers key aspects of the therapy in a consistent, easily understandable manner. Here are samples written by a nurse about patients receiving various forms of peripheral infusion therapy.

IV start	IV started in right lower cephalic vein with a 20G 1 1/4" Insyte; two attempts. The site prior to and postinsertion was unremarkable. 0.9% NaCl and 20 mEq KCl infused at 125 ml/hour without difficulty.	1053 10/31/98 M. Black, RN
IV site problems	IV in left hand infiltrated; approximately 2 cm size area slightly puffy with no discomfort. IV de'd, and warm pack applied.	1214 4/26/98 M. Black, RN
	Patient pulled out IV in left forearm. Small hematoma at site. Pressure dressing applied for 10 minutes. Restarted in right basilic vein with 20G, 1" Protectiv catheter; two attempts. Site was benign before and after insertion. Lactated Ringers' infused at 75 ml/hour without difficulty.	1632 6/1/98 M. Black, RN
	Routine IV site change not done due to limited vein access. No redness, tenderness, or swelling at IV site.	1129 1/11/98 M. Black, RN
Patient refusal	Patient refused routine IV site change. Left hand IV site has no problems. Patient informed of site rotation policy. Patient states, "Leave it alone. It feels fine."	0812 1/4/98 M. Black, RN
Discharge instructions	Patient instructed to apply warm packs if tenderness at IV site persists and to notify doctor if fever develops or IV site becomes more sore.	1323 2/23/98 M. Black, RN

Voicing internal complaints

Never use the chart to defend the actions or inactions of other staff or to discuss problems with coworkers. The chart is an inappropriate place to complain or place blame.

Obliterating entries

Never erase or obliterate entries in a nurse's note or a doctor's orders. If mistakes are completely covered, they become suspect. The proper way to document a charting mistake is to draw a single line through the erroneous entry, initial the error, and write the word *error.*

Methods of charting

To avoid legal risks in charting infusion therapy procedures, you need to understand three common methods of documentation: computer charting, charting by exception, and checklist charting.

Computer charting

Computer charting has solved many problems with timeliness of documentation, but not all facilities use it. Results from one study indicated that the quality of charting improved significantly when computers were used. Entries were clearly expressed, and the number of planned interventions increased.

Using computers to chart opens the nurse to new issues of confidentiality and security. Confidential information visible on a computer screen may not be easily concealed from visitors or unauthorized personnel. Unauthorized acquisition of confidential information must also be addressed, principally by the network administrator and the appropriate administrators for the facility. Because the security of a facility's computer system may be called into question in court, administrators should take all the precautions necessary to maintain tight control over the content in the charting system.

Charting by exception

Charting by exception generally means that only deviations from normal are charted. (See *Charting by exception,* page 32.) This kind of charting can save time and cause fewer problems with conflicting or unnecessary information. On the other hand, it is sometimes easy to omit essential documentation, which makes charting all unusual occurrences or conditions even more important.

In addition, judges and juries may not be familiar with documentation by exception. Consequently, they might expect more detail than is regularly provided in this type of documentation.

Checklist charting

Checklists are an efficient way of charting. (See *Documenting with a checklist,* page 33.) They allow rapid documentation of a wide vari-

Charting by exception

Infusion therapy can be documented properly when charting by exception. Here's an example of IV-related charting for a single day. In the chart, V denotes a variance and N is normal. Note that any section marked with a V requires further documentation.

Cardiovascular — Normal findings: Temperature 97° to 99° F. Vital signs within established ranges. Normal sinus rhythm (nonpaced). No chest pain. Pulses present and strong. Nonedematous. IV infusion or insertion sites show no induration, redness, or warmth.

8A	12N	4P	8P			
V	V	V	Ⓥ	V	V	V
Ⓝ	Ⓝ	Ⓝ	N	N	N	N

ety of common findings and nursing care procedures. Part of the risk of using checklists involves the nurse's failure to complete them. Some sections of a checklist may not apply to a particular patient. These sections should be documented as "not applicable" rather than left blank. It is important to use the checklist as a supplement to the main chart, rather than a self-contained charting method.

If something unusual occurs, it should be documented completely to avoid confusion. For example, on an IV checklist, "Infiltration" may be checked. The nurse should then include a narrative similar to, "IV site in left hand has infiltrated to an area approximately 6 cm in diameter. No redness, blanching, or hardness. Patient states there is slight tenderness at the site." Charting such events completely provides information for other caregivers and helps the nurse to recall the events later.

Informed consent

Informed consent is a legal term that carries with it a number of subtle definitions. Perhaps the concept is best explained as a patient's acquiescence to a certain treatment or procedure after receiving sufficient information to decide whether or not to proceed. Courts typically judge how much information should be given to the patient based on what information any reasonable, prudent doctor would give under the same or similar circumstances.

Consent for a procedure may be oral or written. Failure to provide sufficient information and obtain voluntary and free consent

Documenting with a checklist

Infusion therapy can be documented clearly using a checklist form. Here's an example of documentation by checklist.

IV THERAPY PROCEDURE RECORD

Diagnosis _____ Allergies _____

Status				Restart rationale				Procedures									Comments	Initials
Date/Time	Routine rounds	Site OK	Checks, start, restart	Infiltration	Phlebitis	Mechanical	Peripheral line >72 hr	Site location	Catheter, gauge/type	Site capped	Flush line	Tubing change	Dressing change	D/C line	Patient response	Patient teaching		

has resulted in lawsuits claiming assault and battery as well as negligence. The nurse may or may not be responsible for obtaining a consent, depending on the procedure to be performed.

Obtaining consent

Consent should always be obtained prior to a procedure except in a life-threatening emergency. Although procedures such as inserting PICCs traditionally haven't required special consent, many home health agencies and other facilities now require consent forms for these procedures because they're considered invasive. Consent should also be obtained before surgery and blood transfusions. The facility is responsible for determining which procedures or treatments require separate consent forms.

For a consent form to be valid, it must be granted by a mentally and legally competent individual who can understand and appreciate the consequences of giving or withholding consent. In any case, a consent must be freely given to be valid. A consent obtained forcibly or while a patient is under duress can be declared void.

With certain exceptions, a minor is not allowed to give consent for procedures or treatment. However, the minor may be able to give consent if no one is available to sign the form. In some emergency cases, a facility administrator can sign the form. In the event that an adult's signature is required, the minor would be considered legally incompetent to grant consent.

For adults unable to understand or appreciate the consequences of giving or withholding consent, consent may be obtained through certain other individuals who have the right to make those decisions. These individuals include conservators, guardians, and persons granted with the power of attorney.

Role of the nurse

In the past, doctors have been expected to provide information to patients that would enable them to make informed decisions regarding their care. If a facility requires a written consent form for infusion therapy, the nurse is responsible for educating the patient about the procedure. For example, in obtaining consent to insert a PICC, the nurse would explain the procedure to the patient and give a complete description of what will be done. The nurse should discuss the potential benefits and risks of the procedure. Finally, the nurse should offer to answer questions about the treatment or procedure.

Nurses may also be responsible for obtaining a signature on a consent form for procedures performed by a doctor, such as insertion of a central venous catheter. Unless the hospital or facility has given the nurse a specific responsibility for teaching patients about doctor-performed procedures, nurses are free to reinforce what the doctor has taught. If a nurse is concerned that a patient doesn't understand the planned procedure, she should express those concerns to the doctor or to the person responsible for informing the patient.

Patient education

Patients are becoming more knowledgeable about health issues and are taking greater responsibility for their own medical care. They expect to be kept informed of their condition, treatment, and prognosis. If these expectations are not met, the patient may feel that his rights have been violated. Such feelings often lead to lawsuits.

Except for emergency situations, patients should always be taught beforehand about procedures being done and the medications they're receiving. They should also be taught about adverse effects to be expected from their drug therapy.

The teaching you provide establishes a general sense of rapport and trust between you and your patient. The patient's family may require information to help them cope with a loved one's medical problems or to assist in patient care. To make your patient education efforts effective and to reduce your risk of legal liability, you need to understand and know how to apply the teaching process.

Teaching process

Patient education may involve simple explanations for the need for infusion therapy or detailed instructions about care of the IV site, prevention of complications, and follow-up care. The teaching process requires a thorough assessment of the patient's learning needs. Skills or information must be imparted effectively and followed by competent and appropriate implementation. Finally, the effectiveness of the teaching method must be evaluated based on the patient's response

When educating the patient, use a method of teaching best suited to meet that patient's needs. For example, if a patient is illiterate or has a limited education, he may be unable to understand complicated written literature. In this situation, employ a more visual or auditory method of teaching, such as using a videotape or an audiocassette explaining the procedure. For any teaching method to be effective, it must be appropriate to the person's level of education and to the situation. To avoid lawsuits and to provide safe and competent infusion therapy, explain procedures and treatments, complications that might arise from a treatment or illness, and general issues dealing with the patient's ability to assist in his own recovery.

Assessing learning abilities

In assessing learning abilities, evaluate the patient's readiness for learning. (See *Assessing learning abilities,* page 36.) Numerous factors affect learning, including physical condition, development, location, language, and educational level of the patient.

Assessing learning abilities

When teaching your patient about infusion therapy, it's important to assess his ability to learn. A chart similar to this one can be used to document your assessment of the patient's learning abilities.

ASSESSMENT OF LEARNING ABILITY

Factors	Comments	Assessed by	Date/ Time
1. Language (spoken, written)			
2. Physical/environmental limitations			
3. Level of comprehension			
4. Readiness to learn			
5. Previous education			
6. Cultural beliefs			

Educational goals

☐ Goal:	☐ Goal met
☐ Goal:	☐ Goal met
☐ Goal:	☐ Goal met
☐ Goal:	☐ Goal met

Discharge planning

☐ Home care referral   ☐ Self-care   ☐ Extended care facility

Physical condition

A physical condition that impairs concentration can interfere with learning. For instance, it would be futile to teach complicated concepts to an extremely anxious patient.

Development

A person's cognitive level of development affects a patient's ability to learn. A more experienced or more mature individual may learn more easily than someone less experienced or younger.

Location

The place where the instructions are being given plays a role in readiness to learn. For example, if there are several people in the room, it may be difficult for a patient to concentrate.

Language

Organized information should be presented in the patient's native language. Using another language, even your native language, can greatly interfere with the patient's learning.

Educational level

A college graduate typically can absorb a higher degree of technical and specialized instruction than can someone with less education. Adapt teaching strategies to correspond with the patient's educational level.

Evaluation of learning

Check to see how well your patient and his family understand your instruction during your teaching and when you're finished. Ask questions frequently or have the patient or caregivers summarize what you've taught. Ask them for a return demonstration, and then check that they're able to perform the procedure properly. Be certain that your patient and caregivers understand everything they must do to administer IV therapy safely and efficiently, and then document the teaching you did and the patient's and caregivers' understanding of that instruction.

By managing risk, adhering to standards of competency, using UAPs appropriately, following proper procedures for documentation, obtaining informed consent, and teaching patients, the nurse can protect herself legally while expanding her infusion therapy responsibilities.

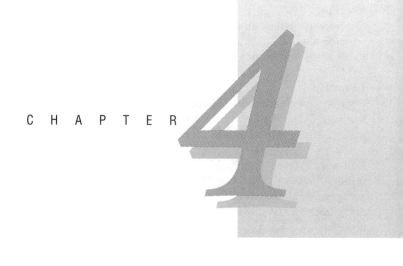

CHAPTER 4

Infusion therapy equipment

Not long ago, infusion solutions came in glass bottles with a rubber stopper and the only way to regulate flow was to adjust a roller device on the tubing. The intervening years have brought a crush of new technologies, heightened in part by an increasingly greater need to protect the patient and nurse from blood-borne pathogens.

To deliver today's infusion therapy, you'll use special connectors, anchoring devices, filters, and numerous kinds of pumps and controllers, to name just a few. This chapter provides an overview of some of the currently available equipment. Types of catheters are discussed in later chapters.

Controllers and pumps

A wide range of increasingly smaller devices are now available for controlling the rate of infusion and reducing the risk of complications. (See *Types of infusion pumps,* pages 40 and 41.) These devices allow for the infusion of IV fluids and medications at precise rates.

They can also monitor the amount of solution infused, prime the IV tubing when needed, and sound an alarm when flow is impeded.

Even though most infusion devices include fail-safe mechanisms to reduce the risk of error, it remains the primary responsibility of the infusion therapy nurse to check that the infusion device is delivering the proper medication in the correct doses at the prescribed rate and in the prescribed volume. The nurse is also responsible for making sure the device used is appropriate for the patient and that it is working properly.

Devices used to regulate infusions include controllers and pumps. Some have special features, including the ability to handle multiple infusions or allow the patient to control his own analgesia.

Controllers

IV controllers are relatively inexpensive and can be used for a variety of infusions, continuous or intermittent. They rely on gravity to assist with the infusion. Controllers can be either nonvolumetric or volumetric.

Nonvolumetric controllers

Nonvolumetric controllers rely on gravity alone to control the rate of infusion, depending on the height of the solution container above the patient, typically 36" (1 m). This height is usually sufficient to overcome venous resistance. These devices use a drop-censoring mechanism to monitor flow and an electric feedback system. When the device detects resistance to flow, it sounds an alarm. The alarm indicates that the controller can't maintain the flow rate, which might mean that the line has infiltrated or become blocked.

These controllers have a low potential for equipment failure. In addition, they require minimal training for staff or patients and their caregivers to operate. However, few controllers can produce sufficient pressure to properly control the flow of heavy or viscous fluids such as blood or to overcome venous pressure caused by the patient simply moving an arm or inadvertently putting pressure in the tubing. In addition, gravity-flow controllers should not be used for central venous lines.

Volumetric controllers

Volumetric controllers also rely on gravity but they also have a vertical peristaltic mechanism that compresses the tubing. This mechanism

(Text continues on page 42.)

EQUIPMENT EXPERTISE

Types of infusion pumps

A number of infusions pumps are available. This chart illustrates and compares some of the pumps currently on the market.

HOMEPUMP, INTERMATE (BAXTER)

Type
Elastomeric pump

Indications
Intermittent and continuous infusions

Advantages
• 50-, 100-, 200-ml size
• Delivers constant rate
• Can attach to belt or rest in pocket so patient can remain ambulatory
• Instruction uncomplicated

Disadvantage
• Fluid may run slowly if not removed from refrigerator 1 hour before infusion

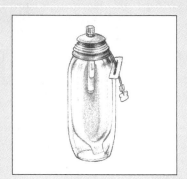

MICROS 4000 (BIOMED)

Type
Bioelectric membrane pump

Indications
Intermittent and continuous infusions

Advantages
• Built-in membrane to filter bacteria and endotoxins
• Good for up to 36 doses over 72 hours
• Heparin in reservoir to maintain patency
• Simple and cost-effective

Disadvantage
• Reservoir holds only 100 ml

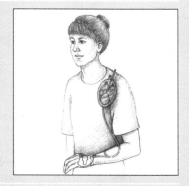

MEDIFUSE (GRASEBY)

Type
Pressure-controlled syringe pump

Indications
Intermittent and continuous infusions

Advantages
• Cost-effective
• No electronics, batteries, rates to set, or drops to count

Disadvantage
• Pump handles only small volumes

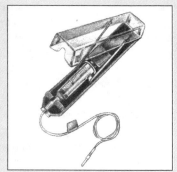

CADD-PLUS, PROVIDER 6000, VERIFUSE, WALKMED 400 (SIMS DELTEC)

Type
Peristaltic action pump

Indications
Intermittent and continuous infusions

Advantages
• Lightweight, portable, battery-operated
• Easily programmed
• Retrievable dosing and infusion data
• Multiple features
• Cassettes last up to 72 hours

Disadvantages
• Patient may have difficulty with programming because of multiple features
• Pump doesn't detect air in tubing
• Pump is expensive
• Some handle only small volumes

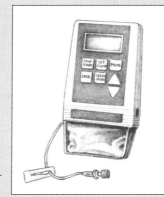

SOLOPAK/PARAGON (SOLOPAK)

Type
Ambulatory infusion pump

Indications
Intermittent and continuous infusions

Advantages
• Easy to fill, store, and carry
• Single-use infusion set
• No noisy motors or batteries

Disadvantage
• Pump handles only small volumes

COLLEAGUE (BAXTER)

Type
Volumetric infusion pump

Indications
Continuous infusions with secondary infusion capabilities

Advantages
• Lightweight, small size
• Event recorder
• Programmable drug library
• Programmable "personalities" for various areas of hospital

Disadvantages
• Pump is expensive
• Patient may find alarm to be loud

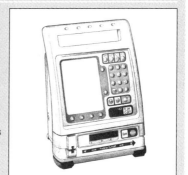

can assist in the flow of solution but can also damage cells if blood or blood products are delivered with the system.

Pumps

Although controllers safely provide for the infusion of a number of IV solutions, they are rapidly being replaced by infusion pumps that use positive pressure to propel solution through the tubing. Infusion pumps permit a level of precision unattainable with controllers. A wide variety of infusion pumps are available, from elastomeric and pressure-controlled pumps to volumetric, syringe, and peristaltic action pumps. In addition, a number of distinctive infusion devices have been developed to handle infusions for patients with special needs.

Elastomeric pumps

An elastomeric pump consists of a bladder reservoir filled with infusate to be delivered. As the bladder collapses, pressure increases and propels the fluid out of the reservoir. The temperature of the infusate can affect the rate of delivery; most pumps require that the solution be at room temperature for accurate delivery.

Elastomeric pumps are designed as single-use, disposable pumps that simplify the patient's need for single-dose infusions of drug solutions. Their small size causes little disruption to the patient's daily activities and so tend to be well-tolerated by active patients.

Pressure-controlled pumps

Pressure-controlled pumps contain a mechanical arm or spring. When tightened, this spring compresses a reservoir containing the solution, which forces the solution out of the reservoir and into the attached tubing. A restriction component of the system controls the rate of flow. Although the mechanism is simple and effective, the range of volumes and flow rates of these pumps is limited.

Volumetric infusion pumps

Volumetric infusion pumps use pressure to move the solution through the tubing at a pre-selected flow rate. They control the flow of the solution completely.

By providing positive pressure, these pumps can overcome resistance caused by filters, viscous fluids, an IV catheter with a narrow lumen, and the resistance created by movement in active patients. To maintain the flow rate specified at the start of the infusion, volumetric pumps increase the pressure of the fluid delivery when resistance builds. The pump will not exert a pressure past a point that could cause rupture of or damage to the IV tubing or catheter.

Syringe pumps

A syringe pump is typically used for the slow but precise infusion of a small volume of IV solution over a long period. For a syringe pump, the nurse places a prefilled syringe in the pump mechanism. The mechanism then presses the plunger at the programmed rate. Such precision offers advantages for infusing small doses of highly potent medications.

Peristaltic pumps

The peristaltic pump is named for the driving force involved—a peristaltic device that propels solution by applying intermittent pressure to the tubing. This device can be either rotary, in which rollers or a disk compress the tubing, or linear, in which one or more "fingers" push against the tubing. As with the volumetric controller, such manipulative action can damage cells if blood is transfused through this pump. Peristaltic pumps are usually used for the infusion of enteral nutritional agents.

Special infusion pumps

Several infusion pumps have been developed recently that allow more precise management of infusion therapy for patients with special needs. These include membrane infusion pumps, patient-controlled analgesia pumps, ambulatory infusion pumps, implantable infusion pumps, special delivery program pumps, and multichannel pumps.

Membrane infusion pumps

A membrane infusion pump, such as a bioelectric membrane pump, is a combination controller and infusion pump. Using gravity and a membrane to propel delivery, the reservoir containing the IV solution (usually under 100 ml in volume) is placed above the tubing. Gravity then moves the solution through the membrane. The membrane filters particulates, bacteria, and endotoxins.

Patient-controlled analgesia pumps

Unlike other infusion pumps, the patient-controlled analgesia pump (PCA) allows the patient to control the infusion; in this case, the delivery of the pain medication, usually morphine. By depressing a button on the pump to initiate a limited infusion of the drug, pain relief can be initiated by the patient. Thus the patient receives the analgesia when needed.

Accidental overdose is prevented because there is an interval during which the PCA pump cannot be activated, usually 6 to 10 minutes after the most recent infusion. PCA pumps result in more complete pain management than with other infusion routes; also, pain is mitigated with less volume of medication infused. PCA pumps are either battery-operated devices activated by the patient pressing a button at the end of a cord, or disposable infusors that contain a collapsible chamber that pushes out the medication after the patient pushes a button on a wrist device.

Ambulatory infusion pumps

Some pumps are compact enough to allow the patient to carry out his normal daily activities without feeling burdened by a pump. Consisting of a small, battery-operated pump, ambulatory pumps are connected to the reservoir of the IV solution with a minimum of tubing. If the volume to be infused is small, most pumps can accommodate the solution in internal storage. If the volume is large, a separate solution container or bag may be required. Either way, the patient is able to go out in public with little disruption or restriction of movement. Ambulatory infusion pumps can provide continuous and intermittent infusion cycles. Some pumps have multiple chambers, allowing simultaneous infusions, each at separate flow rates. Although such diversity is welcome, ambulatory pumps require dedicated administration sets, and battery longevity is affected by the volume, number, and frequency of infusions.

Implantable infusion pumps

Designed for low-volume, long-term infusion in an ambulatory patient, the implantable infusion pump is most often used to deliver narcotics or anesthetics into the epidural or intrathecal space for the management of pain occurring below the level of the fourth lumbar space. The pump component of this system consists of two chambers separated by a flexible membrane. A cannula leads from the pump to an artery, a vein, or an organ such as the liver.

Drugs to be infused are loaded into one chamber. A charging fluid is contained in the second. This fluid changes to a vapor, creating pressure that pushes against the membrane and forces the infusate out of its chamber and into the cannula. When the chamber is refilled, pressure from the chamber pushes against the membrane, which causes the vapor to condense back into a liquid, which stores energy for the next cycle. The pump is refilled every 1 to 3 months by inserting a needle through the skin and into a port in the center of the pump.

These pumps are implanted under general anesthesia. A cannula is then threaded into the appropriate destination vessel or organ. When used for infusing antineoplastic agents for liver tumors, for example, the cannula is threaded through the gastric artery into the common hepatic artery, and then sutured in place. Once the cannula is in place, the pump is sutured into a pocket of subcutaneous tissue in the abdomen or subclavian fossa.

Implanted pumps offer several benefits for patients needing long-term infusions, including:
• extended access to the infusion site
• ability to infuse drugs directly into an organ
• a lower infection rate (because all components are below the skin surface)
• enhanced patient acceptance (because the device isn't plainly visible and doesn't interfere with daily activities).

Such pumps are contraindicated for infusing large volumes, when the patient's body size doesn't permit implantation of the pump itself, and in patients who travel frequently and experience repeated changes in altitude. Because the pump is calibrated for a specific infusion rate at the time of implantation, moving from one altitude to another can increase the infusion rate by as much as 38%.

Numerous patient conditions can affect infusion through an implanted pump. An increase in arterial blood pressure can decrease the flow rate into an artery; a decrease in blood pressure can increase the rate. A fever or a bath in hot water can increase the flow rate by as much as 13%.

Because of these variables in delivery rate, you'll need to closely and regularly monitor these pumps to ensure that the reservoir doesn't run out of medication. With some implanted pumps, you can adjust the rate as needed by increasing the concentration per milliliter. Other pumps feature a remote electronic control you can use to reprogram the rate of delivery.

Special delivery program pumps

Other infusions requiring special delivery programs include TPN. High glucose-concentrated solutions generally need to be started and stopped slowly to allow the body to adjust to the introduction of the solution. Thus certain pumps offer a "ramp-up and ramp-down" mode, with a controlled total time-specified delivery volume.

Current treatment for certain chemotherapeutic agents requires rather sophisticated delivery schedules called circadian rhythm. Predetermined percentages of the drug are delivered at specific times each day over 5 days. For example, 12% of the solution is delivered every night between 9 p.m. and 3 a.m., then 6% is delivered between 3 and 9 a.m., followed by 2% between 9 a.m. and 3 p.m., and ending with the final 4% being infused between 3 and 9 p.m. This pattern is repeated until the reservoir is empty. This regimen permits a higher percentage of infusion to occur at times when the target tumor cells are actively dividing (when the body is at rest) and lower percentages when the tumor cells are not as active.

Multichannel pumps

Many patients currently receive two or more infusions simultaneously. To meet their unique needs, multichannel pumps are now available. These pumps deliver two to four separate infusions at varying rates, volumes, and times. Besides saving space and being cost-effective, multichannel pumps allow home care patients and other patients to remain more active than they might otherwise be without the pumps.

Administration sets

Three types of administration sets are available: primary, secondary, and volume-control sets. Selection of the appropriate set depends on the rate of infusion, the type of solution to be infused, and the type of container holding the solution. (See *Comparing IV administration sets.*)

Primary administration sets carry solution from the container to the catheter by gravity. Most primary sets have one or two Y-sites along the length of the tubing to permit access for secondary infusions or IV push injections. Primary sets deliver 10 to 20 drops/ml of solution and usually have a backcheck valve to prevent backflow of secondary solutions into the primary solution.

Secondary administration sets are used if the patient needs an intermittent additional infusion. The secondary set, which has its own backcheck valve, is connected to the primary set by one of the Y-sites on the primary set.

Comparing IV administration sets

Three main administration sets are available: primary, secondary, and volume-control sets. The illustrations below show the various components of each set.

Primary set

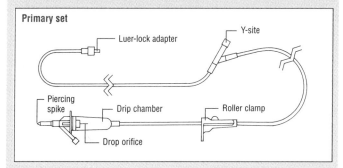

Secondary set

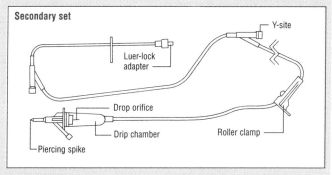

Volume-control set

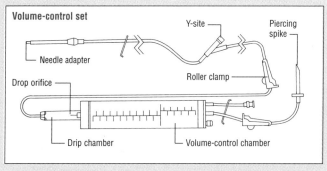

Volume-control administration sets deliver small, precise amounts of solution through the use of a volume-control chamber. The chamber, which attaches to the solution container through a short length of tubing, can be filled with specific amounts of fluid. Once that fluid has infused, no further fluid can be infused without filling the chamber again. Volume-control sets are used mainly for pediatric and critically ill patients who require small amounts of a medication or a well-controlled delivery rate.

Basic components of each type of administration set include:
• spike or piercing pin, inserted into the bag or drug reservoir
• flange, which protects the spike from touch contamination while the spike is being inserted
• drop orifice, which determines the size and shape of the fluid drop
• drip chamber, which houses the drop orifice and is the connection point to the IV tubing
• IV tubing, typically 63" to 98.5" (160 to 250 cm) in length and the main delivery route for the solution
• clamp, a flow-control device on the IV tubing, which uses compression of the tubing to regulate the flow rate
• Y-injection port, which provides an entry point to the IV tubing for infusion of other solutions through the main tubing
• filter, to remove particulates and other matter from the infusate
• luer-lock adapter to attach the IV tubing to the hub of the catheter.

Administration sets are available with two types of drip systems. The macrodrip set delivers large quantities of solution at a rapid rate—10 to 20 drops/ml. The microdrip set delivers small volumes of solution at a slow rate—60 drops/ml. The rate of flow is controlled by a roller or slide clamp on a portion of the administration set tubing.

Filters

Primary or secondary administration sets often include in-line filters, which help to remove pathogens and particulate matter from infusates as well as prevent air from entering the line. The types of pathogens and particulates sifted out depend on the size of the openings within the filter material. The smaller the openings, the more particulates the filter can screen. The size of these openings ranges from 0.2 to 170 microns. For total parenteral nutrition (TPN) solutions without lipids, 0.2-micron filters should be used.

In-line filters

Numerous in-line filters are available for preventing microbes and other contaminants from entering the bloodstream. Like most filters, the filters shown here, manufactured by B. Braun Medical, Inc. (top) and EPS, Inc. (bottom), attach to the IV tubing with a luer-lock connector.

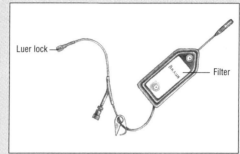

Luer lock

Filter

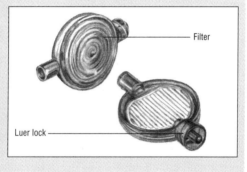

Filter

Luer lock

Larger filters, such as 170-micron filters, should be used for blood and large-molecule infusions. (See *In-line filters*.)

Filters should not be used with:

• infusions of certain large-molecule solutions
• solutions containing chemotherapeutic agents
• solutions containing drugs in dosages below 5 mg.

Use of filters with these solutions can cause the filter to clog, which will stop the infusion, or cause the solutions to lose their effectiveness. Solutions that shouldn't be passed through a filter include lipids and plasma expanders such as dextran. Drugs that shouldn't be passed through a filter include amphotericin B and alcohol.

When filters are used, change them routinely, usually once daily, depending on the manufacturer's recommendations. Frequent filter changes prevent the buildup of microbes and release of endotoxins trapped in the filter, which, as the filter ages and loses its effectiveness, can pass into the patient's bloodstream.

Some filters—typically 0.2-micron filters with positively charged membranes—can remain in place for up to 96 hours. These filters can trap bacteria and endotoxins longer than larger filters and should be used for TPN solutions without lipids. Use 1.2-micron filters for TPN solutions with lipids.

Supplementary devices

With the wide variety of infusion devices available and the increasing number of uses for infusion therapy in less conventional settings comes the need for supplementary devices such as extension sets, connectors, and injection caps.

Extension sets

Extension sets consist of tubing 6" to 12" (15 to 30 cm) in length with a hub on one end (to attach the main administration set) and a male luer-lock adapter on the other end (to attach to the hub of the catheter). This tubing extension allows the infusion therapy nurse to change the administration set and other components safely away from the insertion site, thus reducing the risk of movement of the venipuncture device and the possible resultant complications.

A clamp on the extension tubing prevents air and pathogens from entering the system when changing the main administration set or the injection cap. Although extension sets are widely used in practice, standards developed by the Intravenous Nurses Society recommend limiting the use of extension sets because of an increased risk of infections associated with the manipulation of these devices.

Connectors

Connectors are similar to extension sets and are available in several styles, including loop connectors, T-connectors, and Y-connectors.

Loop connector

A loop connector consists of a horseshoe-shaped piece of tubing that attaches on one end to the IV catheter and on the other to the IV tubing. By looping back on itself, the loop connector allows health care professionals to maintain the system without coming into contact with the insertion site and allows easier access for pa-

Backcheck valves

A backcheck valve is located within the Y-injection site (below, left) or in the tubing just above it (below, right). This valve ensures that the fluid flows in one direction only.

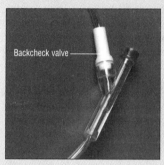

Backcheck valve

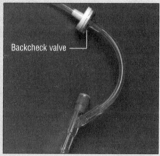

Backcheck valve

tients and caregivers to injection ports and other parts of the administration set.

T-connector

Useful for simultaneous administration of fluids and drugs, this small-bore extension tubing is 3" to 6" (7.5 to 15 cm) long and has an injection cap near its luer-lock adapter. The luer end attaches to the venipuncture device and the opposite end to the IV tubing. This allows another drug or solution to be administered through the injection cap while the primary IV solution infuses. This device can eliminate the need for a second venipuncture device. Using a T-connector or a loop connector can help extend indwelling time and reduce catheter movement during administration set changes and other maintenance procedures.

Y-connector

Y-connectors are specialty extension sets commonly used with controlled-dose pain management or other medications that have serious adverse reactions when given as a bolus. A Y-connector has a backcheck valve on the branch connected to the solution being infused. (See *Backcheck valves.*) If the catheter becomes occluded, the back-check valve prevents medications being infused from backing up into the tubing. Medication-laden fluid that backs up into the tubing can become a potentially harmful bolus if the occlusion resolves and the line suddenly opens.

Injection caps

Injection caps allow for a closed, yet easily accessible system. Most have a luer-lock connection on one end and the port of entry on the other. Newer injection caps provide entry only from a blunt, plastic cannula or luer-lock connection (such as a syringe connection), which reduces the risk of needle-stick injuries.

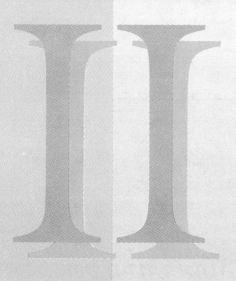

PERIPHERAL AND CENTRAL INFUSION THERAPY

5

Managing peripheral catheter therapy

Few nursing responsibilities require more time, knowledge, and skill than administering peripheral IV therapy, defined as the administration of fluids through a catheter whose tip lies in a vein outside of the body's central circulation, usually in a hand, an arm or, occasionally, a leg. To initiate peripheral IV therapy, you need to assemble the equipment, prepare the patient, insert the venipuncture device, regulate the flow rate, and monitor the patient for adverse reactions.

You also have specific behind-the-scenes responsibilities, such as checking the doctor's orders; labeling solutions and tubings with the date, time, and other information; and documenting nursing interventions related to the therapy being provided.

This chapter reviews the basics of peripheral infusion therapy, including selection of the patient, vein, and device, and insertion and care of a peripheral catheter. It also covers potential complications, patient teaching, removal of the device, and documentation related to peripheral catheters.

Advantages and disadvantages

Peripheral venous therapy can be used for a wide variety of purposes, including to maintain hydration, restore fluid and electrolyte balance, provide fluids for resuscitation, and administer blood, blood components, or nutrient solutions for metabolic support. Peripheral IV therapy can also be used to administer drugs, such as antibiotics, antifungals, antivirals, or narcotics, which can be administered as a bolus injection or through a pump designed for patient-controlled analgesia. Peripheral therapy should not be used for long-term or repeated intermittent therapy.

Selecting a patient

Patients who may benefit from peripheral infusion therapy include those whose therapy will last less than 1 week or will be used intermittently over a short period of time. Patients who require the administration of IV medications or isotonic solutions are candidates for peripheral infusion therapy.

A solution is isotonic if its osmolality falls within the normal range for serum, 240 to 340 mOsm/L. Examples of isotonic solutions include lactated Ringer's and normal saline solution with D_5W. Hypertonic fluids and medications (those greater than 340 mOsm/L) or total parenteral nutrition (TPN) solutions with a dextrose concentration greater than 10% are contraindicated for peripheral infusion therapy. Only 50% glucose boluses are exempt. Standards developed by the Intravenous Nurses Society (INS) allow the infusion of 50% dextrose in peripheral veins during hypoglycemic episodes.

Peripheral infusion therapy may be useful for patients who need irritant drugs or vesicant chemotherapeutic agents, but these drugs are better tolerated through central venous lines.

Selecting a vein

Selecting a vein may be the most important aspect in the success of a patient's infusion therapy. (See *Veins of the forearm and hand,* page 56.) When selecting a vein, the nurse should consider the size,

Veins of the forearm and hand

Most peripheral IV lines are started in a superficial vein of the hand or forearm. These diagrams show the most commonly used superficial veins of the upper extremities.

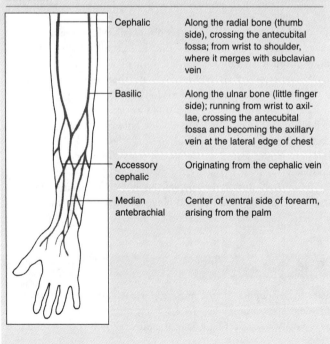

HAND SITES		WHERE IT'S LOCATED
	Dorsal venous arch	Dorsal aspect of the wrist, at the union of the metacarpal veins
	Metacarpal	Between the metacarpal bones on the back of the hand
	Digital	Lateral portion of the fingers

ARM SITES		
	Cephalic	Along the radial bone (thumb side), crossing the antecubital fossa; from wrist to shoulder, where it merges with subclavian vein
	Basilic	Along the ulnar bone (little finger side); running from wrist to axillae, crossing the antecubital fossa and becoming the axillary vein at the lateral edge of chest
	Accessory cephalic	Originating from the cephalic vein
	Median antebrachial	Center of ventral side of forearm, arising from the palm

location and condition of the vein, purpose of the infusion, and duration of the therapy. The most visible veins are not necessarily the most suitable for venipuncture; prominence may occur as a result of a sclerosed condition that interferes with the flow of the solution or the vein may be found in an area that, for a variety of reasons, makes insertion impractical.

As a general rule, distal veins of the hands and arms should be used initially. Subsequent venipunctures should be made proximal to the previous site. Arm veins most often used in peripheral infusion therapy are the basilic and cephalic veins, though metacarpal veins may also be used. Lower extremity veins in adults are used sparingly and only by experienced nurses. In addition, a doctor's order is necessary to cannulate a vessel in a lower extremity. This route should be used only when no alternatives are available.

Veins of the scalp can be used in children in certain circumstances, but the child must be younger than 18 months. Only highly experienced nurses should attempt cannulation of a scalp vein.

The extremity the nurse intends to use should be thoroughly examined and palpated before a site is selected. Use the same finger to palpate veins during every IV insertion attempt. This will help to develop fingertip sensitivity to the feeling of vessels. Palpate for soft, bouncy, unobstructed veins and use them whenever possible. After deciding on a vein, press down and release it to assess its resistance.

Also determine whether the location is suitable for the particular IV therapy. For example, the antecubital site, though highly valuable in an emergency, is less than ideal for home care patients because movement of the elbow may increase the risk of complications at the site of insertion. (See *Comparing peripheral venipuncture sites,* page 58.) The ideal vein for infusion therapy is straight, unused, and located in an area that will be comfortable for the patient and won't be disturbed by movement of the patient's limb. (See *Veins to avoid,* page 59.)

To assure successful vein selection, choose the nondominant arm of the patient whenever possible. Choose a vein above areas of flexion. Avoiding an area of flexion eliminates pistoning, the movement of the indwelling catheter in and out of the insertion site. Select a vein large enough to allow adequate blood flow around the catheter and a site that isn't contraindicated by the patient's plan of care, such as surgery or other procedures to be performed or physical or occupational therapy. Always assess the patient for previous mastectomies, grafts, or fistulas. An order is usually required to use veins in those extremities.

Comparing peripheral venipuncture sites

The veins used for venipuncture vary in size, accessibility, and other factors. This chart outlines major benefits and drawbacks of several common venipuncture sites.

SITE	ADVANTAGES	DISADVANTAGES
Metacarpal veins	• Easily accessible • Lies flat on back of hand • In adult or large child, bones of hand act as splint	• Wrist movement decreased unless short catheter is used • Insertion more painful because more nerve endings in hands • Site prone to phlebitis
Accessory cephalic vein	• Large vein, excellent for venipuncture • Readily accepts large-gauge needles • Won't impair mobility • Doesn't require an arm board in an older child or adult	• Sometimes difficult to position catheter flush with skin • Usually uncomfortable • Venipuncture device located at bend of wrist, so movement causes discomfort or requires hand board
Cephalic vein	• Large vein, excellent for venipuncture • Readily accepts large-gauge needles • Won't impair mobility	• Possible decreased joint movement due to proximity to elbow • Vein tends to roll during insertion
Median antebrachial vein	• A last resort when no other means are available	• Painful venipuncture or infiltration damage possible owing to numerous nerve endings in area • Infiltrates easily
Basilic vein	• Readily accepts large-gauge needles • Straight, strong vein suitable for large-gauge venipuncture devices	• Uncomfortable position for patient during insertion • Penetration of dermis where nerve endings are located causes pain • Vein tends to roll during insertion
Antecubital veins	• Large veins facilitate drawing blood • Often visible or palpable in children when other veins won't dilate • May be used in an emergency or as a last resort	• Difficult to splint elbow area with arm board • Median basilic vein crosses in front of brachial artery • Veins possibly small and scarred if blood has been drawn frequently from this site

Selecting a device

A wide range of peripheral insertion devices are available for use. Most IV therapy infusions are delivered through two basic veni-

Veins to avoid

Selecting the wrong vein for infusion therapy can increase the risk of complications. Avoid the following types of veins whenever possible:
• veins in areas of limb flexion (including the antecubital fossa, a site commonly used in phlebotomy), to reduce the chance of pistoning
• red, swollen, or bruised veins
• sclerosed or hard veins
• small, superficial veins
• veins damaged by infiltration (seepage of a nonirritating, or nonvesicant, solution or medication into the tissue surrounding the vein), extravasation (seepage of an irritating, or vesicant, solution or medication into the tissue surrounding the vein), or phlebitis
• veins in a limb on the same side where a mastectomy was performed or where a dialysis line is present
• veins in an extremity affected by a cerebrovascular accident
• veins near an obviously infected area
• veins of a surgically compromised extremity
• veins of the lower extremities
• veins that have a previous history of being used.

puncture devices: winged infusion devices or over-the-needle catheters (ONCs). (Through-the-needle catheters are not recommended by INS for routine therapy because of risk of puncture or shearing.) According to INS standards, the venipuncture device should be one with the shortest length and smallest diameter that allows for proper administration of the prescribed therapy.

When selecting a device, the nurse should consider the type of therapy to be administered, length of time the device will be needed, type of solution (larger lumen size for blood or blood products), type and number of veins available (particularly in light of the anticipated length of therapy), and the patient's age, size, and activity level. All of these variables may play a role in whether a winged infusion device or ONC is chosen.

Winged infusion devices
Winged infusion devices are available as steel needles and winged ONCs. Large, flexible wings are common to both types and are easily grasped and pinched together during insertion. Once the device is placed within the lumen of the vessel, the wings are flattened against the skin to provide an anchor for easier stabilization.

Steel needles

The steel needle winged device, commonly called a butterfly, does not have a hub. After insertion, the device lies flat on the skin, which makes it easy to secure.

Steel needle winged devices are about ¾" (1.9 cm) long and range in size from 16G to 27G (for gauge). (Needles and catheters are measured using the term *gauge;* the higher the number, the smaller the lumen diameter.)

These devices are thin-walled, extremely sharp, and the easiest of all devices to insert, making them ideal for single IV push injections. However, because the steel needle doesn't bend when the vein does, the risk of infiltration increases the more the patient moves.

Winged ONCs

Several types of winged ONCs are available, including the Intima and the Y-Intima. These devices can be described as more flexible butterfly catheters once the stylet is removed. The Intima has a short, small-bore tubing between the catheter and hub and is especially useful when using hand veins. The Y-Intima has a Y-shaped design and a latex cap to permit intermittent infusions and protection against accidental needle sticks.

ONC devices

The ONC is the most widely used device for peripheral infusion therapy. (See *Comparing venipuncture devices.*) It typically consists of an introducer needle, or stylet, encased in a flexible Teflon or polyurethane sheath. The stylet is removed following successful cannulation, leaving the flexible sheath in place.

The flexibility of ONCs offers active patients greater safety and freedom of movement. Compared to steel needle winged devices, infiltration occurs less often and the catheter can be left in place longer. ONCs vary in diameter, length, design, and composition of materials. Most catheters are radiopaque so they can be seen on X-ray.

Needle and catheter gauges

The type of catheter and diameter of the lumen to be used depends on the patient's age, the purpose of the infusion, and the condition and availability of the veins. (See *Guide to needle and catheter gauges,* page 62.) While catheters may be color-coded according to gauge, never rely solely on color to identify a catheter. Always read the product labeling to ensure proper catheter selection.

Comparing venipuncture devices

Most IV infusions are delivered through two basic devices: winged infusion devices and over-the-needle catheters. These illustrations show samples of the two types.

Winged infusion device
Use: Short-term therapy for cooperative adult patient; therapy of any duration for an infant, child, or elderly patient with fragile or sclerotic veins
Advantages: Easiest venipuncture device to insert; ideal for IV push drugs
Disadvantage: May easily cause infiltration if a steel needle winged device is used

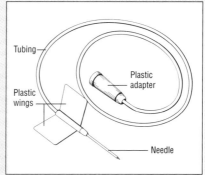

Tubing
Plastic adapter
Plastic wings
Needle

Over-the-needle catheter
Use: Therapy lasting 1 week or less for active or agitated patients
Advantages: Inadvertent puncture of vein less likely than with a needle; more comfortable for patients once in place; contains radiopaque material for easy identification on X-ray (nonradiopaque catheters often used by anesthesia practitioners). Some have protective devices to decrease the incidence of needle sticks among health care providers and also come in winged versions.

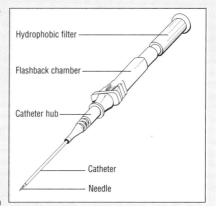

Hydrophobic filter
Flashback chamber
Catheter hub
Catheter
Needle

Disadvantage: Different, sometimes more difficult insertion technique than winged infusion devices

Insertion of a peripheral catheter

The proper insertion of a peripheral access device involves gathering the equipment; preparing the patient, site, and device; and performing the venipuncture.

Guide to needle and catheter gauges

GAUGE	USES	CHARACTERISTICS
16	• Major surgery • Trauma • Large fluid and blood volumes • Rapid infusions	• Insertion painful • Requires large vein • May increase mechanical injury to vein wall • Causes irritation of vein wall
18	• Older children, adolescents, and adults • Administering blood, blood components, and other viscous infusates • Various emergent situations	• Insertion painful • Requires large vein
20	• Children, adolescents, and adults • Suitable for most IV infusions • Appropriate for transfusing blood when rapid rates aren't required	• Commonly used
22	• Infants, toddlers, children, adolescents, and adults (especially elderly adults) • Suitable for most IV infusions	• Easier to insert in small, thin, fragile veins • More difficult to insert into tough skin • Allows slower rates only
24, 26	• Neonatal, pediatric, and elderly • Suitable for most infusions, but flow rates are slower	• For extremely small veins, such as small veins of fingers or inner arms in elderly patients • May be difficult to insert into tough skin

Gathering the equipment

Before preparing the infusion, gather the equipment you'll need, including:

• IV start kit with tourniquet, nonsterile gloves, povidone swabs, alcohol swabs, 2" × 2" sterile gauze, transparent dressing, tape, and a label
• appropriate-sized peripheral catheter
• extension tubing
• infusate
• injection cap
• normal saline flush, 1 to 3 ml
• sharps container.

Preparing the patient

After gathering your equipment, check that a doctor's order has been written outlining solution, medication, dosage, volume, frequency, and rate of infusion. The order should be written legibly and be concise and clear. If it isn't clear or if it doesn't contain all necessary components, contact the prescriber for clarification. Then verify the patient's physical status, including allergies.

Take the time to introduce yourself to the patient. Explain the procedure using easy-to-understand terminology. A confident, friendly approach will help ensure the patient's comfort and cooperation. Your instructions to the patient should include the purpose for the infusion, the basic procedure and what to expect, the effect the IV will have on the patient's activities, and the patient's role in caring for the IV site (such as keeping the dressing clean and dry and avoiding pulling or pinching the IV tubing).

Allow time to answer questions before starting the procedure, and try to allay fears the patient might express. The success of the procedure is, to an extent, influenced by how well-prepared the patient is before therapy begins.

Preparing the device

Preparation for a venipuncture also includes getting the administration and catheter set prepared. Make sure you have a clean working area, a protective barrier for the equipment, and another barrier for the patient's extremity. The area where the procedure is performed should be well lit and have sufficient room to permit the patient and you to be in comfortable positions. Equipment should be placed near the patient for easy access. Always wash your hands with an antiseptic cleaning agent before starting.

To prepare a continuous infusion, first open the administration set and close the clamp, usually a roller or slider clamp. Attach the connecting device (preferably a needleless device). Examine the solution for clarity and freedom from particulate matter, note that it is housed in an intact container, and ensure that it hasn't passed its expiration date. Contact the pharmacist if you aren't completely satisfied with these checks.

Calculate the drip rate according to the drip factor and infusion rate. Verify the calculation with the pharmacist or another nurse. Remove the covering from the spike and the cap from the solution container. Insert the spike into the access area of the container.

Hang the solution on an IV pole or a stable vertical area above the patient. Then prime the tubing to remove all the air. For both continuous and intermittent infusions, attach a cap to the end of an extension set and prime this set.

Preparing the site

Understanding how to prepare a venipuncture site properly is crucial for a successful procedure. Site preparation includes dilating the vein and cleaning the area. Factors that affect vein distention include the patient's age, diagnosis, physical condition, blood pressure, state of hydration, and previous IV sites. (See *Tips on dilating veins.*)

For most patients, the preferred method of engorging the veins in preparation for inserting a peripheral device is the tourniquet, commonly a Penrose drain or piece of latex 15″ to 20″ (38 to 50.8 cm) long and wide enough to prevent it from rolling into a small band. Before using a latex product, check the patient for a history of latex allergies.

The tourniquet should be placed 5″ to 6″ (12.7 to 15.2 cm) above the preferred venipuncture site. A latex strip can be tied on the arm with a loop to allow quick and easy removal. The tourniquet should be applied tightly enough to impede venous return and loosely enough to allow arterial flow. The tourniquet should not be left on for more than a few minutes and should be discarded after use or cleaned thoroughly with an aseptic solution.

A blood pressure cuff can provide a tourniquet-like effect with more control, a particularly useful technique for patients with large arms. To use a blood pressure cuff as a tourniquet, inflate the cuff and then release it to a point just below the diastolic pressure.

After applying a tourniquet, palpate the vein from distal to proximal to determine whether or not anything is obstructing blood flow. If necessary, remove the tourniquet before cleaning the site and reapply it after the site has been cleaned.

After you've put on nonsterile gloves, clean the skin. If hair removal is necessary, clip the hair, don't shave it, prior to cleaning the skin. Shaving can cause microtears and allow bacteria to enter.

To clean the skin, use friction and an antimicrobial solution such as tincture of iodine 1% to 2%, povidone-iodine, or isopropyl alcohol 70%. Use of benzalkonium or hexachlorophene is not recommended.

When using alcohol plus povidone-iodine, use the alcohol first to prevent negating the antimicrobial effect of povidone-iodine.

CLINICAL PEARLS

Tips on dilating veins

Here are some useful tips to help cause venous dilation and make the veins more accessible.

- Use gravity; lower the site below the heart.
- Encourage the patient to tighten his fist or tense his arm muscles, but remind him to relax during insertion.
- Apply warm, moist heat on the extremity for 15 to 20 minutes before insertion.

- Gently tap the vein.
- Use a blood pressure cuff to obtain tourniquet effect.
- Gently rub the extremity in a direction away from the tourniquet.

Clean in a circular fashion, starting from the insertion site and working outward 2" to 4" (5 to 10 cm) from the intended entry site. Repeat, using povidone-iodine. Allow to dry. Do not fan or blow on the area. Avoid blotting the site. (If the patient is allergic to iodine, clean the site with isopropyl alcohol using enough pads to keep cleaning until the last pad used looks clean.)

Some infusion therapy nurses prefer using some form of analgesia prior to insertion. The INS does not recommend routine use of an injectable anesthetic like lidocaine before venipuncture. However, a transdermal analgesic such as EMLA cream may be used for local anesthesia, but it must be applied at least 1 hour before venipuncture.

Inserting the catheter

With the tourniquet in place and the target vein dilated, place the thumb of your nondominant hand below the insertion site and pull the skin away from the site. This maneuver will help to keep the vein from rolling during insertion.

With your dominant hand, grasp the flashback chamber—not the hub of the catheter—or the wings of the needle or catheter device between your thumb and forefinger, with the bevel of the needle upward. Insert the needle into the skin and vein. (See *Inserting a venipuncture device,* page 66.)

In a direct insertion, the needle pierces the skin over a vein at a 30- to 45-degree angle and is then advanced in the same motion into the vein. A steady flashback of blood in the chamber indicates a

Inserting a venipuncture device

When inserting a veni-
puncture device, hold
the device at a wider
angle to penetrate the
skin. Lower the catheter
needle to a 15- to 30-
degree angle, as shown
here, and slowly pierce
the vein. Use the flexibility of your wrist to ensure
proper entry angle.
    Prior to inserting the
device, make sure the
bevel of the needle is up.
The stylet (the introducer
needle) should be re-
moved when the vein
has been properly cannulated. Note the blood return in the flashback chamber, indicating that the catheter has been placed properly inside the vein.

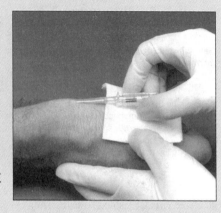

successful vein entry. (See *Absence of backflow?*) When the flashback
appears, immediately reduce the angle of entry. Advance the stylet
slightly to ensure that the catheter tip is inside the vein lumen.

The indirect method is a two-motion approach into the vein.
Stabilizing the vein in the same way and with the needle held in the
same manner as for a direct insertion, enter the skin first at a 30- to
45-degree angle, and then locate the vein. Lower the angle of the
needle, and then enter the vein. The indirect method helps decrease
bruising in small, fragile veins.

Using either approach, you'll feel a slight resistance when entering a vein. Some nurses describe a kind of popping sensation as the
needle pierces the wall of the vein. If the venipuncture is unsuccessful, you may need to try another site. The INS recommends that
only two attempts be made per nurse. Multiple attempts are trau-
matizing to the patient and the nurse.

When the needle is located inside the vein, advance the needle
further, about ¼" (0.6 cm), to ensure that the catheter has been
placed properly. Pull back slightly on the stylet to pull the needle tip
inside the catheter.

To advance the catheter, use one of several methods. When can-
nulating fragile veins, the catheter can be "floated" in by first re-

CLINICAL
PEARLS

Absence of backflow?

If blood backflow stops when you remove the stylet, the cannula might have passed through the opposite wall of the vein. If that happens, you may be able to save the vein by acting quickly. *Never try to reinsert the stylet;* doing so may shear the cannula. Instead, without removing the tourniquet, retract the cannula slightly until blood flashback appears again, indicating that you've pulled the tip back into the lumen. Then quickly advance the cannula into the vein, and promptly remove the tourniquet.

moving the tourniquet, then flushing the catheter with saline after the stylet is removed and advancing the catheter at the same time. This method dilates the vein and permits a safe and easy catheter insertion. Usually though, you'll leave the tourniquet in place and use your nondominant hand to advance the catheter, while keeping the needle stylet in position. Or, continue to stretch the skin with your nondominant hand while using the forefinger of your other hand to push the catheter into the vein. Use your thumb and second finger to stabilize the stylet.

Once the catheter is advanced, never attempt to pull back on it if you meet resistance. This may cause the needle or stylet to tear the catheter. Continue to advance the catheter until the hub touches the skin. Remove the tourniquet.

While putting pressure on the skin over the end of the catheter, remove the stylet and quickly attach the extension tubing, if used, and the cap. Catheters with a protective feature should be advanced and the stylet removed according to the manufacturer's guidelines. (See *Inserting IV lines in specific patient populations,* pages 68 to 71.)

Connecting the administration set
Blood should slowly flow into the extension tubing if the catheter has been placed properly. Once proper placement is confirmed, flush the catheter according to facility policy or begin an infusion by connecting the administration set to the extension. Open the clamp, and observe for fluid flow. Adjust the rate according to the doctor's order. Secure the device according to your facility's policies. Remember, never cover the insertion site with tape.

(Text continues on page 70.)

Inserting IV lines in specific patient populations

This chart highlights key points to remember when starting IV lines in specific patient populations.

PATIENT POPULATION	FINDING A VEIN	TYPE OF CATHETER
Neonatal	• Use a heel warmer to dilate veins. • Check these major veins in the neonate: dorsal metacarpals in the hand, saphenous vein in the foot, and temporal, frontal, and posterior auricular veins in the scalp. • Transillumination can be helpful in identifying veins in neonates.	• 24G over-the-needle catheter; ½" (1.3 cm) to ⅝" (1.6 cm) length most common
Pediatric	• Use veins of hands, forearms, or antecubital fossa for ambulating children. • Avoid using the saphenous vein if the child is ambulating. • Use the nondominant extremity to allow thumb sucking in young children, and crafts or school-work in older children. • Use a warm pack or latex-free tourniquet to help dilate veins.	• 24G, 22G, or 20G • Use the smallest catheter for the vein and the viscosity of the solution. Thin-walled IV catheters provide excellent flow rates, even at smaller gauges.
Elderly	• Use warm compresses to dilate veins, especially if patient is cold.	• Use a small gauge to avoid trauma. • 24G or 22G should be adequate.
Obese or edematous patient	• Use anatomic landmarks to locate veins.	• 22G or 20G • May need longer catheter to

INSERTING THE CATHETER	OTHER TIPS
• Obtain assistance to hold the neonate still. • Take appropriate steps to maintain the neonate's temperature. • Use minimal tourniquet pressure or no tourniquet at all for fragile veins. A rubber band is an excellent size for use in neonates. • Clean the site with alcohol. Iodine tincture may affect thyroid function if absorbed through the neonate's thin skin. • Insert the catheter gently and slowly. • Expect scant blood return in flashback chamber.	• Pad areas under the catheter hub where a pressure sore might occur. • Use minimal tape on fragile skin. • Leave the skin over the cannula tip visible for checking the site. • Use a transparent neonate-sized dressing for visibility. • Use a padded tongue blade or rolled gauze as an arm board.
• Use toys to distract the child during insertion. Bubbles are especially useful for distraction. • Obtain assistance to hold the child still. • Be aware that the younger the child, the less time there should be between explanation of the procedure and starting of the IV. • Use local anesthesia (lidocaine injection or EMLA cream) if your facility's policy allows its use. • Use positioning for comfort techniques whenever possible.	• Pin the arm board to the bed or use neonatal Velcro restraints to limit mobility of the extremity with the IV line. • Secure the site with a padded board if the IV site is over an area of flexion. • Use a sterile transparent semipermeable membrane dressing and, if needed, a clear plastic cup to maintain site visibility. • Secure the tubing to the site, especially in younger children. • Allow toddlers and older children to handle equipment, clean the site, or place a make-believe IV line in a doll (with supervision) to help them better deal with their infusion therapy. • Allow older children and adolescents to participate in their care.
• Use low tourniquet pressure to avoid trauma, especially if the patient is taking an anticoagulant or a steroid. • Avoid areas where valves are located. • Maintain tension on the skin during venipuncture. Consider using the one-handed technique. • Release the tourniquet as soon as blood return is evident.	• Use minimal tape; removing the tape can easily tear the skin. • Consider using a protective polymer solution under the tape around the site. • Use a padded arm board or stretch netting to protect the site.
• Use several tourniquets, progressing distally from the most proximal joint toward the site, to distend veins.	• Avoid circumventing the arm with tape; this may restrict flow and increase edema in the extremity.

(continued)

Inserting IV lines in specific patient populations *(continued)*

PATIENT POPULATION	FINDING A VEIN	TYPE OF CATHETER
Obese or edematous patient *(continued)*	• Displace edema near a vein to the side of the vein or above it to flatten the area. • Use deep palpation to identify hard-to-palpate veins.	pierce tissue or extracellular fluid.
Patient requiring frequent IV insertions	• Allow the patient to assist in locating a vein; he may know his veins better than anyone. • Consider using a warm pack or transilluminator to help locate veins. • Avoid collateral veins, which may be present but aren't appropriate for venipuncture. • Consider using infrequently used veins, such as the basilic vein on the back of the arm or cephalic vein on the upper arm.	• Use small gauge to avoid trauma. • 22G or 24G should be adequate.

Applying a dressing

Venipuncture sites can be dressed with sterile, occlusive gauze, though many infusion therapy nurses now prefer to use transparent, semipermeable membrane dressings to anchor IV devices. Both types of dressings may be used, however.

Gauze dressings include a 2″ × 2″ gauze covering the insertion site and all edges taped to make the dressing occlusive. CDC guidelines state that no ointment should be applied to any catheter site. Gauze dressings should be changed every 48 hours or when they are no longer occlusive.

Transparent, semipermeable membrane dressings allow for continuous observation of the site without removing the dressing. This dressing is applied using aseptic technique and changed when the peripheral catheter is changed or when the edges of the dressing become loose from the skin. After application, press the dressing over the entire area to seal the site. As with gauze dressings, applying ointment to the site is not recommended with this type of covering.

After the dressing has been applied, the tubing should be looped without kinking it and taped securely to the arm. Dispose of used

INSERTING THE CATHETER	OTHER TIPS
• Maintain skin tension during the procedure. • Use areas with the least edema or underlying tissue, such as the dorsum of the hand or palmar surface of the forearm.	
• Pull the skin taut to avoid the skin bunching up on the device. • Use the most experienced staff members to place IV line in these patients.	• Secure the catheter well to avoid repeated venipuncture. • Draw blood for laboratory tests at the same time as the IV line is being inserted, to prevent multiple venipunctures. • Consider alternative access device, such as a midline, peripherally inserted central catheter, tunneled catheter, or port, if frequent access is required or if the patient has veins that are difficult to cannulate. • Consider leaving the catheter in place longer. Observe closely, and follow your facility's guidelines about extending catheter dwelling time.

supplies in a nonpermeable, tamper-proof container. To minimize risk of injury to herself or the patient, the nurse must remember to follow all safety precautions during IV insertion and to follow standard precautions throughout the procedure.

After applying a dressing, place a label on the dressing, indicating the length and gauge of the catheter, date of insertion, and your initials. Place a label on the solution container identifying when the infusion was started, the date of infusion, and your initials. Then label the tubing in the same way.

Maintenance and care

Maintenance care during IV therapy includes regularly changing the dressing and flushing the catheter, changing the IV solution and the administration set, as well as rotating the site.

Changing the dressing

Gauze dressings should be changed using aseptic technique every 48 hours and whenever the dressings become soiled, wet, or loose. Frequency of changing a transparent semipermeable membrane dressing varies by facility and protocol and depends on site rotation and integrity of the dressing. (See *Applying a transparent semipermeable membrane dressing.*)

To change the dressing, wash your hands, put on nonsterile gloves, and carefully remove the old dressing. Assess the site for erythema, temperature changes, edema, and catheter patency. Clean the area around the insertion site with 70% alcohol in a circular motion, from the center outward. Follow this by cleaning in the same manner with povidone-iodine, if the patient is not allergic to iodine. Allow the solution to air dry. Apply a new dressing, and secure the tubing as previously described.

Flushing the catheter

If the peripheral catheter is used for intermittent infusion or bolus injection, flush the catheter with normal saline solution to maintain patency, according to your facility's policy. The volume used is 2 ml or more.

Changing the IV solution

To avoid microbial growth, you shouldn't allow any IV container to hang for more than 24 hours. Before changing the container, obtain a new one and have it ready to be hung. Check it for cracks, leaks, and other damage. Also check it for discoloration, turbidity, and particulates and note the date and time the solution was mixed and the expiration date.

To change the container, wash your hands and then clamp the tubing. Remove the cap from the new container and the spike from the old container, and then quickly insert the spike into the new container. Hang the new container, adjust the flow rate, and discard the old container according to your facility's policy.

Changing the administration set

Change the administration set according to your facility's policy, usually every 48 hours, and whenever you note or suspect contamination. According to the INS, the interval may be extended to every 72 hours if the facility's phlebitis rate is less than 5%. CDC guidelines recommend changing the tubing every 72 hours (24

CLINICAL PEARLS

Applying a transparent semipermeable membrane dressing

Rather than using tape to secure an IV line, you can apply a transparent, semipermeable membrane dressing. Here's how:

1. Make sure the insertion site is clean and dry.
2. Remove the dressing from the package and, using aseptic technique, remove the protective seal. Avoid touching the sterile surface.
3. Place the dressing directly over the insertion site and the hub, as shown. Don't cover the tubing or stretch the dressing, which may cause itching.
4. Tuck the dressing around and under the catheter hub to make the site occlusive to microorganisms.
5. To remove the dressing, grasp one corner, lift, stretch, and peel off.

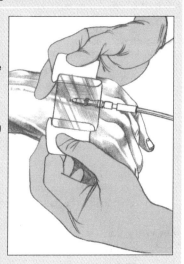

hours for TPN solutions). Whenever possible, change the administration set when you hang a new solution container.

Before changing the administration set, gather a sterile 2" × 2" gauze pad, adhesive tape for labeling, and gloves. Wash your hands, and put on the gloves. Reduce the IV flow rate. Then remove the old spike from the bag or bottle, and loosely place the cover of the new spike over it.

Keeping the old spike upright and above the patient's heart level, insert the new spike into the IV container and prime the system. Place the sterile gauze pad under the catheter hub. Disconnect the old tubing from the catheter hub, being careful not to dislodge or move the device. If you have trouble disconnecting the old tubing, use a pair of hemostats or other device to hold the hub securely while twisting and removing the end of the tubing.

CLINICAL PEARLS

Protecting the IV site

After inserting the peripheral catheter, measures for securing it and applying the dressing should be taken for added protection, especially in home care patients. Many available materials can be used to protect the site. The goal of securing the site is to protect the area from accidental trauma.

The dressing should not constrict the extremity nor be so loose that it doesn't stay in place. For example, for a patient at home, you can use the ankle portion of a sock or part of a leg of clean panty hose. Roller or elastic bandages are not recommended; they limit visualization of the site and can interfere with circulation.

Elastic netting, available in numerous sizes, can be used to secure the site. A size slightly smaller than the patient's extremity typically provides the best protection. Stretch the netting like you would a stockinette prior to application. A clear, plastic shield, which comes in various sizes, may also be used to protect the site.

Using aseptic technique, quickly attach the new primed tubing to the catheter hub. Adjust the flow to the prescribed rate. Label the new tubing with the date and time of the tubing change.

Rotating the site

The IV site should be changed every 48 to 72 hours, with a new sterile, transparent semipermeable membrane dressing applied.

However, rotating an IV site every 2 or 3 days may be difficult in patients who have few acceptable peripheral sites and poor skin turgor. (See *Protecting the IV site.*) In such cases, the dwell time of an existing catheter may be extended based on the following factors:
• condition of the current catheter site, which must be free from redness, swelling, tenderness, leakage, and hardness
• condition of the patient's skin
• type of infusion and its potential to cause vein irritation
• length of therapy remaining. (If the therapy is expected to last more than a week, another type of device should be considered.)

When a catheter is left in place longer than recommended, extra vigilance will be required to detect signs of phlebitis, infiltration, extravasation, and other site complications.

Complications

Numerous complications are associated with peripheral venous therapy, including those relating to the venipuncture, infusion, or medication being administered. (See *Managing peripheral IV complications*, pages 76 to 78.) You can minimize or prevent complications by using proper insertion techniques, carefully monitoring the patient, and scheduling routine site rotations. Thoroughly training the patient or caregiver in aseptic technique and troubleshooting for complications is essential for effective therapy, whether the patient is being cared for at home or in a health care facility.

Teaching the patient

Education of the patient or caregiver needs to start as soon as the treatment is ordered, especially if the patient will be receiving the IV infusion at home. Make sure to explain the reason for the treatment, how to monitor the IV site and maintain a continuous infusion, how to care and use the equipment (including changing solution containers and catheter flushes, if appropriate), potential adverse reactions, how to troubleshoot infusion equipment, possible complications and what to do about them, and how to properly dispose of wastes from infusion therapy procedures.

Removal of a peripheral catheter

IV lines can be discontinued because the therapy is complete, the catheter has been in place for 48 to 72 hours, the site is infected, or improper aseptic technique was used at insertion. When removing a venipuncture device, take care to avoid causing trauma to the vessel or surrounding tissue. To discontinue a peripheral device, you'll need a 2" × 2" gauze pad, tape or another securing device, and nonsterile gloves.

To discontinue an IV infusion, first explain the procedure to the patient. Then wash and dry your hands thoroughly. Stop the pump or clamp the IV line, and then put gloves on. Loosen and then remove the tape or transparent dressing. Withdraw the catheter paral-

(Text continues on page 78.)

Managing peripheral IV complications

This chart characterizes local and systemic complications of peripheral IV therapy and outlines appropriate interventions.

COMPLICATION	SIGNS AND SYMPTOMS	INTERVENTIONS
Phlebitis	Redness or tenderness at tip of device, puffy area over the vein, elevated temperature	*Patient interventions* • Stop infusion and contact nurse. *Nursing interventions* • Remove the device. • Apply warm pack. • Document patient's condition. • Restart IV and infusion, using a larger vein or smaller device to ensure adequate blood flow. • Contact pharmacist for recommendations on diluting medication.
Infiltration	Swelling, discomfort, burning, tightness, cool skin, blanching, slow flow rate	*Patient interventions* • Stop infusion and contact nurse. *Nursing interventions* • Remove the device. • Apply ice or warm pack. • Elevate limb. • Check pulse and capillary refill. • Restart IV and infusion. • Document patient's condition and your interventions. • Check IV site frequently.
Catheter dislodgment	Swelling or leaking at insertion site, catheter backing out of vein	*Patient interventions* • Stop infusion and contact nurse. • Remove catheter, and apply pressure to site. *Nursing interventions* • Reinsert new device, and resume infusion. • Secure catheter.
Catheter occlusion	Decreased flow rate, blood backing up in line, inability to flush catheter	*Patient interventions* • Contact nurse. • Follow directions for flushing line. *Nursing interventions* • If patient cannot flush line, attempt to flush line. • If successful, reattach tubing. If unsuccessful, restart IV. *Prevention* • Apply clamp on extension set when not in use. • Maintain IV flow rate. • Flush line promptly for intermittent medications.
Hematoma	Tenderness or bruising at puncture site	*Patient interventions* • Stop infusion, and contact nurse. *Nursing interventions* • Remove device.

Managing peripheral IV complications (continued)

COMPLICATION	SIGNS AND SYMPTOMS	INTERVENTIONS
Hematoma (continued)		• Apply pressure and warm soaks. • Recheck for bleeding. • Document patient's condition and your interventions. *Prevention* • Choose a vein that can accommodate size of venipuncture device. • Release tourniquet as soon as insertion is achieved.
Venous spasm	Pain along vein, flow rate sluggish when clamp is completely open, blanched skin over vein	*Patient interventions* • Report signs and symptoms to nurse. *Nursing interventions* • Apply warm soaks over vein and surrounding tissue. • Slow flow rate.
Circulatory overload	Discomfort, neck vein distention or engorgement, respiratory distress, increased blood pressure, crackles, positive fluid balance	*Patient interventions* • Stop infusion, and report signs and symptoms to nurse. *Nursing interventions* • Raise head of bed or place patient in sitting position. • Try to reduce patient's anxiety. • Administer oxygen, if available, as needed and ordered. • Notify the doctor. • Administer diuretics as ordered. *Prevention* • Use a pump or controller for more precise infusion. • Monitor infusion closely.
Systemic infection (septicemia or bacteremia)	Fever, chills, and malaise for no apparent reason; decreased blood pressure	*Patient interventions* • Stop infusion, and report signs and symptoms to nurse. *Nursing interventions* • Notify doctor. • Administer medications as prescribed. • Culture site and device, draw blood culture for organism sensitivity. • Monitor vital signs. *Prevention* • Use scrupulous aseptic technique when handling solutions and tubing device. • Secure all connections, and change IV tubing, solution, and venipuncture device as recommended. • Use IV filter.

(continued)

Managing peripheral IV complications *(continued)*

COMPLICATION	SIGNS AND SYMPTOMS	INTERVENTIONS
Air embolism	Respiratory distress, unequal breath sounds, weak pulse, increased central venous pressure, decreased blood pressure, loss of consciousness	*Nursing and caregiver interventions* • Stop infusion. • Place patient in Trendelenburg's position on left side, if possible, with head below feet. • Administer oxygen as ordered, if available. • Call emergency medical service (EMS), and notify doctor. • Document patient's condition and your interventions. *Prevention* • Purge tubing of air completely before infusion. • Use air detection device, such as a pump.
Allergic reaction	Itching or tearing eyes, runny nose, bronchospasm, wheezing, urticarial rash, edema at IV site, anaphylactic reaction	*Patient interventions* • Stop infusion and report signs and symptoms to nurse. • Call 9-1-1 for shortness of breath or tightening in chest. *Nursing interventions* • Stop infusion immediately. • Maintain patent airway. • Call EMS. • Administer antihistaminic steroid, anti-inflammatory, and antipyretic as ordered. • Give 0.2 to 0.5 ml of 1:1,000 aqueous epinephrine subcutaneously, repeated at 3-minute intervals as needed. • Administer cortisone if ordered. • Monitor vital signs. *Prevention* • Obtain patient's allergy history. Be aware of cross-allergies. • Perform test doses prior to administering new medications. • Monitor patient carefully during first 15 minutes of administration of a new drug.

lel to the skin. Be careful not to manipulate the device, which may cause pain.

Cover the site with a 2" × 2" gauze pad and apply pressure for 2 minutes. (Don't use an alcohol wipe because it can cause burning and bleeding.) Then cover the site with a 2" × 2" dressing and secure it with tape. If appropriate, restrict the patient's activity for 10 minutes. Observe for complications.

Documentation

Your documentation about peripheral infusion therapy should include the following points:
• dressing, tubing, and solution changes
• condition of the venipuncture site
• date and time specimens for culture and sensitivity testing obtained and the name of the doctor who ordered the testing.

Documentation about insertion of peripheral infusion device should include:
• date and time of the insertion
• gauge, length, and brand of catheter used
• site of insertion
• number of insertion attempts
• medication or solution used
• rate of infusion
• presence or absence of adverse reactions
• patient teaching performed and the patient's level of understanding.

Documentation about discontinuing an IV line should include:
• time and date of removal
• reason for discontinuing the line
• catheter appearance at the time of removal
• condition of the site at removal
• reactions of the patient to the removal
• pertinent nursing interventions.

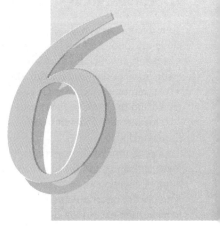

CHAPTER

Managing midline catheter therapy

A midline catheter is typically inserted into a large vein in the antecubital area. Once inserted, its tip lies below the axillary vein. Midline catheters are used for intermediate-length (2 to 4 weeks) infusions. The use of these catheters helps reduce the trauma and costs associated with repeated venipunctures. This chapter covers advantages and disadvantages of use, selection of patient, vein, and device, insertion of a midline catheter, and care of the catheter. Also included are complications, patient education, removal of the catheter, and documentation.

Advantages and disadvantages

When used properly, the midline catheter offers many advantages over traditional peripheral access devices. These advantages include reducing trauma to the patient, longer dwell times, more reliable access, and cost savings.

The use of traditional peripheral catheters requires the nurse to rotate venipuncture sites, which exposes the patient to the pain of repeated venipunctures and leads to a depletion of usable peripheral veins. A midline catheter, because it may need to be inserted only once for an extended period of therapy, avoids repeated venipuncture and helps to maintain the health of peripheral veins.

While a traditional peripheral catheter should be changed about every 48 hours, midline catheters can remain in place up to 4 weeks. This extended dwell time enhances patient comfort and reduces the risk of complications from repeated venipuncture.

Midline catheters are considerably less likely to dislodge from the vein than are traditional peripheral catheters, making infiltration when administering an IV medication or solution less likely. Infiltration can be a particularly serious problem because it interrupts therapy and may cause injury to the patient.

In addition, use of a midline catheter to deliver 4 weeks of antibiotic therapy can reduce the cost of venous access by 75% or more over a traditional peripheral catheter. The savings that can be accomplished by using a peripheral midline catheter are important for cost containment and managed care.

Midline catheters limit the type of solutions that can be administered, however. They should not be used for chemotherapy, central total parenteral nutrition, solutions or medications with a pH below 5 or above 9, or solutions or medications with a serum osmolality exceeding 500 mOsm/L. (See *Understanding osmolality,* page 82.) Avoiding infusions of these agents and solutions through a midline catheter can prevent such complications as phlebitis, thrombosis, and sclerosis.

Selecting a patient

Patients of nearly all ages are candidates for having a midline catheter inserted. Selection depends on the availability of veins, length of therapy, and osmolality of the solution or medication to be infused. Your facility's policy may also dictate selection criteria.

Midline catheters may also be used instead of central venous catheters when stable, short-term venous access is desired. In general, midline catheters tend to be used less frequently than peripherally inserted central catheters.

Therapy planned to exceed 5 days would make the patient a candidate for insertion of a midline catheter. For example, a patient about to receive 7 to 14 days of infusion therapy with a nonirritating antibiotic would be an ideal candidate for placement of a mid-

Understanding osmolality

Measured in milliosmols per liter (mOsm/L), osmolality refers to the number of particles in a liter of fluid. As the particle count increases, the concentration increases and particles in the fluid behave differently. Osmolality and tonicity are frequently used interchangeably. These illustrations show how particles behave in fluids with a normal, high, and low osmolality.

Normal osmolality (isotonic)
Fluids with a normal osmolality (240 to 340 mOsm/L) have a concentration of dissolved particles equal to that of intracellular fluid. Osmotic pressure is therefore the same inside and outside the cells, so they neither shrink nor swell with fluid movement. Examples: D_5W, 0.9% saline, lactated Ringer's and Ringer's solution.

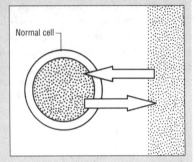

High osmolality (hypertonic)
Fluids with a high osmolality (> 340 mOsm/L) have a higher concentration of particles than intracellular fluid, so osmotic pressure is unequal inside and outside the cells. Dehydration or rapidly infused hypertonic fluids draw water out of the cell into the more highly concentrated extracellular fluid. Examples: dextrose 50%, dextrose 5% in normal saline, and dextrose 5% in lactated Ringer's solution, dextrose 10% to 70% in water, and 3% to 5% NaCl solutions.

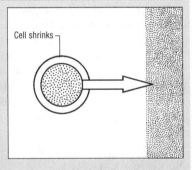

Low osmolality (hypotonic)
Fluids with a low osmolality (< 240 mOsm/L) have a lower concentration of particles than intracellular fluid, so osmotic pressure draws water into the cells from the extracellular fluid. Severe electrolyte losses or inappropriate use of IV fluids can make body fluids hypotonic. Examples: 0.45% NaCl, 0.33% NaCl.

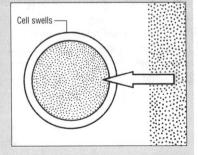

line catheter. In these cases, the catheter should be inserted at the beginning of the therapy.

Selecting a vein

Veins used for midline catheter insertions include the basilic, cephalic, and median cubital veins in the antecubital area. The catheter insertion site may be approximately 1 " (2.5 cm) above or below the antecubital bend and still be an acceptable site for placement. Some patients, like pediatric and elderly patients, may not have suitable hand or forearm veins, but their antecubital veins may still be used for catheter insertion.

If a patient has had repeated venipunctures in this area, the antecubital veins may be unusable. Kinking that occurs during insertion or a catheter that can be threaded only an inch or two into the vein may indicate that the vein is damaged from prior venipuncture. In such instances, another vein should be used.

Selecting a device

You'll need to consider several factors when choosing the most suitable midline catheter for your patient: number of lumens, use of heparin, catheter material, the patient's upper arm length, and catheter size.

When deciding between a single or double lumen, consider whether the patent will be receiving more than one infusion or medication at a time. If, for example, two infusions or three antibiotics are being given, a dual-lumen catheter would be the best choice.

Another important consideration is whether heparin can be used to keep the catheter patent. Some patients are either allergic to heparin or have conditions that contraindicate the use of heparin. If heparin can't be used, a valved catheter should be selected. Valved catheters don't require heparin to maintain patency.

Also consider the patient's sensitivity to specific catheter material. For example, a latex-free catheter should be used for a patient allergic to latex or one who can't tolerate latex products.

Other considerations involved in the selection of the catheter include the need for supplemental insertion equipment and whether the catheter needs to be trimmed before use. Some manufacturers of midline catheters provide insertion trays or kits that include sterile drapes, antiseptic agents, an introducer cannula, an 8" (20 cm) midline catheter, and dressing materials. Other manufacturers sell the catheter and introducer separately. Trimming the catheter may be necessary if the patient's upper arm length is less than 9" (23 cm). Because Groshong catheters can't be trimmed, other catheters should be selected when trimming is necessary.

In addition to choosing the brand of midline catheter, you'll also need to choose the size of the catheter lumen. The catheter size, measured in gauge or French, is usually determined by the size of the available vein or the planned use of the catheter. Use 4Fr or larger to administer or draw blood and a 2Fr to 4Fr for patients with small upper arm veins (to decrease risk of phlebitis). In any case, select a size that will allow sufficient blood flow around the catheter, which will help prevent phlebitis and preserve dwell time.

Midline catheters are 3" to 8" (7.6 to 20.3 cm) long. The length used depends on the age of the patient. Pediatric patients need shorter catheters; adults need longer ones. The catheters are made of either Silastic or polyurethane material. Single- or double-lumen midline catheters are available. Lumen sizes range from 2Fr to 6Fr (approximately 14G to 22G). Some catheters have a built-in extension set to reduce catheter manipulation during routine care and the site irritation that may result. (See *Comparing midline catheters.*)

Some midline catheters have guide wires to help make placement within the vein easier. Most Silastic midline catheters use a guide wire because of the softness of the material, whereas some polyurethane catheters don't need a guide wire because polyurethane is more rigid than Silastic.

Most midline catheters are open at the tip and require the instillation of heparin or saline to maintain patency. Catheters containing the pressure activated safety valve offer an alternative to open lumen catheters. (See *Pressure Activated Safety Valve*, page 86.)

The pressure activated safety valve has a three-way valve in the hub of the catheter that acts to clamp the catheter lumen after infusions or aspirations. The clamp design helps reduce blood backflow into the catheter lumen if the infusion container is empty, which reduces the risk of catheter occlusion. The design also reduces the risk of bleeding or air embolism from accidental disconnections.

Comparing midline catheters

The figures below show two midline catheters and some of their features.

MidCath (Becton Dickinson)
Features:
- Integrated extension set
- Breakaway design for introducer removal
- Available in 20-cm length and 3Fr to 5Fr diameters
- Trimmable
- Latex free
- Single and double lumen catheters available

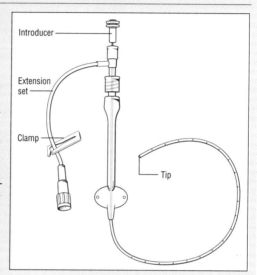

Arrow Midline catheter (Arrow International)
Features:
- Adhesive-backed anchoring device
- Latex free
- Trimmable
- 4Fr and 5Fr diameters available in a 20-cm length
- Peel-away introducer
- Single lumen catheters available

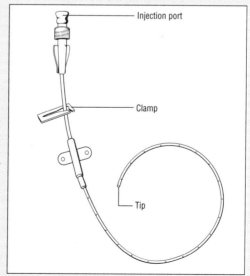

Pressure Activated Safety Valve

The Pressure Activated Safety Valve, built into midline catheters manufactured by Catheter Innovations, acts as an automatic clamp. These illustrations show how the valve works during an infusion, when the catheter isn't being used, and when aspirating.

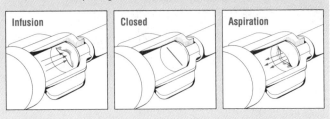

Insertion of a midline catheter

Inserting a midline catheter involves gathering the equipment needed, including the correct catheter. You'll also need to prepare the patient and site, perform the venipuncture and catheter insertion, and apply a dressing.

Gathering the equipment
Before insertion, you'll need an insertion tray. If only the introducer and catheter are available, obtain these additional items:
• two or three sterile disposable drapes
• two pairs of sterile gloves
• alcohol and povidone-iodine swabs to prepare the skin
• two packages of sterile 2" × 2" gauze sponges
• one package of sterile securing strips or a sterile securing device
• one large, sterile transparent semipermeable membrane dressing.

Preparing the patient
The patient's consent and a doctor's order to place a midline catheter may be required in some facilities. Check the policy for obtaining the patient's consent before inserting a midline catheter.

After gathering your equipment, explain the procedure to the patient. Position the patient comfortably in a reclining position, with his arm extended at a 45- to 90-degree angle. Measure the patient's upper arm from the point of planned insertion to two fingerbreadths below the border of the axilla, a distance in most patients of about 7" to 8" (17.5 to 20 cm). The location of the tip of the catheter should not extend beyond 1" (2.5 cm) below the axilla to avoid vessel irritation caused by arm movement. (See *Midline catheter position,* page 88.)

Place a protective pad under the patient's arm. Then apply a tourniquet on the mid–upper arm. Remove the tourniquet once you've found a suitable vein. If necessary, clip the hair 8" to 10" (20 to 25 cm) in diameter around the anticipated insertion site.

An anesthetic agent, such as lidocaine or lidocaine and prilocaine cream (EMLA cream), may be used to numb the site before insertion; just remember that it will take up to an hour for the cream to have an effect. Follow the catheter manufacturer's guidelines before using an anesthetic agent.

Preparing the site

Although variations in insertion techniques exist, an introducer device is usually inserted into the basilic, median cubital, or cephalic vein. This introducer, two sizes larger than the midline catheter, typically has a peel-away feature that allows it to be pulled back out of the patient and then peeled away. This feature lets you remove the introducer without having to separate the catheter from its hub.

After gathering your equipment and preparing the patient, wash your hands and put on a mask, gown, and sterile gloves (preferably powder-free). Then clean the insertion area three separate times with alcohol swabs, starting at the insertion site and working in a circular motion outward until you've cleaned an area 4" to 5" (10 to 12.5 cm) in diameter.

Repeat the cleaning process with povidone-iodine swabs, and allow the solution to air dry. Remove and discard the gloves.

Inserting the catheter

Apply the tourniquet to the upper arm. Put on sterile gloves. Drape the patient's arm with sterile towels or a fenestrated drape, making sure to leave an opening for the venipuncture. The venipuncture site should be one fingerbreadth below or two or three fingerbreadths above the bend of the arm.

Perform the venipuncture with the introducer needle. Insert the catheter according to the manufacturer's directions. Slowly advance the catheter either to the hub or within 1" (2.5 cm) of the hub. If you meet resistance, try placing the patient's arm at a different an-

Midline catheter position

This illustration shows a properly placed midline catheter. Notice that the tip terminates just below the axilla.

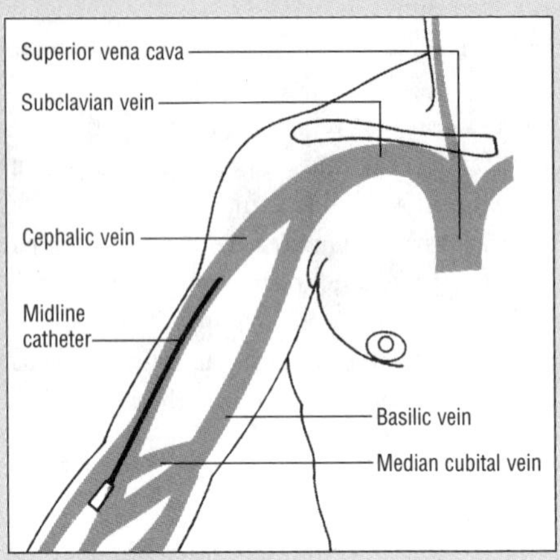

- Superior vena cava
- Subclavian vein
- Cephalic vein
- Midline catheter
- Basilic vein
- Median cubital vein

gle, rotating his wrist, or having him open and close his fist. Applying hot packs to the upper arm may also help.

Remove the tourniquet. If the catheter contains a guide wire, remove it now. Place an injection cap on the catheter hub or connect the IV tubing if you are starting an infusion. Observe the upper arm for swelling as the fluids are infusing. If the catheter will be used for intermittent therapy, flush the catheter according to your facility's policy.

Secure the hub with sterile stabilizing strips, and apply a sterile transparent semipermeable membrane dressing. A 2" × 2" gauze dressing may be used under the initial dressing if drainage is present. Other methods of anchoring the catheter in place include use of a catheter securing device, such as the StatLock or K-LoK devices, which secure the catheter and minimize dislodgment.

Change the dressing within 24 hours, remove the gauze, and assess the site for bleeding, signs of phlebitis, or other complications. Apply a new sterile transparent semipermeable membrane dressing. The stabilizing strips may be changed or, if they're not soiled, remain in place until the next routine dressing change. Note that placing hot packs around the catheter may help prevent mechanical phlebitis.

Maintenance and care

Routine care and maintenance of a midline catheter includes dressing changes and flushing the catheter to maintain patency.

Dressing changes

A sterile dressing change kit and a mask are recommended when changing a midline catheter dressing. These dressings are typically changed every 5 to 7 days. The procedure for changing a midline catheter dressing is similar to that used for changing a central venous catheter dressing. Use of a sterile, transparent semipermeable membrane dressing is preferred over a gauze dressing so that the site can be assessed easily and often. If a gauze dressing is used, it should be changed every 48 hours.

Dressing changes should also include changing the latex injection cap to maintain the integrity of the infusion system and help prevent infection due to a breakdown of the rubber in the cap. Extension sets and stabilizing equipment and strips are also changed at this time.

Flushing the catheter

The peripheral midline catheter must be flushed routinely to prevent blood occlusion and the precipitation of medications. Flush the catheter with normal saline after administering a drug or solution. The recommended volume of normal saline ranges from 5 to 10 ml.

Heparin may also be used, according to policy. The recommended heparin flush volume is 2 to 3 ml of 1:100 U/ml solution.

To keep the catheter patent when no infusions are being given, use the same volumes of either saline or heparin once daily for 3Fr and larger catheters. Smaller lumens should be flushed every 12 hours to avoid catheter occlusion. Follow the manufacturer's guidelines for flushing valved catheters.

Catheter flushes for children require different volumes and heparin concentrations. Pediatric midline catheters are small and become clotted easily. For these patients, a continuous low-volume flush system may be used to keep the vein open. Be sure to refer to pediatric-specific protocols when working with these patients.

Complications

Rare complications of a midline catheter include a sluggish infusion and possibly induration. Other complications include occlusion,

CLINICAL
PEARLS

Assessing for phlebitis

Swelling from phlebitis may be difficult to detect on heavier upper arms. To make detection of phlebitis easier, measure the mid-upper circumference at the time of insertion. Measure it again later if problems are suspected. Comparing the two measurements will help you make a more accurate assessment.

catheter rupture, infection, infiltration, hematoma, air embolus, and thrombus formation. The most common complication, however, is phlebitis, either mechanical or chemical.

MECHANICAL PHLEBITIS. Signs of mechanical phlebitis include redness and tenderness along the catheter track and induration along the vein. When assessing the catheter site for complications, which should be done every 24 hours, inspect the site and gently palpate the path of the catheter along the skin. (See *Assessing for phlebitis*.) Also palpate the approximate location of the catheter tip to detect signs of phlebitis in its earliest stages. If phlebitis is severe, venous inflammation and swelling may impair circulatory return and cause swelling of the arm below the insertion site.

Mechanical phlebitis may be treated with warm compresses two or three times daily. However, if mechanical phlebitis lasts longer than 72 hours or is severe, the catheter should be removed.

CHEMICAL PHLEBITIS. Signs of chemical phlebitis include redness, tenderness, and sometimes swelling above the tip of the catheter, and pain in the axilla when palpating the tip of the catheter or when the arm is moved. If chemical phlebitis occurs, treatment involves removing the catheter.

Teaching the patient

As with all infusion procedures, you should instruct the patient in pertinent aspects of the procedure to enlist his cooperation and enhance the potential for successful therapy. Prior to catheter insertion, teach the patient about the purpose of the infusion device, the location, insertion procedure, follow-up care, and potential complications.

After insertion, patient teaching should focus on dressing procedures, site monitoring, and when to report signs and symptoms of complications. Printed materials that explain the venous access device, site assessment, points of care, and maintenance can help reinforce your teaching.

Removal of a midline catheter

Midline catheters are removed for three main reasons: the patient's therapy is completed, a complication occurs requiring removal, or the catheter is suspected of being contaminated. Before removing the catheter, collect these supplies: clean gloves, antiseptic ointment, $2'' \times 2''$ gauze, tape, and a clean tape measure.

To remove the catheter, put gloves on, stabilize the hub, and begin removing the dressing by pulling it toward the insertion site to avoid putting tension on the catheter. Grasping the catheter hub, gently pull the catheter to begin removal.

When approximately $2''$ (5 cm) of the catheter have cleared the skin line, grasp the catheter below the insertion point and continue removing it. This approach avoids stretching of the catheter and possible breakage. Continue a gentle, constant pulling motion until the entire catheter has been removed. Avoid placing pressure on the insertion site until the entire catheter tip has cleared the skin line.

Use extra caution when removing a catheter that has been in place for a prolonged period. Venous spasm may occur during removal, causing resistance and making removal more difficult. In addition, fibrin might have formed around the catheter, which can also make removal difficult. If you meet resistance when removing a catheter, the removal should be stopped and the doctor notified. *Never stretch the catheter.* Doing so could cause the catheter to break, leading to a catheter embolus.

After the catheter has been removed, apply antiseptic ointment to the insertion site and cover it with the gauze. Tape the gauze in place with tension, to create a pressure dressing. Then assess the catheter tip to make sure the entire catheter has been removed. Measure the length of the catheter to ensure complete removal. Note that Silastic catheters that have been in place for a extended period of time might have stretched while in place and may be slightly longer than the initial length.

Documenting insertion of a midline catheter

When documenting the insertion of a midline catheter, make sure you cover the points shown in this documentation sample.

> Peripheral midline catheter inserted into left median cubital basilic vein using a #4Fr V-Cath 8" catheter (Lot #_____). Catheter advanced without problems. Seven inches of catheter advanced into vein; 1 inch of catheter remains outside insertion point. Patient tolerated procedure well and stated 'that was not bad at all.' Excellent blood return obtained after placement. Catheter flushed with 5 ml normal saline followed by 3 ml of heparin flush solution 1:100 U/ml. Catheter hub stabilized with StatLock device; sterile 2" x 2" gauze over insertion site and IV 3,000 transparent dressing applied.
>
> K McGuire, CRNI.

Documentation

Documentation for the insertion of a midline catheter should cover all aspects of the insertion. (See *Documenting insertion of a midline catheter.*) Aspects that should be documented include:
• specific vein used
• device used (include product, lot number, size, and length)
• length of catheter threaded into vein and amount of catheter remaining outside insertion site
• ease or difficulty when threading the catheter into the vein
• aspiration or confirmation of blood return
• patient tolerance of procedure
• specific dressing material applied
• appropriate flushing of catheter.
    After discontinuing a midline catheter, document:
• the type of device removed and the site it was removed from
• ease of removal or problems encountered
• catheter tip integrity
• length of catheter removed
• dressing application
• patient's response to the procedure.

Managing PICC therapy

Peripherally inserted central venous catheters (PICCs) have become increasingly popular in the last few years. Inserted into a peripheral vein and threaded so that the tip lies within the central vascular system, PICCs have been used for all kinds of patients—from newborns to teenagers to older adults—who need long-term infusion therapy, lack adequate peripheral venous access, are homebound, or require frequent venipuncture to obtain blood for testing. PICCs are also useful for patients receiving chemotherapy, hyperalimentation, analgesics, frequent blood transfusions, dobutamine, antibiotics, or other infusions irritating to the peripheral vasculature.

Qualified personnel who can insert a PICC include certified infusion nurses, registered nurses who have taken a PICC class and successfully completed a preceptorship under the supervision of a clinical expert, and doctors. The number of supervised insertions required for qualification varies from facility to facility.

Once inserted, PICCs are stable enough to remain in place for months at a time, sometimes for a year or more if the line is maintained without complications. In addition, a PICC can handle the infusion of solutions with an osmolality of 600 mOsm/L or more and a pH below 6 or above 8.

This chapter examines advantages and disadvantages of PICC use, how to select a patient for these highly useful catheters, how to choose a vein and catheter, inserting and caring for a PICC, complications, catheter removal, patient teaching, and documentation.

Advantages and disadvantages

PICCs offer several advantages over other catheters. (See *Comparing selected peripherally inserted catheters.*) First, PICCs can be inserted at the bedside or in an outpatient setting rather than solely in an operating or radiology suite. PICCs avoid the need for repeated venipuncture, reduce the risk of phlebitis or infiltration, and are flexible, safe, and comfortable.

In addition, PICCs allow for shorter hospital stays because the patient can continue therapy at home, and compared with central venous catheters, PICCs tend to cause fewer infections. These advantages make PICC therapy more cost-effective overall than central venous catheters.

In some practice areas, such as home care, PICCs are sometimes trimmed so that the tip is located in the midclavicular area. Known as midclavicular catheters, they are peripheral, not central catheters. Organizations such as the Intravenous Nurses Society (INS) either have or are developing position statements on their use.

Like other catheters, PICCs restrict patient activities, such as swimming or strenuous exercise. They also require regular maintenance by trained nurses and patient compliance for routine care. A PICC may cause embarrassment for the patient because the catheter remains visible. A central venous catheter, on the other hand, can be hidden more easily with clothing.

Selecting a patient

Candidates for placement of a PICC include patients with cancer, acquired immunodeficiency syndrome, recurrent infections, sickle cell anemia, multiple trauma, chronic heart failure, Crohn's disease, or cystic fibrosis. A PICC may *not* be a suitable access device for patients with poor antecubital veins, bleeding disorders, or scarring or injury from multiple IV restarts.

PICCs are also not appropriate for confused patients or toddlers because a longer immobilization period is required during the inser-

Comparing selected peripherally inserted catheters

This chart compares tip location, dwell times, and the types of solutions that may be used with midclavicular, midline, and peripherally inserted central catheters (PICCs).

TYPE OF CATHETER	TIP LOCATION	DWELL TIME	DELIVERY OF THERAPIES
Midclavicular	Peripherally inserted with tip placement in proximal axillary or subclavian vein	2 to 3 months	IV fluids, blood products, peripheral parenteral nutrition (PPN), electrolytes, and prescribed medications
Midline	Peripherally inserted with tip placement in proximal portion of extremity	2 to 4 weeks	IV fluids, blood products, PPN, electrolytes, and prescribed medications
PICC	Peripherally inserted with tip placement in superior vena cava	1 year	Total parenteral nutrition, vesicant chemotherapy, and all other fluids

tion procedure and because these patients are more likely to dislodge the catheter.

Because of the limitations on arm movement required for a PICC, children pose a unique challenge for PICC therapy, especially if long-term therapy is anticipated. For children under age 4, an implantable device should be considered rather than a PICC. For children age 4 and older, however, a PICC may be used.

Selecting a vein

Knowledge of vein anatomy is critical for proper insertion of the PICC. For instance, the valves in a vein can impede the advancement of a PICC being inserted. Passage of the catheter in short increments usually alleviates this problem. In general, the preferred insertion sites for a PICC include the basilic, median basilic, cephalic, or accessory cephalic vein.

Because the basilic vein has the widest diameter and greatest blood flow of the upper arm veins, it is the vein of choice for PICC insertion. The basilic vein also has a more direct path to central veins. However, the vein is more difficult to use in patients with more upper arm fat, and it typically lies near the brachial artery and cutaneous nerve, either of which may be damaged during insertion.

The median basilic vein, because of its size and position in the arm, can accommodate a large cannula. The cephalic veins lie near the skin surface and are easy to find during an insertion. Threading the catheter through one of these veins may be more difficult, however. In that instance, changing the position of the arm may make insertion easier.

Selecting a device

Choosing an appropriate PICC for each patient can be challenging. When selecting a catheter, consider catheter design and the characteristics of each type of catheter.

PICCs are made of either silicone or polyurethane. Silicone, a soft and pliable material, can remain in place for a long time without causing irritation, thrombosis, or a breakdown in the integrity of the catheter. In contrast, polyurethane is stiffer but stronger. It has a good flow capacity but may be less compatible with the body. Both catheters are radiopaque so they can be detected on X-ray.

PICCs are available as single- or double-lumen devices and may come with a guide wire to facilitate easier insertion. (See *Types of PICCs,* pages 98 and 99.) Single-lumen catheters can be trimmed to a specific length. PICC diameters range from 16G to 28G for single-lumen; 2Fr to 5Fr for double-lumen. The catheters are approximately 20" to 24" (50 to 60 cm) long.

The choice of a catheter gauge should be based on the size of the vein being used. The catheter should fit snugly into the vessel yet be small enough not to impede blood flow.

Selection also depends on the ability of the patient or caregiver to manage the catheter at home (if appropriate), the length of therapy, type and complexity of treatment, and the nurse's own preference of PICC styles. The financial status of the patient may also play a role in the catheter selected.

Insertion of a PICC

Insertion of a PICC entails gathering the equipment; preparing the catheter, and site; and inserting the catheter, including how to secure the catheter and check tip placement.

Gathering the equipment

Before a PICC is inserted, gather all the necessary equipment. Obtain a catheter insertion kit or obtain these supplies:
• three alcohol swabs
• three povidone-iodine swabs
• injection cap with a short extension tubing (long extension tubing if patient is going to perform the PICC care at home)
• PICC introducer (should be two gauges larger than the PICC) and the PICC
• guide wire (if appropriate)
• local anesthetic (optional)
• sterile and nonsterile measuring tapes
• sterile drapes, forceps, and scissors
• sterile transparent semipermeable membrane dressing
• two pairs of sterile nonpowdered gloves
• three 10-ml syringes
• vial of sterile normal saline solution
• 3-ml vial of facility-approved flush solution
• linen-saver pads
• tourniquet
• sterile 2" × 2" and 4" × 4" gauze pads
• sterile gown and face shield or goggles
• sutures and sterile tape strips.

Extra supplies should be kept handy if accidental contamination occurs or the first attempt is unsuccessful. If powdered gloves are being used, remember to first rinse them with sterile water before proceeding, to prevent talc phlebitis.

Preparing the patient

Check the doctor's order and determine whether the patient has allergies before inserting a PICC. The order should include a post-procedure X-ray to confirm catheter placement. Educate the patient about the reason for the PICC, the insertion procedure, and what will need to be done to care for the catheter. Obtain consent for the procedure, if required and not already obtained.

Types of PICCs

Numerous PICCs are available for use. These illustrations show some of the various types of PICCs.

Per-Q-Cath (Bard)

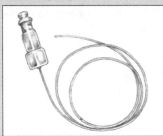

OneCath (Luther)

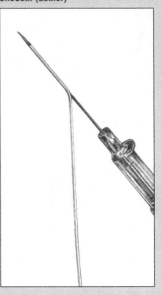

Dual-lumen Per-Q-Cath (Bard)

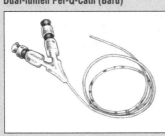

Wash your hands with an antimicrobial soap for 1 minute. Place the patient in a supine or semi-Fowler's position, with the arm extended and abducted at a 90-degree angle. If the patient has a large amount of hair on the arm, clip the hair with scissors rather than shaving with a razor; shaving allows bacteria to migrate into open abrasions and cause infection.

Assess the antecubital fossa. If the area is red, tender, edematous, or draining, select another site. Unless approved by the doctor, do not use an arm on the side of a mastectomy or an arteriovenous fistula. Place a linen-saver pad under the patient's arm, and then place a tourniquet on the upper arm to distend the veins. Select a suitable vein.

Remove the tourniquet, and measure the distance from the planned insertion site to where the tip of the catheter will lie follow-

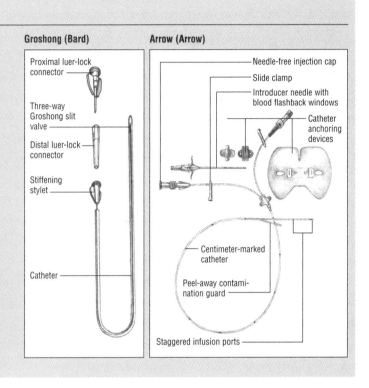

Groshong (Bard)

Proximal luer-lock connector

Three-way Groshong slit valve

Distal luer-lock connector

Stiffening stylet

Catheter

Arrow (Arrow)

Needle-free injection cap

Slide clamp

Introducer needle with blood flashback windows

Catheter anchoring devices

Centimeter-marked catheter

Peel-away contamination guard

Staggered infusion ports

ing insertion. For placement in the superior vena cava, use a nonsterile measuring tape to measure the distance from the insertion site to the shoulder and from the shoulder to the sternal notch. Then add 3″ (8 cm) to this figure.

Preparing the device

Open the catheter insertion kit and drop the sterile items onto the sterile field. Place a mask on the patient, especially if he is immunocompromised. Put on the face mask or shield, sterile gown, and nonpowdered sterile gloves.

Using aseptic technique, withdraw 10 ml of sterile 0.9% saline and fill three syringes. Remove the needles. Take the catheter from the kit, and check that the guide wire is straight and the catheter is intact. Kinks or bends in the guide wire may make removal of the wire difficult after the catheter has been inserted.

If you need to trim the catheter, cut the tip straight across to prevent the catheter from lying flush against the intima of the vein and possibly obstructing the flow of the infusion. Keep in mind that some catheters, like the Groshong, cannot be trimmed.

Using aseptic technique, attach the syringe and flush the extension tubing and cap. Flush the catheter separately with the saline. Place the catheter back in the kit to prevent contamination.

Preparing the site

To prepare the insertion site, clean it with three alcohol swabs, using circular motions from the insertion site outward until you've covered an area about 6" (15 cm) from the site. Extensive cleaning is critical for preventing infection. Continue cleaning for about 2 minutes. Repeat the procedure with the povidone-iodine swabs. Allow the site to air dry. (See *Preparing for PICC insertion.*)

Remove and discard the old gloves, and reapply the tourniquet about 4" (10 cm) above the antecubital fossa. Put on a pair of non-powdered, sterile gloves. Position a sterile drape around the patient's arm and over the tourniquet. Be sure that you can release the tourniquet without contaminating the sterile field.

Inserting the catheter

Palpate the vein and stretch the skin taut. Insert the catheter introducer into the vein at a 15- to 30-degree angle. (See *Inserting a PICC,* page 102.) When blood appears in the flashback chamber, gently advance the plastic introducer sheath without changing needle position until the tip of the sheath is well inside the vein.

Release the tourniquet by grasping the end through the sterile drape. Take care not to contaminate the field. Carefully withdraw the needle while holding the introducer steady. Apply pressure on the vein just above the distal end of the introducer sheath to minimize blood loss.

Using aseptic technique, insert the catheter into the introducer sheath and advance it into the vein. If the vein is small, you may need to keep the tourniquet tied to distend the vein until the catheter has been threaded 3" to 4" (8 to 10 cm) into the vein. You can also help the catheter advance more easily by having the patient turn his head toward the venipuncture site and put his chin on his shoulder.

Preparing for PICC insertion

Proper preparation is critical for a successful insertion of a PICC. This sequence of photos demonstrates the main steps involved in preparing for PICC insertion.

1. Measuring the insertion site.

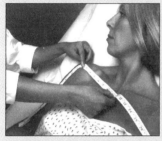

3. Flushing the catheter.

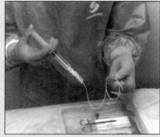

2. Trimming the catheter.

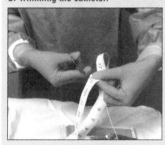

4. Cleaning the site.

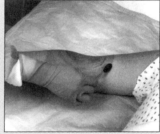

Advance the catheter until about 4" (10 cm) remains externally. Retract the introducer sheath from the vein, leaving the catheter intact. Pull the tabs away from the catheter slowly and smoothly until the sheath is completely split. Gentle movements here are important to prevent dislodging the catheter.

Continue to advance the catheter until about 2" (5 cm) remains externally. Aspirate for blood to determine proper catheter placement. Then flush the catheter with 10 ml of saline solution. With the patient's arm below the level of the heart, remove the syringe. Connect the injection cap with extension tubing to the hub of the catheter.

Securing the catheter
The PICC can be anchored with sutures, sterile tape strips, or catheter anchoring devices to prevent the catheter from migrating or

Inserting a PICC

These pictures show the proper technique for the insertion of a PICC.

1. Check for flashback.

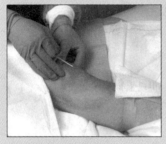

3. Split the introducer sheath.

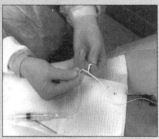

2. Advance the catheter.

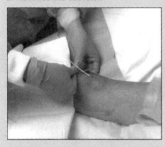

4. Add the connector tubing.

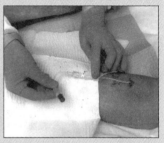

becoming dislodged. After the catheter has been anchored, apply a 2" × 2" gauze pad. Then place a transparent semipermeable membrane dressing directly over the site.

Confirming tip placement

Once the PICC has been inserted, an X-ray is taken to confirm its placement. (See *Proper placement of a PICC.*) Never rely solely on external measurements because internal pathways of the veins vary widely from patient to patient. If the catheter has been placed properly, the X-ray should indicate that the tip of the catheter is located in the upper one-third to one-half of the superior vena cava. After proper placement has been determined, check for blood return again. Then flush the line with 6 ml of normal saline. The PICC may now be used.

Measure the circumference of the upper arm immediately after the catheter is inserted and again during each dressing change, to

Proper placement of a PICC

The following illustration shows the proper placement of a PICC. Note that the tip lies centrally in the superior vena cava.

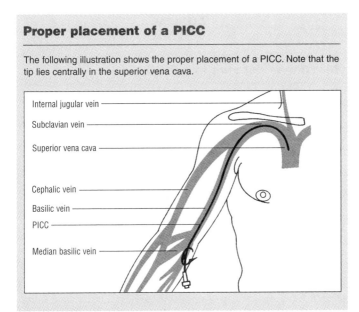

Internal jugular vein

Subclavian vein

Superior vena cava

Cephalic vein

Basilic vein

PICC

Median basilic vein

monitor for signs of swelling. You'll also need to periodically check the external length of the catheter to detect migration.

Maintenance and care

Unlike other peripheral catheters, the site of a PICC doesn't need to be rotated. The catheter can remain in the same vessel from 7 days to 1 year. Maintenance and care of a PICC involve administering medications through the line, changing the dressing (including flushing the catheter and changing the cap), and drawing blood samples for tests.

Administering medications

To administer a medication through a PICC, you'll need to collect three 10-ml syringes, two filled with 3 ml of normal saline solution and one with heparin flush solution (per facility policy). You'll also need gloves, alcohol swabs, and the prescribed medication in a 10-ml syringe.

Before administering the drug, check the doctor's order. Explain the procedure to the patient, and then wash your hands with an antibacterial soap for 1 minute. Check the patient's chart to make sure

CLINICAL
PEARLS

Meeting resistance in a PICC

If resistance occurs when you try to instill a medication, try aspirating and flushing the line with sterile normal saline solution. In some cases, blockages result from the precipitate of a drug and may be treated by instilling another drug to alter pH and bring the precipitate back into solution. If resistance persists, call the doctor for an order for an X-ray (if a kink is suspected) or thrombolytic therapy (if a clot is suspected).

that the placement of the catheter tip has been confirmed by chest X-ray.

Wipe the injection port with an alcohol swab. Flush the tubing with normal saline solution. If you encounter resistance, stop the procedure; the catheter may be blocked. (See *Meeting resistance in a PICC.*) If the port flushes easily, continue flushing. Wipe the injection port again with an alcohol swab, and administer the medication, as ordered. Inject the drug according to the doctor's order, or consult with a pharmacist for the appropriate rate of administration. When the medication has been administered, flush the catheter with the second saline-filled syringe.

Repeat the entire procedure (wipe, flush, wipe, administer) for each medication given. Follow the final saline flush with a heparin flush as your facility's policy allows.

Dispose of all used equipment properly. Wash your hands, and then document the procedure on the patient's chart.

Dressing changes

After 24 hours, you'll need to remove the original dressing and replace it with a transparent semipermeable membrane dressing. Change the dressing every 7 days. The dressing should be changed immediately if it becomes loose, soiled, or wet.

Dressing changes involve gathering the equipment, removing the old dressing, and applying a new dressing. Ideally, routine flushing of the catheter and changing of the injection cap should coincide with dressing changes.

Gathering the equipment

Before changing the dressing, obtain a dressing change kit or gather the following equipment:

• clean, nonsterile gloves and two masks
• sterile nonpowdered gloves
• three alcohol swabs
• three povidone-iodine swabs
• transparent semipermeable membrane dressing
• sterile drape
• sterile tape strips (if catheter isn't sutured or if a stabilizing device such as a StatLock is not used).

Removing the old dressing
To remove the old dressing, wash your hands and explain the procedure to the patient. Position the patient's arm away from his body at a 45- to 90-degree angle. Wear a sterile mask. If the patient is immunocompromised, put a mask on him as well. Put on clean gloves, and then slowly remove the old dressing.

Hold the catheter with one hand while gently pulling the dressing *toward* the insertion site with the other to prevent dislodgment of the PICC. You needn't remove the tape holding the extension tubing unless it's loose. If the extension tubing was placed under the sterile dressing on the previous dressing change, change the tubing. Inspect the site for redness, swelling, or drainage. Dispose of the gloves and dressing according to standard precautions.

Applying a new dressing
New dressings are applied using strict aseptic technique. Prepare a sterile field on a clean, flat surface. Open all sterile equipment and put on nonpowdered, sterile gloves. Place a sterile drape over the patient's forearm, making sure to cover the extension tubing and to leave the insertion site exposed. (See *Changing the dressing,* page 106.)

Clean the site thoroughly with three alcohol swabs. Start at the insertion site and carefully work outward in a circular motion. Repeat with the povidone-iodine swabs. Allow the area to air dry. Take care not to touch the insertion site.

Apply a sterile transparent semipermeable membrane dressing. Label the dressing with the date and time and your initials. Used materials should be disposed of according to standard precautions.

Wash your hands, and document the procedure. Be sure to include a description of the condition of the insertion site and to inform the doctor of complications or other problems.

Changing the dressing

PICC dressings should be changed according to facility policy. The following photos highlight the correct procedure for changing a PICC dressing.

1. Remove the old dressing.

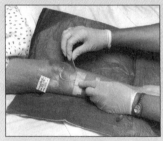

3. Clean the site.

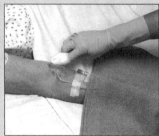

2. Drape the site.

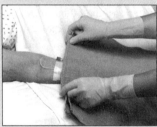

4. Date the dressing after it's applied.

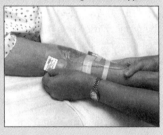

Routine flushing

The procedure for flushing a PICC varies. Check your facility's policies. Flushing isn't needed when the patient is receiving a continuous infusion through a single-lumen catheter. Follow these general guidelines when flushing a PICC.

When a patient has a double-lumen catheter maintained as a heparin lock, flush all lumens with a heparin flush solution every 24 hours. Use normal saline solution only to flush a Groshong catheter.

Check for blood return before flushing to ensure proper placement. Keep in mind that you may not see a blood return if a small gauge catheter is used or if the patient has a low venous pressure.

Recommended concentrations of heparin flush solutions range from 10 to 1,000 U/ml, although 100 U/ml is used most often. The recommended frequency and amount of flush also vary; be sure to follow your facility's guidelines.

In general, flush each unused lumen once daily with 6 to 10 ml of normal saline, followed by 5 ml of 100 U/ml of heparin. Also flush each lumen before and after every use. The maximum daily heparin flush shouldn't exceed 50 U/kg/day.

To flush the catheter, obtain alcohol swabs, the facility-approved flush solution, and a needleless cap, if needed. Wash your hands with an antibacterial soap for 1 minute, and put on clean, nonpowdered gloves. Clean the cap with an alcohol swab, and allow the cap to dry. Inject the flush solution using a needleless syringe. After flushing, maintain positive pressure on the catheter by keeping your thumb on the syringe plunger as you withdraw the needle. This prevents the backflow of blood, which might lead to clotting in the line.

Changing the cap

The frequency of cap changes varies among institutions and the number of times the cap is used. The INS recommends that the cap be changed at least every 7 days.

To change the cap, obtain clean gloves, alcohol or povidone-iodine swabs, and an injection cap. Wash your hands with an antimicrobial soap for 1 minute. Explain the procedure to the patient. Put on the gloves and clean the old cap at its connection to the catheter with a swab.

Clamp the extension tubing with the tubing clamp or a padded clamp, or ask the patient to perform the Valsalva maneuver as you quickly remove the old cap and connect the new cap using aseptic technique. The Valsalva maneuver can help prevent air from entering the line. Document the cap change according to your facility's policy.

Obtaining a blood sample

If the PICC is to be used for drawing blood, it should be a size 4Fr or larger to prevent hemolysis. Obtain an injection cap (if needed), alcohol or povidone-iodine swabs, a 5-ml evacuated tube, appropriate evacuated tubes for the tests being ordered, an evacuated tube holder, and a 20G needle or a needleless blood-collection adapter.

Wash your hands with an antibacterial soap for 1 minute. Put on clean gloves and explain the procedure to the patient. Stop the infusion, and wait 1 minute before drawing blood from the catheter. This prevents IV fluid and medication from mixing with the drawn blood.

For a patient with a double-lumen PICC, you'll draw blood from the lumen not connected to a continuous infusion. Clean the end of the appropriate injection cap with antiseptic swabs. Place a 5-ml evacuated tube into its plastic holder. This tube will be used to collect and discard the filling volume of the catheter, plus an extra 2 to 3 ml. If an evacuated tube isn't available, you can use a 10-ml or larger syringe.

Insert the needle into the injection cap, or, if using a needleless system, attach the syringe directly to the cap. Then withdraw the blood. Note that the first milliliter may be clear because of the previous flush.

When blood stops flowing into the tube, remove and discard the tube. If a needleless system is used, you may need to place an adapter between the syringe and the evacuated tube holder. In some needleless systems, the adapter fits directly into the needleless cap.

Fill the appropriate tubes for the blood tests that have been ordered. When completed, flush the catheter with 10 to 20 ml of sterile normal saline in a pulsatile manner, according to your facility's policy. (See *Pulsatile flushing.*) If the lumen isn't going to be used immediately, flush the catheter with a facility-approved flush solution.

If blood doesn't flow from the catheter and the clamp is open, the tip of the catheter may be resting against the vessel wall. Have the patient raise his arms over his head, turn on his side, or cough or perform the Valsalva maneuver. Flushing the catheter with sterile normal saline may also help to initiate blood flow. If blood fails to flow, the catheter may be kinked or displaced or a thrombus may have formed in the line. Remove the dressing, and examine the site and external catheter. Obtain an order for an X-ray or thrombolytic therapy, as indicated.

Complications

Although PICCs are associated with fewer problems than other central venous catheters, complications can still occur at any time after insertion. Complications of PICC therapy include mechanical phlebitis, bleeding, infection, thrombosis, catheter migration or dislodgment, air embolism, pain, and catheter fracture.

MECHANICAL PHLEBITIS. Mechanical phlebitis is commonly observed within the first 72 hours following insertion and occurs most often when the catheter is inserted in the left arm or when a large-gauge catheter is used. Mechanical phlebitis can also be due to irritation by foreign objects, such as glove powder, lint, or the catheter itself.

Signs and symptoms include pain along the vein track from the point of insertion and a continuous or intermittent red streak over

CLINICAL
PEARLS

Pulsatile flushing

Pulsatile flushing is a technique performed by injecting saline with moderate pressure, stopping, and then resuming again. This sequence is repeated several times and helps to prevent clotting in the catheter by providing more effective clearing.

the catheter pathway. Mechanical phlebitis can be treated by applying warm, moist compresses to the affected extremity for 20 minutes three or four times daily for 48 hours. Limiting the use of the arm and elevating it on pillows are also effective. Treatment is most successful when initiated at the first sign of phlebitis. However, if you note a warm, bright red, cordlike track about ½" (1.3 cm) wide, the phlebitis is advanced and you'll need to remove the catheter.

BLEEDING. Minimal bleeding may occur during the first 24 hours. If blood saturates the dressing, however, inform the doctor. Persistent bleeding may result from anticoagulant therapy, trauma during insertion, or excessive physical activity. Care should be taken during the insertion and maintenance of the PICC to prevent bleeding problems.

INFECTION. Infection in a PICC is usually related to a break in aseptic technique, the length of time a catheter is in place, the number of times the catheter lumen is entered, and inadequate site care. The incidence of sepsis is greater in patients with double-lumen catheters because the lumens of these catheters are usually accessed more frequently.
    Infection is characterized by pain, redness, or drainage at the insertion site. You may also note fever, chills, hypotension, nausea, vomiting, or headache. Antibiotic treatment should begin immediately. If the PICC is the source of infection, the catheter should be removed. To prevent infection, use aseptic technique when changing dressings or manipulating the catheter.

THROMBOSIS. A PICC can become occluded as a result of a thrombus. Poor blood flow around the catheter or the accumulation of fibrin as a result of endothelial trauma can also cause a clot to occlude the catheter. In addition, certain risk factors—such as cancer, sickle cell anemia, or previous pulmonary embolism or deep vein thrombosis— increase the likelihood that thrombosis will develop.

Signs of thrombosis include decreased IV flow rate, resistance when flushing the catheter, or edema in an area distal to the clot (arm, shoulder, supraclavicular area, or neck). The patient might also complain of jaw, shoulder, chest, or ear pain. Infection may follow the formation of a clot because organisms tend to flourish in a thrombus.

If thrombosis occurs, notify the doctor immediately. Once the clot location has been determined, remove the catheter. Infuse anti-coagulant doses of heparin, if ordered. Apply warm, wet compresses locally.

Prevention remains the best treatment, however. Assess the patient frequently for thrombosis, and teach him about the early signs and symptoms of thrombosis and when to report them.

CATHETER MIGRATION OR DISLODGMENT. Once in place, a PICC can migrate, meaning that the tip of the catheter moves forward or backward from its original position in the vein. Vigorous flushing, excessive vomiting, constant coughing, or a poorly secured catheter contribute to catheter migration.

An X-ray should be obtained to confirm tip placement if you're unable to obtain a blood return, if the patient complains of pain, or if you note that the length of external tubing has increased. Careful anchoring of the line and limiting arm movement can help to prevent catheter migration.

PICCs can also become dislodged from the vein, especially by a confused patient or fidgety toddler playing with the dressing or catheter. To prevent the catheter from becoming dislodged, be sure the catheter has been properly secured with tape or sutures.

AIR EMBOLISM. Because the PICC line is inserted below the heart level, air embolism is less likely to occur than in centrally inserted lines. However, whenever the PICC tubing is opened or if air is accidentally injected when priming the line, air can seep into the line and lead to an air embolism. Always use clamps when the line is open to air, such as when changing the cap or tubing. When changing the tubing or inserting a syringe into the system, check that no air enters the tubing or syringe.

If an air embolism occurs, turn the patient onto his left side with his head down, so air can enter the right atrium and disperse through the pulmonary artery. Have the patient maintain this position for 20 to 30 minutes. Notify the doctor, and administer oxygen, as ordered.

PAIN. Pain can occur during any infusion through a PICC but is especially common when the catheter has been inserted in the cephalic or midarm veins. Pain may be caused by a damaged catheter or the chemical properties of the IV solution. Signs of a damaged catheter include obvious leakage of solution at the site during an infusion or flushing or the presence of IV solution on the dressing.

Catheter damage can occur if the catheter is accidentally cut during dressing changes. To prevent this, avoid using scissors near the IV line. Stabilize the PICC before removing the dressing. Pulling the dressing toward the insertion site avoids placing tension on the catheter and possible catheter damage.

CATHETER FRACTURE. Silicone PICCs carry a greater risk of becoming fractured than PICCs made of different materials. Catheter fractures often result from using excessive pressure when flushing the line, flushing the line with a syringe smaller than 10 ml, or using excessive force when removing a PICC line. To avoid fracture, use a 10-ml syringe when flushing. Don't use a syringe smaller than 10 ml. Smaller syringes exert higher pressures and can damage the catheter. Flush gently, and refrain from using too much force when removing the PICC.

If you think the catheter is fractured, place a tourniquet on the patient's upper arm near the axilla to prevent catheter migration. The tourniquet should be tight enough to occlude venous return but not so tight that it closes off arterial circulation. Notify the doctor. Tell the patient that if he feels burning, stinging, or a popping sensation in the area, he should suspect a catheter fracture and should call for help immediately. A homebound patient can use a belt instead of a tourniquet to prevent the catheter from migrating. In any case, the PICC should be replaced or the therapy discontinued.

In some instances, a torn PICC can be exchanged over a guide wire or through a peel-away sheath introducer by a specially trained nurse with a doctor's order. This procedure will vary according to facility policy and state nurse practice acts.

Teaching the patient

Before beginning your patient education for a PICC, assess the patient's and caregiver's physical and cognitive ability to assist in caring for the PICC. Explain what a PICC is and why it's used. Instruct the patient and caregiver to report changes, such as swelling, warmth, redness, tenderness, or pain in the affected arm.

Make sure that the patient or caregiver can explain how to maintain a PICC and can return demonstrate critical skills. Also make sure that the patient or caregiver receives written instructions of all the points you cover in your teaching.

Removal of a PICC

Once therapy is completed, the PICC can be removed. You'll need povidone-iodine swabs, sterile 4″ × 4″ gauze pads, tape measure, suture-removal scissors (if needed), a linen-saver pad, and clean, nonpowdered gloves.

Once you've gathered the equipment, explain the procedure to the patient. Have the patient assume the supine position, making sure the head of the bed is flat and the patient's arm is at a 45- to 90-degree angle to the body.

Wash your hands with antibacterial soap for 1 minute. Place a linen-saver pad under the patient's arm, and don clean gloves. Carefully remove the dressing, adhesive strips, and clip sutures, if present. Stabilize the catheter at the hub with one hand and pull the adhesive dressings toward the insertion site with the other. Avoid stretching the catheter. Instruct the patient to perform the Valsalva maneuver and have him sit up just before removal, to reduce the risk of air embolism.

Using aseptic technique, pull out the catheter slowly and gently until it's completely out of the vein. If resistance occurs, tape the catheter to the skin using slight traction. Wait a few minutes, and try removing the catheter again. Applying warm, moist heat over the catheter track and insertion site for 30 minutes can help ease removal, as can injecting saline while removing the catheter or placing the patient's arm by his side.

Once the catheter has been removed, place a sterile gauze pad on the site and apply manual pressure for 1 minute or until the bleeding stops. Cover the site with a small gauze dressing, and check the site periodically for bleeding. Dispose of used items according to standard precautions, and then wash your hands.

Measure the catheter's length and inspect the catheter closely to make sure it's intact. If part of it has broken during removal, notify the doctor immediately, obtain an X-ray, and monitor the patient for signs of distress. If a piece of the catheter remains in the patient, removal should be done by an interventional radiologist. If the catheter is defective, save the catheter and complete a variance or incident report.

Documentation

Documenting the insertion, care, or removal of a PICC involves notations about a wide variety of events and procedures. Make sure your charting about the insertion of a PICC includes the following information:
• vein and site used
• preparation of the site
• number of insertion attempts made
• complications or difficulties in placing the catheter
• size and length of the catheter from the exit site to the catheter tip
• length of the catheter from the exit site to the hub
• total length of the catheter
• lot number and product code of the catheter
• confirmation by X ray of tip placement
• success of aspiration for blood return
• flushing of the line
• date, time, and type of catheter
• patient teaching performed
• patient's response to procedure.

Documentation for dressing changes and other maintenance care, including removal of the catheter, should cover:
• dates and times of all dressing changes
• upper arm circumference at time of insertion and at removal
• condition of the site
• patient's response to each procedure
• patient teaching performed
• date and time of procedure
• length and appearance of catheter on removal.

8

Managing central venous catheter therapy

Central venous catheters (CVCs) are long catheters inserted into the subclavian or jugular vein and threaded so that the tip is located in the superior vena cava. The femoral vein, rarely used, requires tip placement in the inferior vena cava. At one time, CVCs were used only in critical care settings. Their use today covers all settings, from emergency departments to step-down units to the patient's home.

CVCs are used to deliver drugs and fluids, monitor central venous pressure and cardiac efficiency, and obtain blood for tests when frequent blood sampling is needed and peripheral venous access is limited or otherwise contraindicated. This chapter examines the advantages and disadvantages of CVCs; selection of patients, veins, and catheters for CVCs; insertion of CVCs; catheter and site care; complications; patient teaching; catheter removal; and documentation of a CVC.

Advantages and disadvantages

In general, CVCs allow access to central veins for the infusion of large amounts of fluids or medications and a means to draw blood samples without the need for repeated venipuncture. CVC therapy is superior to peripheral therapy for home care patients because patients find caring for a CVC easier than for a peripheral catheter. For example, a patient with a peripheral catheter would have only one hand free when caring for the line; a patient with a CVC would have both hands free.

In addition, CVCs allow for the infusion of highly osmolar or caustic fluids. These fluids, when infused into a central vein, are rapidly diluted by greater blood flow, thereby reducing the risk of chemical phlebitis. Some CVCs also allow for monitoring of central venous pressure and other pressures.

As with any invasive procedure, however, central venous therapy has its drawbacks. It increases the risk of complications, such as pneumothorax, sepsis, thrombus formation, and perforation of adjacent blood vessels, particularly the carotid artery and the subclavian vein or artery.

Disadvantages of CVC insertion in a neck vein, a common insertion site, include limited mobility of the patient's head, the potential for discomfort, and exposure of the patient to trauma because of the catheter's position. The patient's body image may also be affected by the catheter's presence in such an obvious position as the neck. In addition, insertion costs are higher for CVCs than some other types of central venous access devices, especially if an operating suite is required for insertion. However, some CVCs may prove more economical over time.

Insertion of a CVC into the subclavian vein may be more difficult in a patient on a ventilator or in one who is dehydrated. However, once inserted, catheters placed here are relatively easy to stabilize and maintain.

Selecting a patient

CVCs may be suitable for a wide variety of patients in many clinical settings. The catheters themselves are varied, depending on the use, and fall into two basic categories: nontunneled, for therapy expected to last just a few days or weeks, and tunneled, for therapy expected to last many months. Short-term nontunneled catheters often have one lumen but may have as many as four. Commonly used long-term catheters include Groshong, Hickman, and Broviac tunneled catheters. (See *Comparing central venous catheters.*) These catheters may also have several lumens.

The type of CVC to be used and your facility's policy about CVC insertion determine who may insert a CVC. Generally, short-term catheters are inserted by doctors and specially trained nurse practitioners and physician assistants. Long-term CVCs are usually inserted by doctors in an operating room.

Patients who require the immediate delivery of drugs or fluids and those who need long-term infusion therapy are candidates for central venous (CV) therapy. Nontunneled catheters, used for short-term CV therapy, are used especially when rapid venous access is needed for delivering lifesaving drugs or fluids. Tunneled catheters are preferred for patients who need long-term infusion therapy or drug administration.

Patients who need total parenteral nutrition or long-term chemotherapy and those with chronic diseases are ideal candidates for receiving long-term catheters.

Selecting a vein

Choosing a vein for insertion of a CVC depends on the patient's age, clinical condition, expected length of therapy, type of CVC used, and the skill of the individual performing the procedure. CVCs are usually inserted in the subclavian, internal jugular vein or, occasionally, the femoral vein. These veins are difficult to locate and more prone to complications than are peripheral veins. The subclavian vein is used for most long-term tunneled catheters and percutaneously inserted CVCs.

The right side of the chest is preferred for insertion because the vessel anatomy allows for direct access to the superior vena cava. (See *Neck and chest anatomy,* page 118.)

The internal jugular vein may be used as well. Insertion of a CVC in this vein and applying an occlusive dressing may prove difficult, especially if the patient has a beard. The patient's mobility will be impaired while the catheter is in place. Note also that the vein's proximity to the respiratory system makes accessibility more dangerous. (See *Central venous catheter pathways,* page 119.)

The femoral vein is infrequently used for CVC placement because it carries with it an increased risk of complications, such as thrombo-

Comparing central venous catheters

Each type of central venous catheter (CVC) offers various advantages and disadvantages. This chart compares nontunneled and Groshong, Hickman, and Broviac tunneled CVCs.

CATHETER	ADVANTAGES	DISADVANTAGES
Nontunneled	• Easily inserted at bedside • Cost effective • Easily removed • Easily changed over guide wire • Stiffness aids central venous catheter monitoring • Allows administration of several solutions at once	• Easily dislodged by patient movement • Limited functions • More thrombogenic because of catheter material • Requires sterile dressing changes • Not flexible; may break • Requires heparin flushes when not in use
Groshong	• Valve eliminates need for Valsalva's maneuver • Does not require heparin • Less thrombogenic • Easily repaired • Valve eliminates frequent flushes • Anchored to chest wall so movement is not restricted • Cuff decreases chance of infection • Does not require clamp; reduces catheter damage • Reduced time and cost for maintenance	• Requires surgical insertion • Fragile—can tear or kink easily • Blunt end makes it difficult to clear substances from tip • Requires doctor for removal • Susceptible to infection • May affect body image
Hickman	• Less thrombogenic • Anchored to chest wall so movement is not restricted • Cuff decreases chance of infection • Clamps eliminate need for Valsalva's maneuver	• Requires surgical insertion • Difficult to repair • Open end • Requires doctor for removal • Tears and kinks easily • Susceptible to infection • May affect body image
Broviac	• Small lumen • Less thrombogenic • Anchored to chest wall so movement is not restricted • Cuff decreases chance of infection • Clamp eliminates need for Valsalva's maneuver	• Requires surgical insertion • Open end • Requires doctor for removal • Tears and kinks easily • Small lumen may limit use • Single lumen limits function • May affect body image • Susceptible to infection • Difficult to repair

sis and infection, as well as hampered mobility. The femoral vein is used in emergencies or in patients with superior vena cava syndrome or thrombosis of the internal jugular vein or superior vena cava.

Neck and chest anatomy

A thorough understanding of the location of anatomic structures in the neck and chest is necessary to safely insert and care for a central venous catheter. The illustration below shows major blood vessels in the neck and chest.

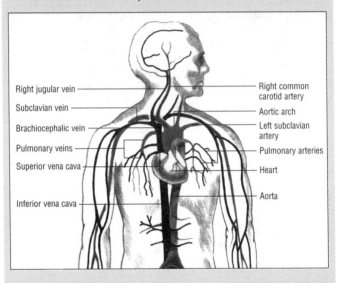

Right jugular vein

Subclavian vein

Brachiocephalic vein

Pulmonary veins

Superior vena cava

Inferior vena cava

Right common carotid artery

Aortic arch

Left subclavian artery

Pulmonary arteries

Heart

Aorta

Selecting a device

The type of catheter selected varies according to its design and the characteristics of the catheter. Some catheters are best used for short-term therapies; others, for long-term therapies.

Two types of catheter—nontunneled and tunneled—are available. Both types are radiopaque. Nontunneled catheters may be made of several different materials, including polyurethane, silicone, and polyvinyl chloride (PVC), depending on the brand of catheter. Because PVC is stiff, these catheters tend to irritate vessel walls and lead to thrombus formation. The use of polyurethane and silicone catheters reduces the risk of those complications.

Although nontunneled catheters are associated with a higher infection rate than are tunneled catheters, some coated nontunneled catheters are now available, including catheters with an antimicro-

Central venous catheter pathways

Central venous catheters (CVCs) are typically inserted into the subclavian or internal jugular vein. The illustrations here show common pathways for inserting a CVC and the catheter tip's location.

Internal jugular

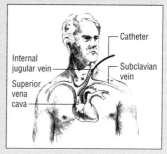

Subclavian (nontunneled)

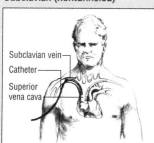

Subclavian (tunneled)

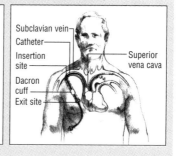

bial coating. Some even have an attachable cuff that acts as a mechanical barrier against microorganisms. These cuffs are most effective when the catheter is left in place for more than 4 days.

Tunneled catheters are usually made of silicone, a material that minimizes irritation or damage to the innermost layer of the vein wall. In addition, tunneled catheters all have a cuff that allows tissue growth at the exit site (in about 2 weeks) to anchor the catheter and keep bacteria from migrating into the catheter tract. In most cases, the cuff is made of Dacron.

Another cuff that can be added, the VitaCuff, contains silver ions that provide antimicrobial action lasting about 3 months. Antimicrobial cuffs are more effective than topical antimicrobial ointment in preventing infection.

Comparing nontunneled catheters

Nontunneled catheters can have one or more lumens. These illustrations show examples of single- and multiple-lumen nontunneled catheters and characteristics of each.

DESCRIPTION

Single-lumen catheter
• Polyurethane, polyvinyl chloride (PVC), or Silastic
• Approximately 8" (20.3 cm) long
• Lumen gauge varies (14Fr to 27Fr)
• Percutaneously placed
• Available features: heparin, antibiotic, and antiseptic coatings
• Antimicrobial cuff available

Multiple-lumen catheter
• Polyurethane, PVC, or Silastic
• Double, triple, or quadruple lumens, exiting at ¾" (2 cm) intervals
• Lumen gauge varies (14Fr to 7Fr)
• Most models have color-coded lumen parts

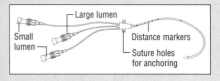

Characteristics of a CVC vary according to whether it's a nontunneled or tunneled catheter.

Nontunneled

Nontunneled CVCs range in size from about 3" to 12" (8 to 30 cm). They may have one or as many as four lumens that vary in size from 14Fr to 27Fr. Selections for a nontunneled CVC should be based on the length needed for each particular patient and the type and duration of therapy required. (See *Comparing nontunneled catheters*.) Multiple-lumen catheters are associated with an increased risk of complications, probably as a result of the manipulation required for multiple-lumen versus single-lumen catheters. Meticulous care of multiple-lumen catheters is essential.

Tunneled

Tunneled catheters surgically inserted into the subclavian vein and then threaded through the subcutaneous tissue exit through the chest wall, usually medial to the nipple. These catheters are used for

INDICATIONS	NURSING CONSIDERATIONS
• Short-term central venous catheter access—days to weeks • Emergency access • Single-purpose therapy: IV therapy, antibiotics, total parenteral therapy, blood transfusion, chemotherapy • Central venous pressure (CVP) monitoring • Blood sampling for diagnostic testing	• Use aseptic technique when caring for insertion site. • Assess frequently for signs of infection and clot formation. • Use air elimination filter to minimize risk of air embolism. • Obtain a chest X-ray to verify catheter placement after insertion. • Minimize patient movement.
• Short-term central venous access • Emergency access • Patient with limited access sites who needs multiple infusions that may not be compatible • CVP monitoring • Blood sampling for diagnostic testing	• Realize that nursing considerations for short-term catheters apply. • Know the gauge and purpose of each lumen. • Use the same lumen for the same task. • Remember to label the lumen used for each task. • Heparinize ports not in use to prevent clotting, according to facility policy.

long-term therapy and may remain in place for several years if cared for properly. If a tunneled catheter becomes damaged, repair kits are available. The most common types of tunneled catheters are the Broviac, Hickman, and Groshong catheters. (See *Comparing tunneled catheters,* pages 122 and 123.)

The Broviac catheter has a smaller lumen than a Hickman or Groshong and is used more frequently in children than adults. Broviac catheters require daily flushing with both normal saline solution and heparin.

The Hickman catheter is basically a modified Broviac catheter with a larger diameter. These catheters are used more often for adults rather than children. A Hickman catheter can be single-lumen or multiple-lumen.

The Groshong catheter has a pressure-sensitive valve at the tip that prevents the backflow of blood into the catheter lumen, a feature not found in the Hickman and Broviac catheters. The valve remains closed at normal vena cava pressures but allows for the easy flow of solutions when positive pressure is applied to the

Comparing tunneled catheters

Three types of tunneled catheters are in common use, the Groshong, Hickman, and Broviac. These illustrations show examples of all three types of tunneled catheters, when they're used, and nursing considerations related to their use.

DESCRIPTION

Groshong catheter
• Silicone rubber
• Approximately 35" (89 cm) long
• Closed end with pressure-sensitive, two-way valve
• Polyester fiber (Dacron) cuff
• Single lumen or multiple-lumen
• Surgically inserted

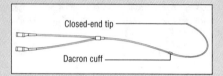

Hickman catheter
• Silicone rubber
• Approximately 35" (89 cm) long
• Open ended with clamp
• Dacron cuff
• Single lumen or multiple-lumen
• Surgically inserted

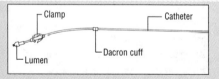

Broviac catheter
• Identical to Hickman but smaller diameter

valve. When negative pressure is applied, blood samples may be drawn.

Because of its valve, a Groshong catheter must be flushed with normal saline solution only. It must never be flushed with heparin. Weekly flushing is sufficient to maintain catheter patency, thus making home maintenance easy for patients and caregivers. Using saline rather than heparin avoids problems for patients with heparin sensitivity or coagulation conditions and is also more cost effective.

INDICATIONS	NURSING CONSIDERATIONS
• Long-term central venous access • Heparin allergy • Infusion of IV fluids, antibiotics, total parenteral nutrition (TPN), blood, or chemotherapy • Blood sampling for diagnostic testing	• Activity restricted until tissue adheres to cuff (2 to 3 weeks). • Dress two surgical sites immediately after insertion. • Use gauze dressing until drainage stops; then use transparent semipermeable membrane dressing. • Handle catheter gently; silicone tears easily. • Have catheter repair kit available. • Check external portion of catheter for kinks or leakage. • Flush with enough saline solution to clear length of catheter. • Encourage patient to participate in use and care of device. • Flush weekly with 0.9% NaCl. • Know purpose and function of each lumen.
• Long-term central venous access • Home IV therapy • Infusion of IV fluids, antibiotics, TPN, blood, and chemotherapy • Blood sampling for diagnostic testing	• Handle catheter gently and check frequently for kinks, leakage, or tears. • Clamp catheter when it is open or becomes disconnected. • Heparinize unused ports, according to facility policy. • Encourage patient to participate in use and care of device. • Two surgical sites require dressing immediately after surgery. • Know purpose and function of each lumen.
• Long-term central venous access • Patients with small central vessels, especially children and elderly patients • Infusion of fluids, antibiotics, TPN, blood, or chemotherapy • Blood sampling for diagnostic testing	• Handle catheter gently and check frequently for kinks, leakage, or tears. • Clamp catheter when it is open or becomes disconnected. • Heparinize unused ports, according to facility policy. • Encourage patient to participate in use and care of device. • Check facility policy before drawing or administering blood or blood products. • Activity restricted until tissue adheres to cuff (2 to 3 weeks). • Two surgical sites require dressing immediately after surgery.

Insertion of a central venous catheter

Insertion of a tunneled CVC is usually done in an operating suite. However, a nontunneled CVC may be inserted at the bedside. You may be asked to assist with the procedure.

Insertion of a nontunneled CVC involves gathering the equipment, preparing the patient and site, and inserting the catheter.

Gathering the equipment

Before insertion of a CVC, gather all the equipment you'll need. If CVC insertion trays are available in your facility, gather a tray and these items:

- sterile towel drapes
- sterile gloves
- sterile gowns
- mask and eye protection
- linen-saver pad
- flush syringes, one with normal saline solution and one with heparin. You'll need saline and heparin flush syringes for each lumen of the CVC.

If your facility doesn't carry CVC insertion trays, gather these supplies:

- povidone-iodine swabs
- 70% alcohol solution
- sterile normal saline solution
- syringe with 25G, 1" needle for lidocaine
- 1% or 2% injectable lidocaine
- suture material
- sterile 4" × 4" gauze pads
- sterile scissors
- sterile transparent semipermeable membrane dressing
- tape.

Preparing the patient

Make sure an informed consent has been obtained from the patient before proceeding with the insertion. Then explain the procedure to the patient, using developmentally appropriate teaching techniques. Include the family and other caregivers as necessary. Tell the patient what role he can play in minimizing anxiety and making catheter placement easier.

Teach the patient how to perform Valsalva's maneuver and have him give a return demonstration before the CVC is inserted. (See *Valsalva's maneuver.*) Valsalva's maneuver helps reduce the risk of air embolus following insertion.

You'll also need to determine if the patient is allergic to iodine or local anesthetics. If analgesic ointment will be used, remember that to be effective, the ointment must be applied at least 60 minutes before the procedure.

Once you've obtained a consent, instructed the patient in doing a Valsalva's maneuver, and determined allergies, place the patient on

CLINICAL
PEARLS

Valsalva's maneuver

Valsalva's maneuver increases intrathoracic pressure in the central veins from a normal 3 to 4 mm Hg to 60 to 70 mm Hg. The increased pressure reduces the risk of an air embolus during catheter insertion and removal and when the catheter lumen is open to air without being clamped. An easy method of increasing intrathoracic pressure is to have the patient exhale against a closed glottis (airway).

Instruct the patient to take a deep breath and hold it. Tell him to bear down—as though he is having a bowel movement—for 10 to 12 seconds. Then have the patient exhale slowly and calmly. The patient should practice this technique once or twice so he'll be able to perform the maneuver during central venous catheter insertion.

his back or, for chest or neck insertions, in Trendelenburg's position (if his condition permits). In Trendelenburg's position, the central veins dilate, thus reducing the risk of air embolus during insertion. Place a linen-saver pad under the patient's shoulder and neck (or groin if the femoral site is used).

If the catheter is being inserted into the subclavian vein, place a towel roll between the patient's scapulae to allow easier access to chest vessels. If the jugular vein is the anticipated site of insertion, turn the patient's head to the opposite side and extend the neck to expose anatomical landmarks there more clearly.

Preparing the site

After you've assembled the equipment and completed your patient teaching about the procedure, expose the intended insertion site.

Remove hair in a 5" (12.5-cm) area around the catheter insertion site. Clip the hair with scissors, hair clippers, or an electric shaver; don't shave the hair with a razor. Shaving causes microabrasions and as a result, increases the risk of site infection. Avoid use of depilatories as well. These agents can cause allergic reactions.

After the hair has been removed, rinse the area with normal saline solution. Then wash the area with soap and water to remove body oil and dirt. Wash your hands with an antimicrobial soap. Provide masks, protective eyewear, and sterile gowns as appropriate for all personnel involved in the procedure, according to facility policy.

Open the sterile CVC insertion tray. Put on sterile gloves. Have the patient turn his head away from the site. Drape the insertion site with sterile towels, creating a wide sterile field.

Clean the area over the insertion site with povidone-iodine swabs. Clean in a circular motion from the intended site of insertion outward 2" to 4". If the patient is allergic to iodine, use alcohol or 2% tincture of iodine instead. Allow the antiseptic to dry before inserting the catheter.

Inserting the catheter

Because doctors generally insert CVCs, you'll assist as necessary during the procedure. You'll also need to support the patient throughout the procedure, using touch and verbal communication. Let the patient know what to expect as the procedure progresses.

After the site has been prepared, the insertion site is anesthetized and the catheter is inserted using the Seldinger technique. (See *Seldinger technique.*) The catheter is inserted over the guide wire and threaded into position; then the guide wire is removed.

When the guide wire is removed or the end of the catheter is opened to air, instruct the patient to perform Valsalva's maneuver. Monitor the patient throughout the procedure for complications.

If the catheter is advanced beyond the superior vena cava into the right side of the heart, arrhythmias may occur. Observe the patient for irregular pulse, shortness of breath, chest pain, palpitations, dizziness, fainting, or loss of consciousness. Also note that during Valsalva's maneuver, the pulse rate declines. Patients with cardiac problems may be at an increased risk at this time for decreased cardiac output. Monitor the patient for shortness of breath, dizziness, or chest pain—all signs of decreased cardiac output.

Place an injector cap on all lumens. Connect a syringe to each of the catheter ports, and aspirate each lumen for blood. Irrigate the lumens with normal saline solution. For intermittent drug administration, flush the lumen with heparin. When withdrawing the needle from the injection cap, use keep positive pressure on the plunger to prevent the back flow of blood into the catheter. Keep unused lumens clamped, if indicated.

Securing the catheter

Once inserted, the catheter may be sutured in place. If it isn't, sterile adhesive strips can be used to secure the catheter. After the catheter is secured, apply an occlusive dressing using sterile 4" × 4" gauze pads or a sterile transparent semipermeable membrane dressing. One advantage of using a transparent semipermeable membrane dressing is that it allows the site to remain visible for continuous assessment.

Seldinger technique

The Seldinger technique can be used when inserting a central venous catheter over a guide wire. These illustrations show the step-by-step process of the Seldinger technique.

Locate the vein to be cannulated. Then insert a small (18G) needle into the vein.

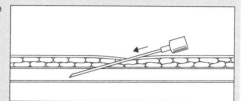

Pass the guide wire through the needle, and thread it into the vein.

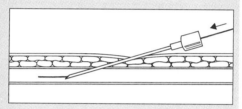

With the guide wire remaining in place, withdraw the needle.

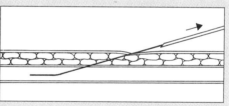

Advance the catheter over the guide wire into the vein. Rotate the catheter as you advance it over the guide wire.

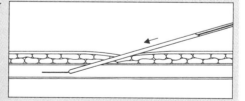

With the catheter in place, carefully re-move the guide wire.

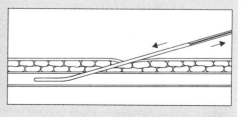

After the dressing has been applied, label it with the time and date of the insertion; also note the length of the catheter.

When the CVC is being used for IV infusions, label all ports to indicate what medications or solutions are being infused. These ports shouldn't be used for other solutions to prevent inadvertently mixing incompatible medications or fluids. Monitor the site for bleeding or signs of infection. Expect serosanguineous drainage for the first 24 hours.

Confirming tip placement
After the catheter has been inserted and the dressing applied, prepare the patient for a chest X-ray to determine catheter tip placement. Once proper tip placement has been verified, the catheter may be used.

Maintenance and care

Caring for a CVC involves a wide variety of functions, including dressing and catheter changes, flushing the catheter, and obtaining blood samples from it.

Catheter changes
Nontunneled CVCs are generally changed every 3 to 7 days, sometimes longer in patients who were initially difficult to catheterize. When a nontunneled CVC is left in place longer than 7 days, the risk of complications and infection increases, even with meticulous site care and frequent dressing changes.

Tunneled catheters can remain in place for months and may not need to be changed at all, depending on the duration of therapy.

Dressing changes
Dressings covering a CVC decrease the risk of local or systemic infection. Dressings for all nontunneled and newly inserted tunneled catheters should be changed routinely. As the site heals and cuff epithelialization occurs, tunneled catheters may need to be cleaned with soap only. Two types of dressings are used: sterile gauze and sterile transparent semipermeable membrane dressings.

Gauze dressings must be applied using aseptic technique and changed every 48 hours or, if the integrity of the dressing is compromised, immediately. Apply tape or other adhesive material over the gauze to guarantee that the dressing is occlusive. If the site could become easily contaminated from respiratory secretions or drainage, don't use a gauze dressing; it can become a site for bacterial growth.

Transparent semipermeable membrane dressings allows rapid and continuous inspection of the site. Transparent semipermeable membrane dressings should be changed every 3 to 7 days or whenever the integrity of the dressing is compromised. Avoid using tape on these dressings because it can interfere with visualizing the site and may compromise the integrity of the dressing. Note that if a transparent semipermeable membrane dressing is placed over gauze, it must be considered a gauze dressing and changed every 48 hours.

Gathering the equipment

Before changing a CVC dressing, gather a pair of nonsterile gloves, tape, and a CVC dressing kit. If a kit isn't available in your facility, you'll need to also collect these supplies:
• sterile 4" × 4" gauze or transparent semipermeable membrane dressing
• alcohol sponges or swabs
• sterile and nonsterile gloves
• povidone-iodine swabs
• povidone-iodine ointment
• protective skin barrier (optional)
• sterile barrier
• mask for yourself and the patient, if indicated. Check your facility's policy.

Removing the old dressing

The first step in changing a CVC dressing is to remove the old one. Before you do that, explain the procedure to the patient and determine whether he has any allergies, especially to iodine. Then wash your hands with an antimicrobial soap. Open the dressing kit, if available, or set up a sterile field with a sterile barrier and cleansing swabs. Put on nonsterile gloves and a mask.

Ask the patient to turn his head away from the catheter site. Also have the patient put on a mask, if necessary. Carefully remove the old dressing, pulling toward the insertion site to prevent accidental dislodgment. Check the site for redness, swelling, pain, and exudate. Note the appearance of sutures.

Discard the soiled gloves and dressing according to standard precautions, and then wash your hands with an antimicrobial soap.

Applying a new dressing

To apply a new dressing, first put on sterile gloves. If the catheter is tunneled, palpate the catheter cuff to verify proper placement. Remember that the hand you use to palpate is no longer sterile.

Clean the insertion site and surrounding skin with an alcohol swab or sponge. Starting at the exit site, work outward in a circular pattern, covering an area 3" to 6" (7.5 to 15 cm) in diameter. Repeat twice using a clean swab each time. Never wipe the exit site with a used swab. Allow the alcohol to remain on the skin for 60 seconds.

Wipe the catheter from the proximal end to the distal end with an alcohol wipe. Clean the site with povidone-iodine swabs, again in a circular motion, covering the same area as you did with the alcohol. Repeat twice using a clean swab each time. Allow the site to dry, but don't fan it. Fanning iodine may increase the risk of site contamination.

Povidone-iodine ointment may be applied to the insertion site, according to your facility's policy. Apply a dressing using sterile gauze and tape or a transparent semipermeable membrane dressing. Secure the tubing to the skin. If the tubing is long, loop it carefully to avoid kinks, and then tape it securely to prevent accidental displacement.

Label the dressing with the date and time of the dressing change and your initials. Discard used supplies according to standard precautions. Then remove your gloves and dispose of them in the same way. Wash your hands with an antimicrobial soap.

Routine flushing

You'll need to regularly flush the CVC to maintain its patency. In general, CVC lines should be flushed before and after administering medications, when an IV infusion is discontinued, if the catheter is in place but not being used, and after drawing blood.

When using heparin, use the lowest possible concentration. This concentration varies from 1 to 10 U/ml in infants and up to 10 to 100 U/ml in children and adults. Follow your facility's policy for heparin concentrations.

The volume of flush solution also varies from facility to facility. Typically, the volume of flush equals twice the volume capacity of the cannula and add-on device, an amount that varies with the catheter being used. As always, follow your facility's policy about flush volumes.

Gathering flush supplies

Before you flush the catheter, collect these items:

• nonsterile gloves
• 10-ml syringe with normal saline solution (preservative-free solution for infants)
• 10-ml syringe with heparin flush solution
• alcohol or povidone-iodine swabs.

Flushing the catheter

To flush the CVC after withdrawing blood for tests, administering medications compatible with heparin, and discontinuing IV fluid therapy, and to maintain catheter patency, you'll need to explain the procedure to the patient, wash your hands with an antimicrobial soap, and put on nonsterile gloves.

Clean the injection cap with an alcohol or povidone-iodine sponge. Insert the syringe with normal saline solution or heparin and flush the catheter. Maintain positive pressure on the syringe plunger while withdrawing the syringe from the injection cap. Clamp the catheter, if indicated. Discard the used supplies according to standard precautions; then wash your hands with an antimicrobial soap.

To flush a CVC either before or after administering medications and solutions incompatible with heparin, follow the SASH (**s**aline, **a**dministration of medication, **s**aline, **h**eparin) procedure. After explaining the procedure to the patient, washing your hands, and putting on nonsterile gloves, clean the injection cap with an alcohol or povidone-iodine sponge.

Insert a syringe filled with normal saline solution, aspirate for the free flow of blood, and then flush the catheter. Clean the injection cap with an alcohol or povidone-iodine sponge, and allow the cap to dry. Administer the medication or solution through a needle or needleless adapter that has pierced the injection port.

Clean the injection cap with an alcohol or povidone-iodine sponge, and allow the cap to dry. Insert a syringe filled with normal saline solution, and flush the catheter. Clean the injection cap again, and allow it to dry.

Insert a syringe filled with heparin, and then flush the catheter. As always, maintain positive pressure on the syringe plunger while withdrawing the syringe from the injection cap. Again, clamp the catheter, if indicated. Discard the used supplies according to standard precautions, then wash your hands with an antimicrobial soap.

Changing the cap

You'll need to change injection caps on the CVC at least once a week and each time blood is drawn. Caps used several times daily may need to be changed more frequently. Also change the cap if the integrity of the cap is questionable. Repeated cap puncture increases the risk of infection and of embolization from pieces of rubber that have broken off from the cap.

To change the cap, you'll need nonsterile gloves, alcohol sponges, a new injection cap with a luer-lock design, and a padded, nonserrated clamp, if the CVC doesn't have a clamp.

Explain the procedure to the patient, and wash your hands with an antimicrobial soap.

Clamp the catheter midway between the cap and the insertion site with a padded or nonserrated clamp. If the catheter can't be clamped, have the patient perform Valsalva's maneuver when the cap is being changed.

Open the package with the new cap and place it on a flat surface, keeping the cap's connection end sterile. Then put on nonsterile gloves. Clean the old injection cap with alcohol at its connection to the catheter hub. Remove the used injection cap from the lumen, and attach the new one, using aseptic technique and making sure to insert it securely. Don't use tape to secure the cap.

Unclamp the catheter, and flush it according to your facility's policy. Clamp the catheter, if indicated. Discard the used equipment and gloves according to standard precautions, and then wash your hands with an antimicrobial soap.

Obtaining a blood sample

Although facility policies vary, the responsibility to draw blood specimens from a CVC usually rests with the nursing staff. Here's how to obtain an accurate specimen, as well as ensure accurate CVC functioning.

To obtain a blood sample from a CVC, gather this equipment:
- alcohol or povidone-iodine swabs
- nonsterile gloves
- normal saline solution in a sterile 10-ml syringe to flush the catheter after blood is drawn
- heparin flush solution
- sterile injection cap, if necessary
- blood collection tubes, as needed
- Vacutainer with needle or needleless attachment. (See *Using a Vacutainer.*)

Using a Vacutainer

You may need to collect blood periodically from a central venous catheter using a Vacutainer. To do so, unclamp the catheter lumen and pierce the injection cap with the Vacutainer (top). Advance the collection tube farther into the Vacutainer, and collect the amount of blood required (bottom).

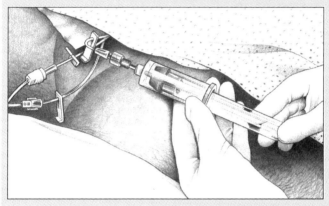

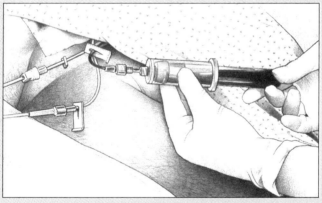

After collecting needed equipment, explain the procedure to the patient, wash your hands with an antimicrobial soap, and put on nonsterile gloves. Then, if the CVC is being used to infuse fluids, clamp the tubing with the tubing clamp or a nonserrated clamp covered with tape, to prevent tubing damage.

Disconnect the tubing, and insert the luer end of a sterile needle onto the end of the tubing, to maintain sterility. Place the new injection cap on the end of the catheter. Make sure all ports of a multiple-lumen catheter are clamped and that all infusions are turned off, to avoid mixing the infusate with the blood specimen. If the CVC is used for intermittent infusions, use the distal port.

Clean the injection cap with alcohol or povidone-iodine. Allow the cap to dry completely. Place a 5-ml blood collection tube into the Vacutainer. Insert the Vacutainer needle or adapter into the port's injection cap.

Collect the first tube of blood, which you'll discard. Insert and then remove tubes as needed for the tests ordered, making sure each time to remove only the amount of blood needed for that specific test. Check with laboratory personnel to determine what those amounts are.

Remove the Vacutainer, and label all specimen tubes. Clean the injection cap again with alcohol or povidone-iodine. Briskly flush the catheter with normal saline solution. As always, maintain positive pressure on the syringe plunger while withdrawing the syringe from the injection cap. When flushing a small-gauge Silastic CVC, flush gently to avoid damaging the catheter.

If you need to reconnect the infusion after flushing the catheter, do so at this time, then restart the infusion. If the catheter isn't being used for an infusion, flush it with heparin flush solution, according to your facility's policy. Use positive pressure when withdrawing the syringe. Then clamp the catheter, if indicated.

If you encounter difficulty withdrawing blood from the catheter, check that the catheter is not kinked or clamped. If it isn't, have patient turn on his side, cough, raise his arms over his head, perform Valsalva's maneuver, or turn his head to the side where the catheter is inserted. Then flush the catheter with normal saline solution, and try drawing blood again. If you still can't obtain a specimen with a Vacutainer, try using a syringe to obtain the sample.

Complications

Complications can occur at any time during infusion therapy through a CVC. (See *Complications of central venous catheters.*) Traumatic complications, such as pneumothorax, typically occur during catheter insertion but may go unnoticed until afterward. Systemic complications, such as infection, typically occur later in therapy. Other complications include cardiac tamponade, air embolism, thrombosis, and others.

Complications of central venous catheters

Central venous catheters (CVCs) are prone to numerous complications. The table below lists possible complications, their causes, and ways to prevent them.

COMPLI-CATION	CAUSES	NURSING INTERVENTIONS	PREVENTION
Pneumo-thorax, hemothorax, chylothorax, hydrothorax	• Puncture of lung with needle on guide wire • Puncture of large blood vessel during insertion of catheter • Puncture of lymph nodes with leakage of fluid • Infusion of IV fluid into intrapleural space by dislodged, misplaced, or infiltrated catheter	• Notify doctor. • Remove catheter or assist with removal. • Administer oxygen, as ordered. • Prepare for and assist with chest tube insertion. • Document your actions.	• Assure clear visualization of central veins during insertion by placing towel supports between scapulae. • Never start an IV infusion until placement is confirmed by X-ray. • Assess for early signs of fluid infiltration. • Instruct patient on all aspects of care to gain full cooperation. • If patient is unable to cooperate, consider sedation or insertion of line in the operating room.
Cardiac tamponade	• Perforation of heart wall with catheter	• Give oxygen, if ordered. • Prepare patient for emergency surgery, if ordered. • Monitor patient continuously. • Keep emergency equipment available.	• Ensure patient immobilization during insertion. • Assess for signs and symptoms of cardiac tamponade. • Don't start infusion until placement is confirmed by X-ray.
Air embolism	• Valsalva's maneuver not performed when catheter is inserted, when lumen is open to air, or when catheter is removed • Cutting or breaking catheter by mishandling or trauma	• Clamp catheter immediately. • Turn patient onto left side with head down so air can enter right atrium and disperse through pulmonary artery; have him maintain position for 20 to 30 minutes. • Administer oxygen, as ordered.	• Teach Valsalva's maneuver for use during insertion and removal. • Tape tubing so physical trauma from manipulation doesn't occur. • Use locking devices for all connections. • Use infusion control device with air detection capability.

(continued)

Complications of central venous catheters *(continued)*

COMPLI-CATION	CAUSES	NURSING INTERVENTIONS	PREVENTION
Air embolism *(continued)*	• Accidental disconnection of injection cap from lumen • Improper removal of air from IV tubing when purging the system	• Notify doctor. • Document your actions.	• Instruct patients and caregivers on proper technique for irrigating line and changing cap. • Purge all air from tubing before connecting to CVC lumen.
Thrombosis	• Thrombogenic catheter material • Infusion of irritating fluids • Sluggish flow rate • Patient's hematopoietic status • Preexisting cardiovascular disease • Repeated or long-term use of same vein	• Notify doctor. • Remove catheter, if ordered. • Infuse anticoagulant doses of heparin, if ordered. • Verify thrombosis with diagnostic test results. • Apply warm, wet compresses locally. • Don't use limb on affected side for venipuncture. • Document your actions.	• Maintain flow with infusion pump or flush at regular intervals. • Consult with health care provider before insertion; if possible, use a less thrombogenic material. • Use positive pressure when flushing CVC lumens. • Dilute irritating solutions prior to infusion. • Flush catheter completely between medication administration.
Infection	• Failure to maintain aseptic technique during catheter insertion and care • Failure to comply with dressing change protocol • Failure to change wet or soiled dressings in a timely manner • Contaminated infusate • Multiple access to central line	• Obtain culture from site. • Redress aseptically. • Use antimicrobial ointment locally, as ordered. • Treat systemically with antibiotic or antifungal agents, depending on culture results and doctor's orders. • Draw central and peripheral line cultures; if results show the same organism, catheter is primary source of sepsis and should be removed. • Culture tip of device, if removed. • Assess for other infection sources.	• Use aseptic technique during insertion and maintenance of line. • Change dressing in accordance with facility policy or when soiled or wet. • Inspect all IV solutions for contamination (cloudiness, particulate matter). • Change IV fluids as mandated by facility policy.

Complications of central venous catheters *(continued)*

COMPLI-CATION	CAUSES	NURSING INTERVENTIONS	PREVENTION
Infection *(continued)*		• Monitor patient's vital signs closely, especially temperature. • Document your interventions.	• Manipulate catheter as little as possible.
Dislodgment	• Manipulation of catheter by patient • Repeated manipulation of catheter by staff • Catheter improperly secured at site • Loosening of sutures securing catheter	• Apply pressure to site. • Apply antimicrobial ointment and occlusive dressing to site. • Monitor vital signs. • Inspect catheter and note length. • Notify doctor and prepare for possible reinsertion. • Document your interventions.	• Loop catheter and tape securely to patient's chest. • Use clothing that hides catheter on children or confused patients. • Avoid pulling on catheter. • Properly anchor catheter with sutures or sterile adhesive strips. • Use extreme care when the patient is moving, ambulating, or exercising with short-term CVC in place.

Besides these complications, CVCs can become damaged by frequent manipulation, high-flushing pressures, or physical damage from scissors or improper use of serrated clamps. When this occurs, blood can flow backward through the damaged area and infusate can leak out of the damaged area onto the dressing. In addition, air or bacteria can enter the catheter at the damaged site and cause an air embolus or catheter infection.

Damaged CVCs can be repaired temporarily by replacing the damaged portion of the catheter with a blunt-tipped needle. This is a temporary fix and should be performed only by specially trained personnel. (Permanent repair kits are also available.)

Teaching the patient

When teaching about CVC therapy, keep in mind that the patient and caregivers should play an active role in planning the patient's care. They need to understand the purpose of the CVC as well as its benefits and potential risks.

Patients on long-term therapy need to learn how to manage the CVC. Teach the patient about flushing, changing the injection cap and dressing, and administering medications and fluids. Following the instructions, have the patient give a return demonstration of critical techniques.

You'll also need to teach the patient how to recognize and handle problems that might occur with the CVC. In addition, you should consult with Social Services personnel and the patient's doctor about arranging follow-up visits at home, if indicated. (See *Home care instructions for central venous catheters.*)

Removal of a central venous catheter

Although registered nurses may remove nontunneled CVCs, only a trained doctor or nurse practitioner may remove a tunneled catheter. Before removing the catheter, examine the patient's X-ray reports (if available) showing the catheter's placement. That way, you can follow the path of the catheter during removal.

Before removing the catheter, teach the patient how to perform Valsalva's maneuver. Place the patient in Trendelenburg's position to increase intravascular pressure in the central veins and decrease the risk of an air embolism. If the patient can't tolerate this position, place him in the supine position.

To remove a CVC, you'll need to gather this equipment:
- sterile and nonsterile gloves
- suture removal kit or implements
- 2" × 2" gauze pad
- tape
- alcohol or povidone-iodine swabs
- povidone-iodine ointment
- culture material, if necessary
- disposal bag
- sterile barrier.

After collecting needed equipment, explain the procedure to the patient and wash your hands with an antimicrobial soap. Open the sterile barrier and place the sterile dressing on it. Place povidone ointment on gauze pad. Put on nonsterile gloves and a mask.

If the infusion is running, clamp it. Then remove the old dressing, pulling toward the insertion site. Discard the dressing and your gloves according to standard precautions. Put on sterile gloves.

Home care instructions for central venous catheters

When a patient will care for a central venous catheter at home, you'll need to review this teaching guide with the patient and caregivers.

- Keep the catheter capped at all times.
- Never use pins, scissors, or any sharp objects around catheter.
- When showering or bathing, keep entire catheter covered with clear plastic wrap.
- If a small amount of blood is noted in the catheter (especially Groshong), flush it using the method indicated by the nurse. (Blood may back up into the catheter with heavy lifting or straining.)
- If the catheter should break or leak fluid, use a clamp without teeth and clamp it between the break or tear and the insertion site. Call the health care provider immediately.

- If redness, swelling, drainage, or pain occur around the catheter site, call the health care provider.
- If chills or fever over 100.5° F occur, call the health care provider at once.
- Keep the catheter tubing secured to the chest with tape to avoid accidental pulling.
- If the catheter becomes dislodged or pulled out, apply pressure over the area to stop bleeding and call the health care provider.
- If the catheter cannot be flushed, call the health care provider.
- If the injection cap becomes dislodged, clamp the catheter with a nonserrated clamp (Groshong does not need to be clamped), wipe the end of the lumen with an alcohol or povidone-iodine sponge, and apply a new cap.

- Dress children or confused patients who may pull at the line with clothes that button in the back and keep the catheter covered at all times. Never leave these patients alone when they are undressed.
- Make sure all caregivers (such as school nurse, day care staff, companions) are taught about the catheter.
- If chest pain; face, neck, or arm swelling on the side of the catheter; shortness of breath; shoulder or neck pain; irritability; palpitations; lightheadedness; or fainting occur, call the health care provider or seek emergency care if these symptoms are severe.

Clean the site with alcohol or povidone-iodine. Inspect the site for signs of drainage or inflammation.

Using the suture removal set, clip the sutures and remove them. Instruct the patient to perform Valsalva's maneuver while the catheter is withdrawn. Remove the catheter in a slow, even motion as you follow its exit path. If resistance is felt, stop the removal process immediately and contact the doctor.

When the catheter has been removed, immediately place sterile gauze with povidone-iodine ointment on the site and apply pressure. Pressure helps initiate hemostasis. The ointment helps to seal the insertion site. Place an occlusive dressing over the area, and leave it in place for 24 hours. Thereafter, change the dressing every 24 hours until the site is fully healed.

Inspect the catheter to see if part of it has broken off during removal. If so, notify the doctor immediately and observe the patient for signs of distress. If a culture has been ordered, use sterile scissors and cut approximately 1" (2.5 cm) off the distal end of the catheter and place it in a culture tube. Then label and send the culture tube to the laboratory.

Discard the used equipment and gloves according to standard precautions, and then wash your hands with an antimicrobial soap.

Documentation

Proper documentation for CVC insertion and maintenance varies with the procedures being performed.

When documenting the insertion of a CVC, make sure to note this information:
- informed consent
- date, time, and site of insertion
- name of health care provider inserting the catheter
- catheter length and type, including number of lumens
- problems encountered
- X-ray confirmation of catheter before initiation of IV infusion
- response of the patient to the insertion
- patient teaching about the insertion.

When documenting maintenance care of a CVC, make sure to note this information:
- dressing and cap changes and other maintenance care
- presence of blood return
- complications noted
- steps taken to resolve complications
- appearance of insertion site.

When documenting the removal of a CVC, make sure to note this information:
- date and time of catheter removal

- position of the patient
- use of Valsalva's maneuver during removal
- appearance of the insertion site
- integrity of the catheter
- type of dressing applied
- use of povidone-iodine ointment
- whether culture was obtained
- response of the patient to the removal procedure.

C H A P T E R

Managing vascular access port therapy

A vascular access port (VAP) is a reliable alternative for patients requiring long-term central venous access. Surgically implanted (usually in the chest wall) and able to remain in place for months or years, the port consists of a rigid reservoir with a self-sealing rubber septum. The tip of an attached catheter is located in a central vein. To gain access to the venous system, the septum must be punctured. Only nurses who have successfully completed VAP training are allowed to access or provide site care for a VAP.

VAPs allow repeated intermittent access—as many as 2,000 times, depending on the size of the needle—without loss of integrity. Special noncoring needles are used to access a VAP. This chapter explains advantages and disadvantages of a VAP; how to select a patient, vein, and port; inserting a port; port care; complications; patient teaching; port removal; and documentation.

Advantages and disadvantages

One of the VAP's most important advantages lies in the fact that the device doesn't require site care, other than a monthly flush when not in use. This makes the VAP ideal for patients unable to care for an external catheter and who have no reliable caregiver.

Implanted ports also decrease the number of home care visits needed for routine dressing changes. The only time a dressing is needed on the VAP is when an access needle is in place.

Because the port, buried beneath the skin, is protected from water, bacteria, and irritants, patients can continue engaging in activities they normally enjoy. Children can play without fear of damaging an external catheter, and adults can carry on their day-to-day activities without the embarrassment commonly associated with external venous access devices.

A major disadvantage of a VAP is the anxiety associated with repeated needle sticks for entry into the port. Using an anesthetic cream such as a combination of lidocaine and prilocaine can reduce the discomfort and help alleviate this fear, particularly in children. Patients who remain anxious about this aspect of VAP therapy may be better suited to receive an external device such as a Hickman catheter.

Another disadvantage of VAPs relates to the possibility that, once the needle is in place, its tip may become dislodged if the tubing is tugged on and cause infiltration of the infusate.

Selecting a patient

Implanted VAPs are indicated when intermittent, long-term (more than 3 months) vascular access is needed, usually in patients with limited peripheral venous access due to frequent venipunctures and in those with thrombosed or sclerotic veins. The devices are also useful for obese patients whose peripheral veins are obscured by adipose tissue, patients receiving chemotherapeutic agents over the long term, and HIV-positive patients receiving several IV antibiotic or antiviral medications. Be aware, however, that patients who are immunocompromised will need vigilant care and monitoring for signs of infection of the port pocket. Infections there may require removal of the port.

Patients requiring repeated blood sampling and the administration of blood products, IV antibiotics, narcotic analgesics, and other medications may benefit from having a VAP. VAPs may also be useful for short-term total parenteral nutrition (TPN) and fluid replacement therapy.

A VAP may not be suitable if long-term, continuous infusions such as TPN are required because an access needle would need to remain embedded in the device continuously. The needle would also need to be changed periodically. In these cases, an external, long-term catheter would be a better choice.

VAPs are also contraindicated in patients with sepsis or uncontrollable coagulopathy. Other conditions making it difficult or impossible to implant a VAP include thrombosis of the subclavian or innominate (brachiocephalic) veins or superior vena cava, cardiac tamponade, or chest wall tissue too thin to support the device.

Selecting a vein

Vein selection hinges on the ease of access to the superior vena cava, the desired location for the VAP tip. The subclavian and internal jugular veins generally prove ideal for gaining access to the superior vena cava.

The cephalic, basilic, or brachial veins can also be used, as can the femoral vein. The femoral vein is particularly useful when the patient has currently or had at some point superior vena cava syndrome or a thrombosis of the internal jugular or subclavian vein. (Superior vena cava syndrome can occur when the superior vena cava becomes occluded by a thrombus, catheter, or fibrin.) When the femoral vein is used, the tip of the catheter should be located in the inferior vena cava, not the superior vena cava.

Keep in mind that a patient might have an implanted port that isn't used for venous access. For instance, a patient may have an arterial access port or a port that gains access to the peritoneal cavity. All ports should be clearly marked so that IV medications aren't inadvertently infused into body cavities, a potentially deadly event.

Selecting a device

Selecting a port involves assessing the patient's needs, the design of the VAPs available, and the characteristics of each type of VAP.

When selecting a VAP, consider the long-term needs of the patient, the patient's age or vein size, allergies to port components, and other factors. For instance, if the patient is a small child or very thin adult, a low profile port is likely the best choice because of its smaller height (½") and greater stability.

Consider a dual-lumen VAP if the patient will be receiving continuous infusions or two or more IV drugs. Dual-lumen ports consist of two separate ports and are attached to a catheter with two separate lumens, an advantage for administering more than one fluid or medication or for having blood drawn. For instance, many doctors dedicate one lumen for drawing blood and the other for administering medications. A dedicated line for drawing blood reduces the chances of medications or fluids mixing with the blood sample. It also reduces the need for interrupting an infusion.

VAP reservoirs are usually made of plastic or titanium, though some are made of stainless steel. (See *Selected vascular access ports,* page 146.) Plastic ports produce the fewest radiographic artifacts on a magnetic resonance image (MRI). If an MRI may be required at some point, a nonmetallic port should be considered.

Stainless steel and titanium are both more durable than plastic and easily visible on an X-ray. Most reservoirs lack corners, which allows thorough flushing of the catheter and helps to prevent the build-up of "sludge," a combination of thrombus and residues of blood product or medications.

VAPs designed for peripheral placement are smaller in diameter and lighter than traditional chest wall devices. Peripheral ports can be used as chest wall devices for emaciated patients or small children.

The size of the catheters used with VAPs ranges from 6Fr to 10Fr for single lumen and 10Fr to 13Fr for double lumen. Catheters are usually made of silicone, though some manufacturers make both silicone and polyurethane catheters for their ports. Silicone and polyurethane are radiopaque, so placement can be verified by fluoroscopy or X-ray. The catheter either comes already attached to the reservoir or is part of a two-part system connected after insertion. The length of the attached catheter ranges from about 20" to 30" (50 to 75 cm). The catheter must be trimmed to fit so the tip lies in the superior vena cava and doesn't extend into the right atrium.

VAPs come in both single- and double-lumen styles and are classified according to height. A port can be either a high- or a low-profile port, depending on the height of the reservoir, usually ½" to 1" (1.3 to 2.5 cm) high. (See *Anatomy of a vascular access port,* page 147.)

Selected vascular access ports

A number of vascular access ports (VAPs) are currently available. The illustrations below show several VAPs and some of their more prominent features.

P.A.S. Port
(SIMS Deltec)
Type: Titanium, top entry port
Features:
• Low profile
• Catheter connector integrated with port for easy assembly
• Peripheral insertion

Plastic Low Profile Port
(Arrow International)
Type: Plastic, top entry port
Features:
• Low profile
• Central insertion required
• Arrow Blue FlexTip, designed to decrease vessel trauma

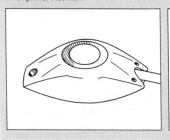 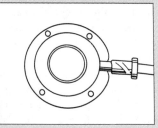

Celsite
(Braun)
Type: Titanium, top entry port
Features:
• Smaller and lighter than most ports
• Peripheral or central (shown) insertion
• Single (shown) or dual port

Vital-Port
(Cook Incorporated)
Type: Titanium or polysulfone (shown), top entry port
Features:
• Available with single or dual (shown) chambers
• Central insertion required

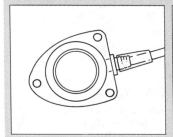 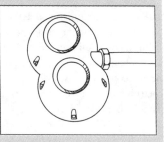

Low-profile VAPs are more difficult to access but are usually more stable when implanted. A low-profile port is suitable for patients with a thin or normal-sized chest wall.

EQUIPMENT EXPERTISE

Anatomy of a vascular access port

A vascular access port (VAP) contains a self-sealing septum for repeated, leak-proof puncture. The diagram here shows a cross-section of a VAP with a noncoring needle in place. The self-sealing septum holds the needle upright. Note that the port reservoir accepts fluid from the needle tip and allows it to flow into the outlet tube leading to the catheter.

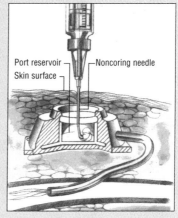

High-profile VAPs allow easier access but are less stable. Because the septum on a high-profile port is easily palpable, a high-profile port would be ideal for an obese patient.

In some VAPs, the septum is recessed to facilitate identification. The septum in other VAPs is dome-shaped to make it easier to locate.

Entry into most VAPs is gained using a noncoring needle (discussed later in this chapter) inserted perpendicular to the septum. For some VAPs, however, you'll enter through the side. (See *Side-entry vascular access port,* page 148.)

Recent advances in design technology have led to the development of highly sophisticated VAPs. The CathLink, for instance, a product from Bard Access Systems, has a funnel-shaped metallic body leading to a small entry port. (See *CathLink 20 implanted vascular port,* page 149.) The port can be entered using a standard over-the-needle type catheter. The hemostatic diaphragm of the CathLink leads directly to the catheter and doesn't have a reservoir, which eliminates the need for a special access needle and permits a greater flow rate than conventional VAPs. Because of its low-profile design, the CathLink can be used as a chest or peripheral port.

Side-entry vascular access port

Although in most vascular access ports, the needle is inserted through the top, in a side-entry port, the needle is inserted through the side of the port. Note that the angle of entry is nearly parallel to the port reservoir.

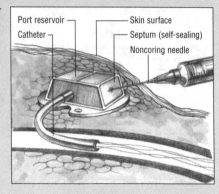

Port reservoir — Skin surface
Catheter — Septum (self-sealing)
Noncoring needle

Insertion of a vascular access port

VAPs are typically inserted by a surgeon or interventional radiologist in an operating room or interventional radiology suite. Inserting a VAP involves gathering the equipment, preparing the patient and site, and implanting the port.

Gathering the equipment
Insertion of a VAP requires the following items:
• appropriate VAP insertion trays
• normal saline solution for flushing the device and catheter
• 3- to 5-ml heparinized flush solution (100 U/ml)
• sterile gloves and gowns
• head and foot coverings and masks for everyone involved in the insertion
• local anesthetic agents and appropriate syringes and site preparation materials.

Preparing the patient
Before VAP insertion, check that the patient has completed an informed consent form. Explain the risks and benefits of VAP insertion, including steps in the insertion procedure, patient responsibilities during and after the procedure, and potential complications.

EQUIPMENT
EXPERTISE

CathLink 20 implanted vascular port

The CathLink 20 port, shown here, lacks an internal reservoir, which decreases the possibility of complications by reducing fibrin residue buildup. Note that this port is being punctured with a 20G over-the-needle peripheral IV catheter. Traditional noncoring needles shouldn't be used with this type of port.

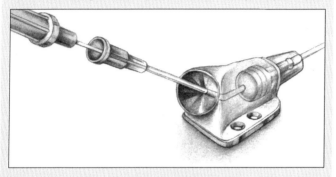

Answer all questions frankly, and make sure the patient understands other therapy options available.

Place the patient in Trendelenburg's position to fill the chest veins for greater ease in insertion of the catheter into a central vein. Keep the patient informed about what's being done throughout the procedure and what to expect next.

Preparing the site

The doctor will prepare the site with a povidone-iodine solution or a similar, facility-approved cleansing solution. After the povidone-iodine solution dries, sterile drapes are applied and a local anesthetic administered. Some patients may require conscious sedation or general anesthesia.

Implanting the port

Insertion of either a single- or dual-lumen VAP involves making two incisions, one to create a subcutaneous pocket that holds the port and another to insert the catheter into the vein. The port is implanted completely beneath the skin and against a bony structure for stability. Ports implanted in the chest, the most common site, are usually placed over the anterior ribs or the right infraclavicular fossa.

After a central venous catheter has been inserted and its tip threaded into the superior vena cava (or inferior vena cava for catheters inserted into the femoral vein), a trocar is used to tunnel the other end of the catheter to the port site. The port's base is sutured to the fascia, and the catheter is attached to the port.

After insertion, tip placement is confirmed by fluoroscopy. The port's stability, patency, and ability to handle various flow rates are also tested. Incisions in the chest wall are then sutured closed, leaving no external parts of the port or catheter. If implanted correctly under the skin, the VAP is easy to palpate. (See *Proper catheter and needle positions.*)

If the port will be used immediately after insertion, a needle used during surgery should be left in place to handle infusions and reduce the discomfort associated with site access. Swelling and tenderness at the site may exist for 72 hours after the procedure, during which time palpation of the device may be more difficult and more uncomfortable for the patient.

Using a venous access port

Using a VAP involves accessing the site using aseptic technique, administering bolus injections or infusions appropriately, obtaining blood samples as needed, and flushing the port when indicated.

Accessing a VAP

For nearly all ports, you'll use a noncoring needle to access the port for bolus injections, infusions, or drawing blood. A noncoring needle has a deflected or angled point, which slices the septum and, when removed, allows the septum to seal shut. (See *Comparing noncoring and hypodermic needles,* page 152.) Traditional needles shouldn't be used to enter a port because coring and leakage can occur after only a few accesses, rendering the device ineffective.

Noncoring needles typically come in 19G, 20G, and 22G and are ½" to 2" long. Larger noncoring needles, specifically 14G and 16G, are now available for high-flow infusions.

A straight noncoring needle may be used for bolus injections. A right-angled noncoring needle with an attached extension set can be used for either a bolus injection or an infusion. (See *Right-angle noncoring needle,* page 153.) Take care in selecting the most appropriate-sized noncoring needle for the patient. Most VAPs are designed to withstand up to 2,000 punctures with a 22G noncoring

Proper catheter and needle positions

The position of a vascular access port and the catheter tip is critical for successful therapy. These illustrations show the catheter tip placement in the superior vena cava with the port placed in a subcutaneous pocket in the forearm (below, left) or, more commonly, the chest (below, right). Note that the port is sutured to the fascia beneath the subcutaneous tissue and is implanted so that palpation is easy (right).

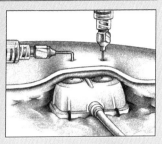

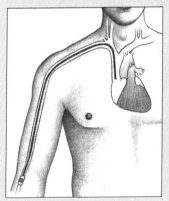

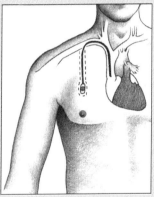

needle. A larger needle may be used if viscous fluids such as blood are being infused or if the fluid needs to be infused at a high rate. Use of a larger needle than necessary reduces the overall life of the device.

Careful attention must be given to syringe size when working with VAPs. The smaller the syringe, the greater the pressure placed on the port. Excessive pressure can cause the VAP to separate at the point of attachment or cause a fracture in the catheter lumen, especially if the lumen is partially occluded.

Bolus injection

Many drugs can be administered in a bolus injection, even through a VAP. Bolus injections through a VAP require that you gather necessary equipment and then administer the bolus.

Comparing noncoring and hypodermic needles

Because hypodermic needles can tear the septum of a vascular access device, always use a noncoring needle. These illustrations compare a noncoring needle with a traditional hypodermic needle. Note the deflected point on the noncoring needle that prevents coring of the septum.

Noncoring needle   **Hypodermic needle**

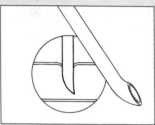 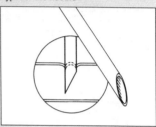

Gathering the equipment

Before administering the bolus, gather the following items:

- noncoring needle
- three 70% isopropyl alcohol swabs or pads
- three povidone-iodine swabs
- syringe with 3 to 5 ml of heparin solution (100 U/ml)
- 10-ml syringe with normal saline solution
- 7" extension set, if needed
- prescribed drug
- 2" × 2" sterile gauze dressing
- sterile towel
- tape
- mask and sterile gloves.

Administering a bolus injection

To administer a bolus injection, first explain the procedure to the patient. Wash your hands; then palpate the port to assess its depth and size. If you have trouble palpating a deep port, use a long needle (1½") when attempting entry. If the patient is anxious about the needle stick, especially if the port is newly inserted, apply an ice pack for 1 to 2 minutes to numb the skin over the port. A topical anesthetic, such as 0.1 to 0.15 ml of 2% lidocaine solution or a transdermal cream having anesthetic properties, may be used. Re-

EQUIPMENT EXPERTISE

Right-angle noncoring needle

The noncoring needle used for gaining access through a vascular access port (VAP) varies with the type of port involved. For a top-entry VAP, you may use a right-angled needle, shown here. This type of needle is attached to an extension tubing, which should be primed with normal saline solution before use.

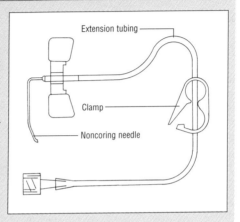

Extension tubing

Clamp

Noncoring needle

member that for a transdermal analgesic cream to be effective, it must be applied an hour before the procedure.

Wash your hands again, set up your equipment on the sterile field, and then put on a mask and sterile gloves. Attach the syringe of saline to the extension set and then to the noncoring needle. Make sure all air has been primed out of the system.

Clean the site with the alcohol swabs, followed by the povidone-iodine swabs. Clean from the port outward in a circular pattern until you've cleaned an area about 2" (5 cm) in diameter around the port. Allow the povidone-iodine to dry completely before attempting entry into the port.

Stabilize the reservoir between your thumb and forefinger. Hold the noncoring needle like a dart, and position it at a 90-degree angle over the septum. Push the needle straight through the skin and septum until it hits the needle stop. Don't insert the needle at an angle; doing so may damage the septum.

Check for needle placement by aspirating for blood return. If you can't obtain a blood return, have the patient cough, turn, raise his arms, or take a deep breath. If you still don't get a blood return, remove the needle and access a different site. Repeated needle sticks in the same spot can cause skin erosion over the septum and possibly infection.

Steadily inject 5 ml of the saline flush solution. If you can't inject the solution, the needle tip may not be in the correct position. Check that the needle tip is advanced to the needle stop and try to inject the solution again.

After the saline flush, clamp the extension tubing, remove the saline syringe and attach the medication syringe. Then inject the prescribed drug.

Flush the tubing and port with 5 ml of saline solution between each drug administration to reduce the chance of drug incompatibility. Remember to clamp the extension tubing each time you change syringes, then flush the tubing with 3 to 5 ml of heparin flush solution, according to your facility's policy.

To remove the needle, stabilize the reservoir between your thumb and forefinger. Then grasp the noncoring needle and pull straight up and out. Don't twist or turn the needle.

Because removal of a noncoring needle sometimes meets with resistance from the septum, some nurses have been stuck by the needle coming down on the hand stabilizing the port. Numerous devices have been manufactured specifically to prevent needle-stick injuries from noncoring needles. For instance, one device consists of a cuplike container that protects the nurse's hand as the needle is removed with a hemostat. Another consists of a pair of plastic blades that slide between the patient and the needle. The blades stabilize the port and lift the needle out of the port. Both devices avoid the need for the nurse to touch the needle, thus helping to prevent needle-stick injuries.

After withdrawal of the needle, you may note a slight serosanguineous discharge at the insertion site. Place a small 2" × 2" sterile gauze dressing over the site. Dispose of used supplies according to standard precautions.

Infusions

VAPs can be used to infuse a wide variety of solutions, including nutrition solutions, blood products, and solutions for fluid replacement. For infusions through a VAP, use an infusion pump with a pressure rating lower than the pounds per square inch rating of the port, to prevent disconnection of the catheter. In addition, always use luer-lock connections to prevent tubing disconnection and air embolism.

To start an infusion through a VAP, you'll need to gather the equipment to prepare the site and then administer the infusion.

Gathering the equipment

Gather this equipment prior to initiating an infusion through a VAP:

- sterile gloves and mask
- three 70% isopropyl alcohol swabs or pads
- three povidone-iodine swabs
- 10-ml syringe of normal saline solution
- right-angled noncoring needle
- extension set with luer lock and clamp, as needed
- sterile towel
- IV solution and administration set
- infusion control device
- sterile adhesive strips
- 2" × 2" sterile gauze
- sterile transparent semipermeable membrane dressing.

Administering an infusion

After gathering the needed equipment, explain the procedure to the patient. Then wash your hands and examine and palpate the port pocket and catheter track for swelling, redness, or tenderness. The presence of those signs, after the postoperative swelling has subsided, indicates system leakage.

After assessing the site, wash your hands, and assemble the solution container and tubing. Prime the tubing. Using aseptic technique, prepare sterile supplies on the sterile towel. Then put on a mask and sterile gloves.

Prepare the area using alcohol and povidone-iodine swabs. Using sterile technique, immobilize the port and insert the needle through the skin at a 90-degree angle until it touches the needle stop at the back of the port reservoir.

Using the saline-filled syringe, aspirate for a blood return. Flush the catheter and clamp. If aspiration or flushing proves difficult, reposition the patient and try again. Stop the procedure and notify the doctor if aspiration and flushing fails to prompt a blood return.

Stabilize the needle at its hub using sterile adhesive strips to prevent rotation. The right-angle bend of the noncoring needle should sit as close to the skin as possible, to allow for more stability. Use a sterile 2" × 2" gauze under the needle for additional support, if necessary.

Apply a transparent semipermeable membrane dressing. (See *Securing the needle,* page 156.) Make sure the port site is visible to assess for edema, erythema, drainage, bleeding, or bruising.

Securing the needle

When starting a continuous infusion, secure the right-angle noncoring needle to the skin. If the needle hub isn't flush with the skin, place a folded sterile dressing under the hub (right). Secure the needle and tubing, using the chevron taping method (below, left).

Apply a transparent semipermeable membrane dressing over the entire site (below, right).

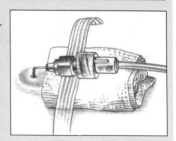

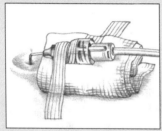

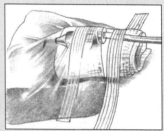

Connect the IV tubing to the needle's extension set. Unclamp the administration set and extension tubing, and begin the infusion. Tape the tubing and extension set securely to avoid placing tension on the tubing and accidental needle dislodgment.

Throughout the infusion, monitor the site for infiltration, especially if administering a vesicant drug. If the patient complains of stinging, burning, or pain at the site, discontinue the infusion and implement appropriate measures.

In addition, after a VAP has been accessed for an infusion, the device should be examined at least every 8 hours. When infusing vesicant chemotherapeutic agents, monitor the site hourly.

For prolonged use of the port, the noncoring needle should be changed at least every 7 days. A sterile occlusive dressing should be changed every 3 to 7 days, according to your facility's policy, or immediately if it becomes loose, soiled, or wet. Injection caps on needleless systems (if used) and extension tubings should be changed when the noncoring needle is changed.

Drawing blood samples

When drawing blood from a port, you'll access the port as usual. If a solution is being infused, stop the infusion, clamp the extension set, and disconnect the tubing. Wear gloves and, as always, follow standard precautions. Obtaining a blood sample from a VAP involves gathering the appropriate equipment and and then drawing the blood for testing.

Gathering the equipment

To obtain a blood sample, gather these items:

- nonsterile gloves
- 70% isopropyl alcohol or povidone-iodine swabs
- 1 10-ml syringe (empty) and 2 filled with normal saline solution
- syringe with 3 to 5 ml of heparin flush solution (100 U/ml)
- 19G or 20G noncoring needle
- extension set with luer lock and clamp
- injection cap, if needed

Obtaining the sample

Before obtaining blood from a VAP, explain the procedure to the patient, wash your hands, and put on clean gloves. Clean the needleless injection cap or extension set hub with alcohol or povidone-iodine. Then take these steps:

Attach a 10-ml syringe, withdraw at least 5 ml of blood, and then discard the syringe. Using another 10-ml syringe, withdraw the amount of blood needed to perform the test. Don't use a Vacutainer. Use of a Vacutainer creates a negative pressure within the catheter lumen and may cause it to flatten, making aspiration difficult. If you're drawing blood from the extension set hub, clamp the set each time you change syringes.

After withdrawing the blood, flush the port immediately with 5 to 20 ml of normal saline. Clean the injection cap or extension set hub, and then reconnect the tubing. Restart the infusion, if appropriate.

If the infusion won't be continued, flush the tubing with 3 to 5 ml of heparin flush solution (100 U/ml). To avoid the backflow of blood into the lumen during the flush, clamp the extension set at the same time the last 0.5 ml of heparin is injected, keeping positive pressure on the plunger as the needle is withdrawn. Cap the tubing, as needed, or remove the noncoring needle from the port.

Flushing a vascular access port

Flushing is part of the routine care of a vascular access port. First, locate the port by palpating the area (below, left). After preparing the site, access the port with a noncoring needle (below, center). When flushing, stabilize the needle and maintain positive pressure (below, right).

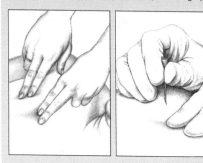
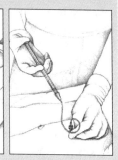

Maintenance and care

When VAPs aren't in use, they need to be flushed to prevent the formation of clots and occlusion of the catheter or port. Flushing a VAP regularly maintains patency and can prevent occlusion. (See *Flushing a vascular access port.*) To flush the port, first access it as usual with a noncoring needle and aspirate for blood return. If you encounter difficulty in obtaining a blood return, try repositioning the patient. (See *Troubleshooting a vascular access port.*)

Flush the catheter with 5 ml of normal saline solution using the pulsatile flush technique, which helps to clean fibrin residue from the lumen and reduces the risk of fibrin sheath formation.

Follow with 3 to 5 ml of heparin flush solution (100 U/ml), according to your facility's policy. As with any flush, maintain positive pressure when removing the needle from the port. If the port is attached to a Groshong catheter, use 10 to 20 ml of normal saline solution as a flush, not heparin.

Dual-lumen ports, which have a medial and a lateral port, have special maintenance requirements. Use care when flushing a dual-lumen port. Excessive pressure during flushing may cause the port to separate. Make sure to access and apply dressings to each port separately, taking care to label the medial and lateral ports correctly.

Troubleshooting a vascular access port

Numerous problems can occur with a vascular access port (VAP), most of which relate to an inability to flush the port or obtain blood or to palpate the port. Use this chart when troubleshooting a problem port.

POSSIBLE CAUSES	INTERVENTIONS
Kinked tubing or closed clamp	• Check tubing or clamp.
Catheter lodged against vessel wall	• Reposition the patient. • Raise the patient's arm on the same side as the catheter. • Have the patient cough, sit up, or take a deep breath. • Attempt to infuse 10 ml of saline solution into the catheter. • If still unable to flush VAP, regain access using a new sterile needle.
Incorrect needle placement or needle not advanced through septum	• Regain access to the device. • Teach the patient or caregiver to push down firmly on noncoring needle device in septum and to verify needle position by aspirating for a blood return.
Clot formation	• Assess patency by attempting to flush the VAP while the patient changes position. • Notify the doctor to obtain an order to administer urokinase, if facility permits. • Teach patient or caregiver to avoid forcibly flushing VAP.
Catheter migration or port rotation (Twiddler's syndrome)	• Notify the doctor immediately.
Deeply implanted port	• Use deep palpation to palpate port. • If the patient or caregiver is unable to access port, make a home care visit and access port. • If the home care nurse is unable to access port, another nurse can make an attempt. • Use a 1½" or 2" noncoring needle to access VAP.

Rotating ports during prolonged therapy may increase the life of the port's septum.

Flush each port separately once a month with heparin flush solution, to avoid occlusion. Be aware of the schedule for flushing the dormant port if one port is being used for a prolonged infusion.

Complications

A patient with a VAP faces most of the same risks associated with traditional tunneled or nontunneled central venous catheters. Complications of VAP use range from insertion-related problems such as hematoma to occlusion, infection, air embolism, extravasation, and VAP displacement. This section examines each type of complication and its treatment.

INSERTION-RELATED COMPLICATIONS. Normally, implantation of a VAP results in a small bruised area at the port site that usually disappears within a few days. The formation of a hematoma, however, can result in pain and make palpating the port difficult and painful.

Other insertion-related complications include brachial plexus injury, pneumothorax, perforation of thoracic blood vessels, thoracic duct injury, and air embolism. Monitor the patient during the immediate postoperative period for signs and symptoms of hematoma or other insertion-related complications: pain, sensory abnormalities, weakness on the affected side, shortness of breath, diminished breath sounds or unequal expansion on the affected side, hypotension, chest pain, tachycardia, cyanosis, and confusion.

For a hematoma, apply cold to the site several times a day until the swelling diminishes. Pneumothorax, thoracic duct injuries, and other serious complications require immediate action. Notify the doctor, administer oxygen as ordered, prepare for insertion of a chest tube, as appropriate, and provide other supportive measures as indicated.

OCCLUSION. A VAP can become blocked when a clot or fibrin sheath forms or when a drug or lipid solution precipitates. A blood clot occluding the catheter or a fibrin sheath forming at the tip of the VAP can be caused by inadequate flushing, pump malfunction, or the patient's hypercoagulable state, among other factors. In such cases, the catheter should be declotted with thrombolytic therapy. (See *Using urokinase for catheter occlusion.*)

VAP occlusions can also be due to compression of the catheter, a condition known as pinch-off syndrome. (See *Pinch-off syndrome,* page 162.) Regardless of the cause, VAP occlusion may lead to edema and tenderness on the side of the patient's body in which the port is located, or to resistance when flushing or aspirating.

To help prevent VAP occlusions, use extreme care when taking blood samples from a patient's port. The catheter should be flushed

Using urokinase for catheter occlusion

Thrombosis of a vascular access device (VAP) or its attached catheter usually involves administering anticoagulation therapy. The drug used most often is the thrombolytic agent urokinase. To administer urokinase through a VAP, follow these steps:

- Clean the needleless injection cap with an antiseptic solution such as povidone-iodine.
- Attach a 10-ml urokinase-filled syringe to the needleless cap on the end of the extension set or the noncoring needle. The usual dosage is urokinase 5,000 U/ml in an amount equal to the VAP volume, plus 0.2 ml.
- Unclamp and slowly instill the prescribed amount.
- Reclamp the extension tubing, remove the syringe, and attach an empty 5-ml syringe. Wait 5 minutes, then attempt to aspirate 4 to 5 ml of blood. If unsuccessful, repeat aspiration attempts every 5 minutes, for up to 30 minutes if necessary. If the catheter isn't open within 30 minutes, cap it and let the urokinase work for 30 to 60 additional minutes before attempting aspiration again. A second instillation may be necessary. Remember to be patient; in most instances, the procedure will prove effective. If a second instillation does not clear the thrombosis, obtain an X-ray to rule out occlusions from something other than a clot.
- After aspirating 5 ml of blood, clamp the catheter and remove the syringe. Connect a 10-ml syringe filled with normal saline solution. Gently flush with saline; then reclamp the extension tubing.
- Restart the infusion or flush the port with a heparin solution, according to your facility's policy.

well with saline, using a pulsatile flow technique. This rinses the internal lumen of the port reservoir and catheter and prevents fibrin buildup. Instill the usual volume of heparin using the same technique.

In addition, use care when administering drugs known to form precipitates, including diazepam, calcium gluconate, and phenytoin. Be sure to flush the catheter before and after administering these medications. Be aware of potential drug and solution incompatibilities for the patient's prescribed therapies.

If you suspect a blockage is caused by drug precipitate, notify the doctor. Some facilities use hydrochloric acid or sodium bicarbonate to break up the precipitate. Lipid occlusions can sometimes be cleared with ethyl alcohol.

INFECTION. VAP-related infections occur in as many as 30% of patients with a VAP. Erythema, or skin redness, may be the first sign of a VAP infection. Infection can result from poor access technique, excessive movement by the patient while the noncoring needle is in place, repeated use of the same port entry site, or hub or infusate contamination. In addition, port infections may stem from infections else-

Pinch-off syndrome

Pinch-off syndrome results from repeated compression of a central catheter, placed percutaneously into the subclavian vein, when it gets caught between the clavicle and the first rib. An uncommon complication, pinch-off syndrome can ultimately cause fracture of the catheter and catheter embolization. Look for these signs of pinch-off syndrome:

• port works only when a patient is in a specific position, particularly when the patient rolls his shoulder or raises the arm on the side where the port is located
• recurrent pump alarms
• difficulty aspirating blood
• a sluggish infusion.

Temporary occlusions can be corrected by having the patient cough, perform Valsalva's maneuver, or change position. If the occlusion is corrected *only* by raising the arm or shoulder, obtain a chest X-ray to determine positioning of the catheter on the VAP.

The severity of the pinch-off is often assigned a grade, ranging from 0 (no distortion) to 3 (catheter fracture or transection). Catheters with grade 2 or 3 pinch-off should be removed.

where in the body, such as the lung or bone. Left untreated, VAP infections may lead to bacteremia, a potentially life-threatening complication of VAP use.

Preventing VAP infection requires strict attention to sterile technique during insertion and routine care duties. If the port is the suspected source of infection, blood cultures should be taken, usually from both the port and a peripheral site in the opposite arm. If blood cultures indicate bacteremia, the port may need to be removed, particularly if antibiotics fail to control the infection within 72 hours or if symptoms recur after antibiotic therapy.

AIR EMBOLISM. An air embolism can occur anytime an infusion is given through a central venous catheter. During breathing, intrathoracic pressure drops below atmospheric pressure, which causes a negative pressure in central veins. This negative pressure acts like a vacuum and can draw air directly into a vein if the port or catheter is open to air. Signs and symptoms include chest pain and shortness of breath with accompanying cyanosis. Examination may reveal hypotension and a weak, rapid pulse. Untreated, air embolism can lead to shock and, eventually, cardiac arrest.

If an air embolism occurs, immediately close off the source of air into the vascular system and place the patient in a left-sided Trendelenburg position. Notify the doctor, monitor vital signs, and administer oxygen, as ordered.

Preventing an air embolism includes closing the clamp on the extension set when changing injection caps or tubing, using air-eliminating filters on IV tubing, changing solution containers before they're completely empty, adequately purging air from IV tubing, and using luer-lock connectors to prevent accidental opening to air. Also make sure to educate the patient about the signs, symptoms, and prevention of air embolism.

EXTRAVASATION. If the patient complains of a burning sensation at the port site, the needle might have become dislodged from the port, causing infiltration or extravasation of the drug or solution being infused. Edema may develop under the arm or in the neck area. Extravasation of vesicant drugs can cause severe local tissue damage.

Treatment varies with the type, concentration, and volume of medication infused. Follow your facility's policy for treating extravasation, stop the infusion, and notify the doctor for antidote orders. Then confirm that the noncoring needle remains in its proper position.

VAP DISPLACEMENT (TWIDDLER'S SYNDROME). If the patient manipulates the port through the skin, a common occurrence in pediatric patients and confused or highly anxious patients, the VAP may rotate or the catheter may migrate out of the original tip position. Signs of a displaced port include difficulty with infusion, movement of the port when entered with a noncoring needle, leakage at the site, or a burning sensation in the area.

If displacement is suspected, obtain an X-ray to determine tip location. The catheter may be repositioned under fluoroscopy or, if that's not possible, the entire port may be removed and a new one inserted, depending on the severity of the displacement. To avoid displacement, teach the patient the importance of not pulling on or otherwise manipulating the device.

Normal growth of the patient may also lead to displacement of the catheter. Because VAPs are considered long-term central access devices, a pediatric patient who has a port for months or years may outgrow the tip placement. In a growing child, periodically confirm tip location.

Teaching the patient

For successful patient teaching about VAPs, keep the information simple and provide written material for the patient's review. Assess the patient's knowledge about central venous therapy, and use this assessment as a guide to further his knowledge about VAPs. Videotapes commonly provided by VAP manufacturers may prove helpful.

Reassure the patient that a VAP doesn't restrict activities and requires little maintenance except when the port is in use. Explain the frequency of catheter and port flushing, and tell him to make an appointment for flushing of the device if the VAP hasn't been used for more than 4 weeks. Teach the patient how to flush the VAP.

Explain the signs and symptoms of local and systemic infection, extravasation, and other complications; also explain what should be done if those signs or symptoms occur. Instruct the patient to wear a medical alert bracelet or carry an identification card informing all health care providers about the VAP. Tell the patient that if he undergoes an invasive procedure, such as dental work or surgery, prophylactic antibiotics may be needed.

If the VAP is used at home for periodic infusions, make sure the patient or caregiver knows how to access the port. Before discharge, have the patient practice the procedure. Emphasize that he should feel the needle hitting the reservoir bottom before initiating the infusion or injection.

Teach the patient how to confirm needle placement with a blood return and how to change the dressing. The patient should return demonstrate both procedures. Include in your instructions measures to prevent the needle from becoming dislodged and the name and number of the person or facility the patient should contact if problems or questions arise.

Provide the patient with written material that includes clear descriptions of the port, including the type, brand name, location, gauge, length of catheter and access needles, insertion date, condition at discharge, and the environment in which the line was placed and by whom. Instruct the patient to keep this information handy and present it to health care providers when necessary.

Removal of a vascular access port

A VAP is removed surgically when the required treatment has been completed or is no longer necessary. A surgeon removes the port by sharp dissection through the old incision.

If purulent drainage is present, the port will need to be cultured to identify the organisms on its surface. If the patient develops signs of bacteremia, treatment should be based on culture results. Following removal of the port, monitor the patient carefully for air embolism or other complications. Check the site for redness, swelling, or drainage. Keep the patient supine to maintain positive intrathoracic pressure and allow the catheter tract to close.

Teach the patient the signs and symptoms of air embolism. Change the dressing and inspect the site every 24 hours until it has begun to heal. Keep in mind that the longer the port was in place, the longer it may take for the insertion site to completely close.

Because removal is often done in an outpatient surgical center, instruct the patient or caregiver to watch for signs of redness, swelling, drainage, or fever.

Documentation

When caring for a patient with a VAP, you'll need to document:
- each step taken when accessing a port or removing a needle
- drugs or fluids infused
- presence of a blood return
- needle size
- dressing changes
- appearance of access site
- patient's response to the procedure
- patient teaching done
- presence of complications and what steps you took to handle them
- short- and long-term goals of VAP therapy and nursing interventions for each.

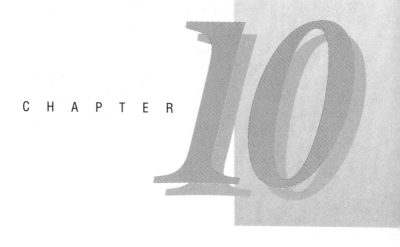

Managing alternative access routes

Today's infusion therapy professionals deal with more than peripheral and central intravenous infusions and injections; they also handle infusions and injections through a number of other routes, including epidural, intraosseous, intraperitoneal, and subcutaneous. This chapter examines each of these infusion routes in detail.

Epidural infusions

Epidural infusions are used in pain management. When opioids are given by the epidural route, they diffuse across the covering of the spinal cord and mix with the CSF. Then they bind with opiate receptors, blocking the transmission of pain signals to the thalamus. When local anesthetics are administered, they block the movement of pain signals from the dorsal root ganglion to the spinal cord.

Uses of epidural access devices
Epidural access devices are used mostly as a means to administer analgesics. To produce analgesia for the chest and upper abdomen, the

catheter is placed between the fifth and eighth thoracic vertebrae. Placing it between the second and fourth lumbar vertebrae provides analgesia to the lower abdomen and legs.

Epidural catheters may be used for patients with acute postoperative or chronic pain. Analgesics administered postoperatively by the epidural route may result in better mobility and increased lung expansion because the patient has less pain with inspiration.

Epidural access devices can also be used for patients with intractable pain that has failed to respond to conventional analgesic therapy and for patients with chronic pain from cancer.

Epidural analgesia delivery should be avoided in patients with a low platelet count, a coagulation disorder, a local infection, an epidural space compromise (identified by myelography), CNS structural pathology, spinal arthritis or deformity, hypotension, marked hypertension, or an allergy to the prescribed drug.

Analgesics given through an epidural access device *must be* preservative-free because of the risk of nerve damage from the preservatives. The most commonly used drugs for epidural analgesia include morphine sulfate, hydromorphone, fentanyl, sufentanil, and bupivacaine.

Lipid-soluble drugs—such as fentanyl, sufentanil, and bupivacaine—cross the dura or lipid membrane of the spinal cord readily and provide rapid onset of analgesia. Water-soluble drugs—such as morphine and hydromorphone—cross the dura more slowly, resulting in slower onset. These drugs are also retained longer in the CNS, so are useful for prolonged analgesia. Combinations of an opioid and a local anesthetic such as bupivacaine offer the analgesic effects of both drugs while allowing lower dosages of each and thus reducing the risk of adverse effects.

Selecting an epidural access device

Four main types of epidural access devices are available: short-term external catheters, long-term or tunneled catheters, subcutaneously implanted ports, and implanted pumps. The type of device chosen depends on the patient and clinical needs.

Short-term external catheter

Epidural catheters are placed percutaneously in the epidural space. A needle is inserted into the epidural space, located outside the dura mater and beneath the ligamentum flavum, connective tissue that binds adjacent vertebrae together. (See *Epidural catheter placement,* page 168.) A catheter is then threaded through the needle and advanced into the space.

Epidural catheter placement

An epidural catheter may exit directly over the spine or it may be tunneled subcutaneously to an exit site on the patient's side or abdomen. This cross-sectional view shows the internal structures of the CNS with a catheter inserted into the epidural space.

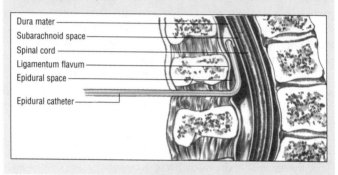

Dura mater
Subarachnoid space
Spinal cord
Ligamentum flavum
Epidural space
Epidural catheter

Short-term epidural catheters are inserted by an anesthesiologist or nurse anesthetist. Other types of epidural access devices are surgically inserted by specially trained medical personnel. The catheters are used to manage acute postoperative or short-term chronic pain, often for patients who need therapy for less than 1 month. They're also used for a short time, usually 3 to 7 days, to test the effectiveness of therapy in patients prior to the implantation of a permanent access device. Short-term epidural catheters are quicker, easier, and less costly to insert than permanent devices. However, they're also associated with a higher rate of mechanical problems.

Long-term indwelling catheter
Long-term or tunneled catheters are composed of kink-resistant silicone tubing and a Dacron cuff. The catheter is tunneled under the skin from the epidural space and exits through the anterior chest wall or abdomen. Tunneled catheters provide longer dwell times; they're more stable and less prone to infection than short-term catheters.

Implanted subcutaneous port
Used for intermittent or continuous infusion of analgesics for patients with chronic pain, the implanted subcutaneous port consists of a portal body attached to an internal long-term catheter. The portal body has a 60-micron filter inside the reservoir, which prevents pieces of the septum from entering the epidural space if an ac-

Implantable infusion pump

An implantable infusion pump, often used for epidural infusions, has no external pieces. This illustration shows an implantable pump in place.

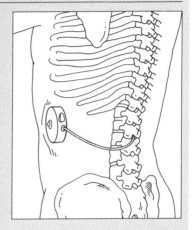

cidental coring of the septum occurs. Even so, a noncoring needle should always be used for gaining access to this port.

Implanted pumps

Of the most commonly used epidural access devices, the implanted reservoir offers the lowest risk of infection because it's a closed system. (See *Implantable infusion pump*.) The most commonly used implanted pumps—Pfizer's Infusaid and Medtronic's Synchro-Med—are disk-shaped and made of lightweight titanium. They have a self-sealing silicone septum through which access is gained by a noncoring needle.

They each have their own power supply—Freon in the case of Infusaid, and a lithium battery in a SynchroMed. The Infusaid pump requires a refill of medication every 3 to 4 weeks. The SynchroMed is refilled every 16 weeks. Follow the manufacturer's directions for the use of either pump.

Irrespective of the pump used, take great care when accessing the device to refill it. Some pumps have an additional catheter access port near the edge of the pump for bolus injections. Inadvertent injection of medication into this port can cause a potentially fatal overdose.

Administering an infusion or bolus injection

Procedures for administering a medication through an epidural catheter vary according to your facility's policies and your state's nurse practice act. To administer a bolus injection or continuous infusion, first gather the supplies, wash your hands, and explain the procedure to the patient. Obtain the patient's vital signs, including respiratory rate.

Put on sterile gloves and a mask. Clean the injection cap with povidone-iodine, and allow the solution to dry completely. Insert the needle of an empty syringe into the injection cap, and attempt aspiration to assess for the absence of blood or CSF. If you aspirate blood or more than 1 ml of clear fluid, stop the procedure and notify the doctor.

For a bolus injection, replace the syringe with the medication-filled syringe, and inject the medication into the catheter at the prescribed rate.

For a continuous infusion, attach the tubing or filter to the medication container and purge all air from the system. Be aware that all epidural infusions require the use of a 0.2-micron filter without surfactant for drug administration. Always use luer-lock connections to the catheter. Then attach the tubing to the infusion pump and program the pump to deliver the infusate at the prescribed rate. Remove the syringe from the catheter, and connect the pump tubing or filter to the catheter. Begin the infusion at the prescribed rate. Finally, label the medication container, tubing, and catheter "For epidural use only," to avoid inappropriate use of the catheter.

Dispose of all used equipment according to standard precautions.

Maintenance and care

Nursing care of the epidural catheter includes care of the exit site, changing the injection cap. Keep in mind that alcohol should not be used to prepare the site or access the device; alcohol may cause nerve damage if it migrates into the epidural space.

Caring for the exit site

Proper management of the exit site of an epidural access device is important for avoiding infection and other complications. To care for the exit site, gather the supplies, wash your hands, and explain the procedure to the patient.

Then put on a mask and clean gloves, and carefully remove the old dressing. Assess the site for redness, drainage, swelling, or pain; if present, notify the doctor. Change to sterile gloves.

Using friction, clean the site with povidone-iodine swabs three times and allow the solution to dry. Use a circular cleaning motion, working outward from the exit site 2" or 3" (5 to 7.5 cm). Apply a sterile gauze or transparent semipermeable membrane dressing, as ordered. Then coil the catheter and secure it with tape. Dispose of all used equipment according to standard precautions.

Changing the injection cap and filter

Injection caps and filters are changed every 48 to 72 hours. To change the injection cap and filter, gather the supplies, wash your hands, and explain the procedure to the patient. Put on sterile gloves and a mask.

Connect the new injection cap to the new filter, and flush the entire system with sterile preservative-free normal saline solution. Clean the connection between the catheter and the filter with a povidone-iodine swab.

Remove the old filter and injection cap, and then, using aseptic technique, screw on the new filter and cap securely. Dispose of all used equipment according to standard precautions.

Complications

Complications of an epidural access device include those related to the device itself and those related to the potential for adverse effects of the analgesic used. Problems associated with epidural devices include infection, epidural fibrosis, tissue erosion, fluid leakage, and catheter migration.

INFECTION. Meningitis, epidural abscess, and infection of the pump pocket are possible infections associated with the use of epidural access devices. Signs of infection include decreased effectiveness of the medication; tenderness, pain, redness, or drainage at the exit or implant site; fever; neck stiffness; headache; vomiting; an elevated WBC; and altered sensory or motor responses in the lower extremities. Infections are treated with antibiotics and, possibly, removal of the epidural access device. To prevent infections, use rigidly applied infection control techniques whenever caring for a patient with an epidural access device.

EPIDURAL FIBROSIS. Patients with an epidural access catheter in place for more than 12 months and in whom analgesia has become inadequate to meet their needs might have developed fibrosis, a buildup of scar tissue around the catheter. In addition to decreased effectiveness of the analgesics, other signs of epidural fibrosis include increased resistance when injecting a drug, pain on injection, or a bulge at the site of catheter entry following injection.

Increasing the concentration of the drug and decreasing the volume of the injectate may temporarily improve analgesia. Intrathecal catheters may be preferred over epidural catheters when long-term placement is anticipated; fibrosis doesn't occur with intrathecal catheters. The epidural catheter may need to be removed because symptoms of epidural fibrosis tend to steadily worsen over time.

TISSUE EROSION. Erosion of the subcutaneous tissue over the port or reservoir site may occur if the patient lacks healthy tissue over the implantation site. Tissue erosion usually occurs as a result of malnutrition, general wasting, deterioration of the patient's overall health, shallow placement of the port, or poor local circulation.

When tissue erosion occurs, look for wound edges that separate and a port or reservoir that becomes visible through the skin. Treatment includes the removal of the implanted device, antibiotic therapy, and wound care.

FLUID LEAKAGE. Leakage of CSF can occur if the epidural catheter punctures the dura during insertion or if the catheter migrates and punctures the dura. CSF leakage causes a decline in pressure within the spinal canal and may result in a prolonged and pounding headache, typically felt in the front of the head and worsening when the patient tries to sit or stand.

Alert the doctor if you think the catheter has migrated to the subarachnoid space because the patient could be subjected to an overdose of the analgesic ordered. Encourage the patient to maintain bed rest and take additional analgesics and fluids to manage the pain until it subsides.

As the dura heals and seals the puncture (usually within 48 hours), the headache will subside. If it continues, the doctor may order caffeine injections or a blood patch treatment, which involves withdrawing about 10 ml of the patient's blood from a peripheral vein and injecting it into the epidural space. When the epidural needle is withdrawn, the patient is instructed to sit up. As the blood clots, it usually seals off the leaking area. Blood patches can relieve a headache almost immediately.

CATHETER MIGRATION. An epidural access device can migrate out of position or become otherwise dislodged. Look for decreased effect-

iveness of the drug and, if the catheter has migrated into the subarachnoid (intrathecal) space, signs and symptoms of drug overdose:
decreased respiratory rate, unilateral analgesic effect, hypotension,
nausea, and weakness in the extremities. Keep in mind that, if analgesics meant for the epidural space are administered into the intrathecal space, signs of overdose can occur at much smaller doses,
approximately one-tenth the epidural dose.

Check for the catheter's position by monitoring its external
length and aspirating the catheter. If you aspirate blood or more
than 1 ml of CSF, the catheter needs to be repositioned.

Teaching the patient
Teaching the patient about an epidural access device can be extremely important in assuring a successful outcome of therapy, particularly for long-term devices. Describe the device thoroughly, using illustrations for the internal placement within the epidural space.

In addition, describe the potential problems associated with the
epidural device. Explain the purpose and effects of epidural analgesia
as well as the potential adverse effects of the analgesics used. Teach
the patient how to effectively manage his pain, care for the exit site,
administer the medication, and operate the infusion pump. Emphasize the need for strict adherence to infection control procedures and
for daily assessment of the exit site.

Removal of an epidural catheter
The removal procedure for an epidural catheter varies with the type
of access device used. A qualified registered nurse may remove a
temporary epidural catheter. A tunneled or implanted device is removed by a doctor. A sterile dressing will be left over the site. Monitor the site for fluid leakage, redness, swelling, or tenderness.

Documentation
Your documentation for an epidural access device should include
the following:
• type of catheter
• date and time for all procedures performed
• dose, volume, and rate of administration for all drugs administered
• type and amount of solution used to flush the catheter
• description of aspirate
• site care
• effectiveness of the analgesics used
• patient teaching

- informed consent (for insertion)
- patient tolerance of the procedure
- complications and nursing actions for those complications.

Intraosseous access

The intraosseous route provides access into the bone marrow, offering immediate access for the rapid administration of fluids and medications in emergency situations in which gaining venous access proves impossible. Fluid injected directly into the bone marrow drains rapidly into the central venous channel and enters the systemic circulation through smaller veins. (See *Intraosseous infusion sites.*)

Care of a patient with an intraosseous access needle includes an understanding of the uses and types of devices, insertion techniques and devices (including the bone injection gun), care of the intraosseous access needle, complications, patient teaching, removal of the intraosseous access needle, and documentation.

Uses of intraosseous access needles

Intraosseous access allows for immediate, temporary access to bone marrow in life-threatening situations until ordinary vascular access can be obtained. Intraosseous access has a high success rate for therapy and a low rate of complications.

Intraosseous access needles can be used for infants, children, or adults when emergency venous access can't be established within the first 5 minutes of care. The needle should be removed as soon as a standard venous access device has been inserted.

Using the intraosseous route is sometimes preferred over instillation of emergency drugs through an endotracheal tube. Only atropine, epinephrine, lidocaine, and naloxone can be instilled through an endotracheal tube, and no fluids or blood products can be administered that way.

Intraosseous administration can also prove useful when administering regional anesthesia in the treatment of certain orthopedic conditions in which venous access fails or isn't feasible.

Intraosseous access needles shouldn't be inserted in an infected area, into a bone in which intraosseous access has been previously attempted, or into open fractured bone or a known bone tumor lesion. Use of an intraosseous access needle is contraindicated in patients with bone disorders such as osteoporosis.

Intraosseous infusion sites

A common intraosseous infusion site is the anteromedial surface of the proximal tibia, about 1" (2.5 cm) below the tibial tuberosity, as shown (right). Alternative sites include the distal tibia, distal femur, and iliac crest. The upper anterior portion of the sternum is rarely used because injection there can cause complete bone perforation. Because bone marrow acts as a noncollapsible vein, drugs infused into the marrow cavity (below) enter the circulation rapidly through an extensive network of medullary sinusoids.

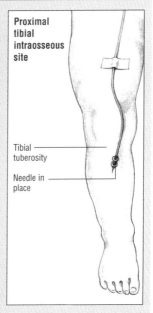

Proximal tibial intraosseous site

Tibial tuberosity

Needle in place

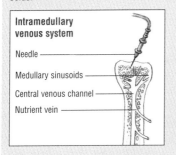

Intramedullary venous system

Needle

Medullary sinusoids

Central venous channel

Nutrient vein

Selecting an intraosseous access needle

A number of needles can be used to gain access to the bone marrow, the selection of which is based on the age and size of the patient. Disposable needles specifically designed for intraosseous access are usually used. Other types of needles include steel hypodermic, spinal, trephine, sternal, and standard bone marrow needles.

The sharp obturator on an intraosseous access needle protects the tip, and circular screw-type threads help the needle to penetrate the bone. To improve the success rate of intraosseous administration, needles should have the following features (found in commercially available intraosseous devices and in some bone marrow aspiration needles):

- short shaft, to avoid accidental dislodgment
- stylet, to prevent the needle from becoming plugged with bone
- large bore
- rigidity
- handle that secures the stylet during insertion.

Initiating an intraosseous infusion

Intraosseous access needles are inserted only by specially trained doctors, nurses, and emergency personnel. To initiate an intraosseous infusion, you'll need to gather your equipment, prepare the patient and site, and start the infusion.

Gathering the equipment

Before starting an intraosseous infusion, gather:

- povidone-iodine swabs
- sterile gloves
- appropriate-sized intraosseous access needle with obturator
- 3- to 5-ml syringe and 1% lidocaine
- normal saline flush solution
- infusion syringe or IV administration set
- medication and solution
- sterile tape
- sterile gauze or transparent semipermeable membrane dressing
- infusion pump or controller, as indicated.

Preparing the patient

Time constraints may radically limit your ability to properly prepare for an intraosseous infusion. However, preparation is important for a successful insertion. Begin by explaining the procedure to the patient or caregiver.

Determine the most appropriate site for the patient. Recommended sites in children include the distal or proximal tibia and the distal femur. The distal tibia is the preferred site because of the thin covering of bony cortex over the area and because access is easier on the flat area of the bone proximal to the malleolus. To find the proximal tibia site, measure one or two fingerbreadths below the tibial tuberosity on the anteromedial surface.

Access to the distal femur is more difficult because the bone has a heavy padding of muscle and fat. Sternal insertions are not recommended in children because of the risk of penetrating the mediastinum. Avoid insertion of intraosseous needles into the epiphyseal plates in children.

Recommended sites for insertion in adults include the iliac crest or sternum, the distal end of the radius in the forearm, the proximal metaphysis of the humerus, and 1" to 1½" (3 to 4 cm) proximal to the distal tip of the lateral or medial malleolus. The needle can also be inserted into the ulnar styloid, the distal epiphysis of the second metacarpus, or the distal epiphysis of the first metatarsus.

Preparing the site

To prepare for insertion of an intraosseous device, wash your hands and gather necessary supplies. Set up a sterile field using aseptic technique. If an extremity will be used for the intraosseous access needle insertion, secure it in a comfortable, stable, dependent position. Restrain the limb of a pediatric patient.

Clean the skin over the site vigorously with povidone-iodine swabs, starting in the center and working outward about 2″ (5 cm). Repeat, and then allow the solution to dry.

Inserting the device

After you've gathered your supplies and prepared the patient and site, you'll need to carefully insert the needle. Put on sterile gloves. If ordered, anesthetize the skin with 1% lidocaine injected down to the periosteum. Quickly advance the needle through the skin to the bony cortex. In children, angle the needle away from the joint space to avoid hitting the epiphyseal plate.

Insert the needle further, into the marrow cavity, using firm pressure and a downward screwing or rotating movement. You can feel the needle pass through the bony cortex and into a soft and hollow area, the spongy bone. You'll know when you've reached the bone marrow when you feel a soft "pop" and a decrease in insertion resistance. In addition, the needle will stand upright without support when inserted into the bone.

When you believe the tip of the needle is located in the bone marrow, remove the obturator from the needle, attach a 5-ml syringe, and aspirate some bone marrow to check placement. Replace the syringe with one containing normal saline solution; then flush the cannula to confirm needle placement and to clear the cannula of blood and bone particles. There should be no resistance when flushing the needle.

Remove the flush syringe and connect the needle to a standard syringe or IV administration set. Clean the site again with povidone-iodine swabs. Secure the needle with sterile tape. Make sure to securely tape the infusion syringe or IV tubing to prevent accidental dislodgment or a rocking motion of the needle. Apply a sterile gauze or transparent semipermeable membrane dressing.

To minimize pain in a conscious patient during the initial infusion of fluid, withdraw 2 to 5 ml of bone marrow and then slowly inject 2 to 5 ml of 1% lidocaine over 60 seconds.

Bone injection gun

A bone injection gun can insert an intraosseous access device rapidly. These illustrations show how the gun is used. Note that the gun is locked in position (right). After triggering, the gun's housing becomes separated from the trocar-needle (below, left). After removal of the stylet, a syringe (below, right) or standard IV tubing is attached to the needle.

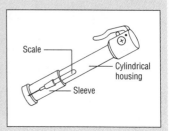

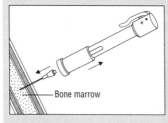

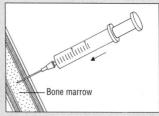

If the first intraosseous access attempt is unsuccessful, use another bone for any subsequent attempt, to prevent leakage of infused fluid into the original puncture site.

Using a bone injection gun

Bone injection guns are available that insert a needle into the bone marrow automatically. The use of a bone injection gun, such as the BIG, manufactured by BIG-TEIC Ltd. Science Park Technion, allows intraosseous access in adults. (See *Bone injection gun*.)

The BIG, a gunlike device that inserts a 15G trocar needle into the bone marrow at high speed, is propelled by a powerful, charged coil. To insert an intraosseous access needle using the BIG, first set the depth (measured in centimeters) of penetration needed. Injections into the proximal tibial metaphysis should penetrate to a depth of 2.5 cm; into the medial malleolus, 2 cm; into the lateral malleolus or distal metaphysis of the radius, 1 to 1.5 cm.

After the injection site is prepared, place the front end of the BIG perpendicular to and against the site. Hold the BIG firmly, and pull out the safety pin. Press the trigger. Manually separate the stylet trocar from the needle cannula, leaving the needle in the bone. Connect the needle to either a syringe or to standard IV tubing, and begin the infusion. Secure the needle, and apply dressings as for a standard intraosseous access needle.

Maintenance and care

Routine maintenance and care of an intraosseous access needle involve flushing the needle and infusing drugs or solutions through it. Before starting the infusion, you'll need to flush the access needle with normal saline solution to confirm access and to clear the needle of blood and bone material.

Medications or fluids may be infused through the needle by gravity or infusion pump. The needle size and density, and the size of the bone marrow cavity, affect the rate of flow. Solutions of normal saline have been administered through a 13G intraosseous access needle by gravity at rates as high as 600 ml/hour and by an infusion pump at rates as high as 2,500 ml/hour.

Complications

Principal complications associated with the use of intraosseous access needles include improper needle placement, needle obstruction, and osteomyelitis. Other complications associated with this device include subcutaneous abscess and osteomyelitis.

IMPROPER NEEDLE PLACEMENT. If the needle isn't placed properly, it may result in subperiosteal effusion, indicated by swelling, lack of an aspirate, inability of infusate to flow properly, or signs of extravasation into the surrounding subcutaneous tissue.

NEEDLE OBSTRUCTION. The intraosseous needle can become obstructed from pieces of bone marrow or blood clots. Obstructions are more likely to occur if an infusion is delayed or the needle isn't flushed after placement. Signs of obstruction include lack of an aspirate and an inability of the infusate to flow properly.

OSTEOMYELITIS. The longer an intraosseous access needle is left in place after 24 hours, the greater the risk of osteomyelitis. Risk of osteomyelitis is also increased when the patient has already acquired an infection elsewhere in the body.

Signs and symptoms of osteomyelitis include fever, pain, leukocytosis, and limitation of movement of the affected limb. In addition, look for drainage, swelling, or redness or other discolorations at the insertion site.

Teaching the patient

Patient teaching about an intraosseous access needle, even in an emergency, can prove important for enlisting the patient's cooperation and allaying fears of the patient, family, or caregiver. Explain the purpose, risks, and benefits of the procedure and treatment.

Removal of an intraosseous access needle

The intraosseous access needle should be removed within 24 hours of insertion. To remove the needle, close the clamp on the infusion administration set and turn off the infusion pump, if indicated. Wash your hands, and put on clean gloves. Stabilize the site by holding the surrounding skin. Then withdraw the needle, and cover the site with a dry, sterile gauze dressing.

After the needle has been removed, inspect the site and change the dressing every day until there is no further drainage, which usually disappears within 48 hours. Watch for signs and symptoms of site infection, and report redness, swelling, exudate, or pain.

Documentation

Once the insertion procedure has been completed, document the following in the patient's record:
• date and time procedure was completed
• type and size of needle or cannula inserted
• site location
• number of attempts required for successful insertion
• type and amount of flush solution used
• type and amount of drug or solution administered, including dose, volume, and rate of administration
• patient's response.

Intraperitoneal access

Intraperitoneal catheters, used for short- or long-term peritoneal dialysis or for administering chemotherapy, are generally placed in the low pelvic area, below the umbilicus. Intraperitoneal catheters and ports must be inserted surgically by a doctor.

Uses of intraperitoneal access devices

Intraperitoneal access devices are used to deliver intraperitoneal dialysis or regional chemotherapy for ovarian, gastric, or bladder cancer or extrahepatic disease with peritoneal seeding (metastatic disease dispersed in the peritoneal cavity). Intraperitoneal chemotherapy enhances each drug's ability to kill cells at the tumor site and reduces systemic drug effects. The catheters may also be used to drain fluid from the peritoneal cavity in patients with malignant ascites.

Selecting an intraperitoneal access device

The design and characteristics of intraperitoneal access devices vary with the use. The devices include short-term catheters, long-term catheters, and subcutaneous intraperitoneal ports.

Short-term catheters

Made of a rigid material, short-term intraperitoneal catheters are designed for one-time, acute use only. They may also be used for chemotherapy if the treatments are administered less frequently, perhaps once a month. In such cases, the catheter would need to be inserted each time. Short-term catheters can be inserted at the bedside by a doctor and used immediately and are less expensive and easier to remove than other intraperitoneal access devices.

Short-term catheters aren't without their risks, however. For instance, organ perforation can occur because of the rigidity of the catheter. Other risks include more patient discomfort, a greater risk of dialysate leakage, and migration of the catheter out of the intraperitoneal cavity. Peritonitis with long-term use can also occur; reinserting the catheter at each treatment reduces this risk.

Long-term catheters

Long-term intraperitoneal catheters are made of silicone and polyurethane material and usually have one or two cuffs that contain material that accelerates tissue growth around the catheter. The growth of tissue aids catheter stabilization, blocks the penetration of microorganisms, and prevents leakage of fluid.

The catheters decrease the risk of organ perforation when inserted during a laparotomy and also allow for intermittent treatments over a long period. Removal also doesn't require surgery.

Long-term intraperitoneal catheters must be inserted surgically, however, and home care must be managed by the patient. Compared with an implantable port, these catheters have a higher rate of infection. They may also cause an altered body image due to the presence of an external catheter.

Subcutaneous intraperitoneal ports

A subcutaneous intraperitoneal port consists of a portal body, central septum, reservoir, and catheter. Portal bodies are made of several materials, including stainless steel, titanium, plastic, or polysulfone, or a combination, and contain a self-sealing silicone septum that can withstand 1,000 to 2,000 needle punctures. Catheters are available in silicone or polyurethane and usually have radiopaque strips or tips to allow verification of location under fluoroscopy.

The catheter tip has several openings at the distal end to allow the infusion or drainage of fluid. Two attached Dacron cuffs anchor the catheter within the peritoneal cavity. The catheter is inserted through a small incision near the umbilicus into the peritoneum, with the catheter tip placed in the right or left pelvic gutter. The remaining catheter is tunneled subcutaneously to the portal body over the right or left lower rib cage. Its placement is verified by an assessment of catheter patency.

Because the port lacks an external catheter, it doesn't require home care management and causes little change in body image. In addition, the port also reduces the risk of infections and perforated organs when compared to an external catheter because the port is inserted in surgery.

Port implantation is contraindicated if infection is present or if the patient doesn't have enough body tissue to support the device. Port placement is also not recommended for obese patients because of the difficulty in gaining access to the port. Nor is implantation in a patient's chest recommended following radiation therapy to the chest or after a mastectomy. Subcutaneous intraperitoneal ports also tend to be more expensive than external catheters and don't allow for high-pressure irrigation, forced irrigation, or manipulation to dislodge or loosen clots.

Initiating an intraperitoneal infusion

Peritoneal infusions consist of three phases of treatment: infusion time, during which the dialysate or chemotherapeutic agent flows into the peritoneal cavity; dwell time, during which the instilled fluid remains in the peritoneal cavity; and drain time, during which the dialysate or chemotherapeutic agent flows out of the peritoneal cavity. Some chemotherapeutic agents may be left in the peritoneal cavity.

To initiate an intraperitoneal infusion, you'll need to gather the equipment, prepare the patient and intraperitoneal access device, and administer the infusion.

Gathering the equipment
You'll need the following items before beginning the infusion:
- Y-type dialysis administration set
- drainage bag
- warmed dialysate or chemotherapy agent
- povidone-iodine solution
- povidone-iodine swabs
- two pairs of sterile gloves
- two or more masks and a gown
- sterile 4″ × 4″ gauze pads and tape
- two water-resistant sterile barriers or drapes.

Preparing the patient and device
To begin, explain to the patient what you'll be doing. Weigh the patient, obtain his vital signs, and measure his abdominal girth.

Wash your hands, and put on a gown, mask, and sterile gloves. Open the Y-type administration set and attach the single output line to the drainage bag. Close the roller clamps on the tubing. Remove the cover from one tubing spike and insert this spike into the dialysate or other bag of solution.

Open the roller clamp between the dialysate (or other solution) and the patient, and then prime the tubing. After expelling the air, close the roller clamp. Open the roller clamps to the drainage bag, and prime this section of tubing as well. Close all clamps.

Next, create a sterile field using the sterile barrier or drape. Prepare your supplies on the field: gauze pads and povidone-iodine solution and swabs. Have the patient put on a mask. Place a second sterile barrier under the catheter's extension tubing. Remove and discard the used gloves according to standard precautions, and then put on a new pair of sterile gloves.

Administering the infusion
Administration procedures vary somewhat, depending on whether you're infusing through a catheter or an implanted device.

Infusions through a catheter
Using strict aseptic technique, clean the catheter's connection site with povidone-iodine. Remove the cap from the catheter's extension tubing and connect the catheter tubing to the administration set. Secure the connection with adhesive tape. Use tape to secure a loop of the tubing to the patient's abdomen, to prevent catheter movement.

Open the clamp on the catheter's extension tubing and on the administration set tubing to allow the dialysate or other solution to flow into the peritoneal cavity. Record the infusion start time. The roller clamp on the drainage bag should remain closed to prevent the infusate from accidentally flowing into the bag.

After the solution is instilled, close the clamps on the infusion line and the catheter's extension tubing, to keep air out of the tubing and peritoneal cavity. Keep the solution in the cavity for the prescribed dwell time. To allow the solution to come into contact with all surfaces of the peritoneum, you may need to turn the patient.

At the end of the dwell time, open the roller clamps leading to the drainage bag and the catheter's extension tubing, to drain the peritoneal cavity. Turning the patient may help the fluid drain. As the fluid flows into the drainage bag, document its volume and color. Report abnormalities to the doctor. Repeat the infusion, dwell, and drain cycles as prescribed.

When you finish the full infusion, clean the catheter or tubing connection with povidone-iodine. Disconnect and discard the tubing according to standard precautions. Disinfect the open rim of the catheter, and then place the sterile cap on it. Replace the dressing on the exit site, and secure the catheter.

Infusions through an implanted port

To gain access to a peritoneal port, first locate it by palpating through the skin. Clean the skin with antiseptic swabs, and allow the solution to air dry. Put on sterile gloves, a mask, and a gown.

Hold the port edges with the nondominant hand for stability; then puncture the port with a normal saline-primed noncoring needle with extension set or similar access device. Anchor the needle by placing sterile tape or adhesive strips across the hub of the needle and then wrapping the strips around the hub in a chevron pattern.

Using a saline-filled syringe, verify placement by attempting to aspirate fluid. Then flush the port with normal saline solution. Once you've accessed the device, connect the administration set to the extension tubing and initiate the infusion as you would for a catheter.

Keep in mind that intraperitoneal chemotherapy can vary according to the agent used. Some protocols suggest that the drug remain in the peritoneal cavity, allowing the fluid to be absorbed into the portal circulation.

Maintenance and care

After an intraperitoneal catheter has been implanted for dialysis, flush the catheter with 500 ml of a heparinized dialysate solution every 2 or 3 hours for 3 days. Then fill the catheter with 5,000 U of heparin (1,000 U/ml), and cap it off. A healing-in period of 2 weeks allows the catheter to seal so that leakage won't occur.

Maintain port patency by routinely flushing the port with 5 to 10 ml of normal saline solution. Flush the port with 20 ml of a compatible solution before and after administering medications. When removing a noncoring needle from the port, maintain positive pressure on the plunger. The pressure of fluids delivered through the intraperitoneal access device shouldn't exceed 40 pounds per square inch, to avoid breakage of the catheter or separation from the portal body. Change the dressing daily until the site is healed.

Complications

Complications of intraperitoneal access devices include microbial and chemical peritonitis, exit site infections, occlusions, and fluid leakage.

MICROBIAL PERITONITIS. Microbial peritonitis is caused by bacterial contamination of the catheter, principally by *Staphylococcus epidermidis* and *S. aureus.* The contamination typically occurs during insertion or by manipulation of the delivery system. Symptoms of microbial peritonitis include fever, abdominal pain or tenderness with or without rigidity or guarding, cloudy peritoneal fluid, an increase in the amount of peritoneal fluid, and increased WBC counts. Because microbial peritonitis is life-threatening, strict adherence to aseptic technique is critical. If microbial peritonitis is suspected, send the intraperitoneal fluid for culture and sensitivity testing and begin antibiotic therapy.

CHEMICAL PERITONITIS. Chemical peritonitis is an inflammation of the peritoneal lining as a result of irritation by a chemotherapeutic agent. Signs and symptoms of chemical peritonitis typically occur soon after the drug is infused. These symptoms—abdominal pain, fever, and chills—may persist for some time. Take precautions to prevent or manage the pain to avoid having to reduce the dosage or discontinue use of the agent. Obtain a sample of peritoneal fluid for culture and sensitivity testing to verify chemical peritonitis.

EXIT SITE INFECTION. Exit site infections occur from contamination of the exit opening, usually by skin flora. For the first 2 weeks following insertion, clean the site daily with an antiseptic solution (usually povidone-iodine) and cover it with a sterile gauze dressing. The patient may use clean technique at home. If the site appears infected, culture it and treat the infection with a topical antimicrobial preparation. Change the dressing frequently.

OCCLUSION. Occlusions of an intraperitoneal device are usually caused by the formation of fibrous sheaths or fibrin clots inside the catheter or around the tip. These sheaths or clots can block inflow or outflow. Don't use heparin or urokinase to dissolve these blockages. Thorough irrigation of the catheter with normal saline before and after treatment may help prevent catheter occlusion. Forceful irrigation using a push-pull technique may also help to loosen fibrin plugs. Don't carry out high-pressure irrigations on the implanted port because of the danger of breaking or dislodging the catheter. If the catheter or port remains occluded, it must be surgically replaced.

FLUID LEAKAGE. Peritoneal fluid may leak around the catheter for the first two weeks after insertion. After the site has healed, fluid leakage may be related to cellulitis or infection of the tunneled tract, which will require removal of the catheter.

Teaching the patient
Teach the patient the purpose, use, and care of the catheter or port. Tell the patient to avoid taking a shower or tub bath until the exit site is healed (about 4 to 6 weeks). Explain how to self-administer the therapy, including how to assist in drainage of the peritoneal cavity, which may include using Valsalva's maneuver to increase the intra-abdominal pressure. Show the patient how to flush the catheter or port. Explain the signs and symptoms of peritonitis, and tell the patient to report fever, chills, abdominal tenderness, generalized spasms, shortness of breath, nausea, cloudy peritoneal drainage, and redness, swelling, tenderness, or drainage at the catheter exit site.

Removal of an intraperitoneal access device
To discontinue a short-term catheter, drain the peritoneal cavity completely, if indicated (for example, after dialysis). Wash your hands and wear a mask and gloves. Remove the dressing and skin sutures, if present. Then change to sterile gloves and remove the catheter. If the exit site is large, be aware that a suture or sterile ad-

hesive strips may be required to close the site. Apply a topical antibiotic preparation and sterile dressing. Inspect the site daily until it's healed. The discontinuation of a long-term catheter or a port must be done by a doctor.

Documentation
Once intraperitoneal catheter care and infusion have been completed, document the following:
• vital signs, weight, abdominal girth
• assessment of the exit site
• color of catheter drainage
• specific solution or drug administered, including volume, dose, and rate of administration
• drugs added to dialysate
• patient's response to the procedure and education provided.

Subcutaneous access

In subcutaneous fluid administration, a needle or catheter is placed in the subcutaneous tissue, producing effects comparable to use of the IV route. Nurses knowledgeable about this access and prescribed therapy and who demonstrate competency in operating electronic infusion devices may start and manage subcutaneous infusions.

Uses of a subcutaneous access device
Continuous subcutaneous infusions may be used for many purposes, including managing pain in patients unable to take oral medications or who have poor venous access and require parenteral narcotics. Subcutaneous access can also be used for patients who are expected to require subcutaneous injections intermittently for more than 48 hours, for those on long-term insulin therapy, for patients needing iron chelation therapy with deferoxamine mesylate, and for those needing tocolytic therapy for treating preterm labor.

Morphine and hydromorphone are often administered subcutaneously in the home. When providing subcutaneous narcotic infusions for pain management, note that, although plasma concentrations of subcutaneous and IV narcotic infusions are similar at 24 hours, the plasma concentration of the subcutaneous infusion at 48 hours falls to about 78% of an IV infusion. For that reason, a dosage adjustment may be required on the 2nd day of administration.

Subcutaneous access devices don't require flushing and can be quickly inserted. This route is ideal for short-term pain management when venous access is limited or absent. It allows for rapid titration of narcotic doses and, when used for patient-controlled analgesia, provides a sense of control for the patient.

Subcutaneous access devices require frequent changes of the catheter site and limits on the amount of fluid that can be infused each hour. The devices also require skilled nursing and pharmacy support and the use of a costly infusion pump and supplies. Tissue irritation and induration may occur at the insertion site, particularly with high drug concentrations.

Selecting a subcutaneous access device

Devices used for maintaining subcutaneous access typically include either a 25G to 27G subcutaneous butterfly needle, a Sof-set (a Teflon catheter plus an adhesive antibacterial disk), or a 24G Teflon over-the-needle catheter. Select the smallest gauge and shortest length needle or cannula necessary to establish subcutaneous access.

Initiating a subcutaneous infusion

Initiating a subcutaneous infusion involves gathering needed equipment, preparing the patient and the site, and inserting the device.

Gathering the equipment

Before initiating a subcutaneous infusion, gather these supplies:
- povidone-iodine swabs
- subcutaneous butterfly needle or subcutaneous access infusion kit
- extension tubing, as needed, and gloves
- prefilled medication container or cassette and infusion pump
- transparent dressing, tape, and foam pad, as needed.

Preparing the patient and site

First, explain the procedure. Selection of the insertion site is based on the patient's mobility and comfort. The subclavicular region or the upper chest area is preferred for mobile patients. Other sites include the abdomen (at least 1″ [2.5 cm] below or to either side of the umbilicus for insulin), thigh, and upper arm. Sites should be free of irritation and away from bony prominences and the waistline.

Wash your hands; then prepare the infusion set. Attach the needle or cannula and tubing through a luer-lock connector to the pump's reservoir. Prime the tubing according to the pump manufacturer's directions. Verify that the pump is programmed correctly.

Inserting the device

Clean the site with a povidone-iodine swab. Pinch the skin around the insertion site to form a bulge, and then insert the needle or cannula. The angle of insertion varies with the type of needle used. For instance, a butterfly needle is inserted at a 45-degree angle. For a cannula, you'll press the wings against the skin with one hand and gently withdraw the needle with the other. You'll then apply a foam pad over the site with the window over the catheter entry area and the catheter port accessible through the opening.

For a butterfly needle, anchor the wings, if needed. Then cover the site with a transparent semipermeable membrane dressing.

For either device, tape the tubing to the skin to secure the needle or catheter during movement. Turn on the infusion pump.

Maintenance and care

Change the insertion site, infusion set, and dressing every 3 days; more often if complications occur. Indwelling catheters for insulin delivery may remain implanted for up to 1 week.

Complications

Irritation at the insertion site may occur, especially if the infusion rate exceeds 2 ml/hour. (The normal infusion rate is 1 to 2 ml/hour; drug concentrations are calculated based on this goal.) Patients receiving continuous infusions of opioids may experience subdermal toxicity, characterized by the development of raised, indurated subcutaneous plaques at the needle site. These plaques are accompanied by acute pain, tenderness, erythema, ecchymosis, and focal pruritus. The plaques generally do not resolve with time; once a plaque develops, further plaques inevitably occur at every subsequent needle site within 24 to 48 hours. Undetected interruptions of an infusion because of needle displacement or occlusion may lead to diabetic ketoacidosis in a patient receiving insulin and increased pain in a patient receiving narcotics for pain management.

Teaching the patient

Focus on the patient's knowledge and ability to manage a subcutaneous infusion at home. (See *Troubleshooting subcutaneous access devices,* page 190.) Teach the patient about preparation and insertion, insertion sites, indications for receiving the medication, adverse effects of the drug and actions to take, dosage (including basal and bolus doses), infusion frequency or rate, signs and symptoms of site infection, site rotation (every 3 days), and use of the pump.

CLINICAL
PEARLS

Troubleshooting subcutaneous access devices

When teaching patients how to troubleshoot potential infusion problems with their subcutaneous access devices, use this chart as a guide. The chart describes the cause of problems associated with subcutaneous access devices and the actions needed to rectify the situation.

PROBLEM	CAUSE	ACTION
The skin is red and tender or fluid leaks from the insertion site.	The medication is irritating the tissue or the needle has been in the site for too long.	Remove the subcutaneous needle or cannula. Rotate to a new insertion site.
The skin appears normal but fluid is leaking from the insertion site.	The tissue is not absorbing the medication fast enough. The infusion rate should not exceed 1 to 2 ml/hour.	Rotate the needle more often to a new site.
Needle insertion is painful and may meet with difficulty.	The tissue in the insertion site may be inflamed.	Use a different insertion site. Record recently used insertion sites to avoid reusing the same site before the tissue can heal.

Removal of a subcutaneous access device

To remove a subcutaneous access device, loosen the dressing, hold the surrounding skin, and remove the device. Wipe the skin with alcohol, and apply a sterile 2" × 2" gauze dressing or sterile adhesive strip. Dispose of used supplies according to standard precautions.

Documentation

For a patient receiving a subcutaneous infusion, document:
• time and date of the procedure
• brand, type, gauge, and length of the access device
• site of insertion and assessment of the previous insertion site
• medication administered, including the basal and bolus doses, volume, rate, and concentration
• patient's response to the procedure
• patient teaching provided.

III

SPECIAL
INFUSIONS

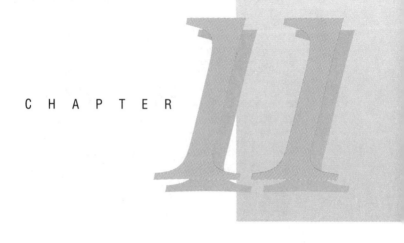

Administering blood and blood products

Transfusing blood or its various components is a complex and demanding procedure that poses significant risks for the nurse and patient. To administer a blood transfusion safely and effectively, you need to understand fully the various aspects of this specialized therapy. This chapter covers the various types of blood products available, compatibility testing, blood administration devices, transfusion administration, complications, patient teaching, and documentation for a transfusion.

Selecting a blood product

Blood transfused into a patient may be the patient's own blood (called an autologous transfusion), donated blood (banked blood), or a commercially prepared product. The type of blood product used depends on the particular needs of the patient and the severity of the condition for which the transfusion is being given.

Autologous transfusions

The term *autologous transfusion* refers to the collection, filtration, and reinfusion of the patient's own blood. Autologous transfusions can be used to replace blood lost during elective surgery (in which case the blood is donated by the patient starting weeks before surgery), nonelective surgery (in which case the blood is withdrawn immediately before surgery), and emergency blood salvage during or after major surgery, such as thoracic or cardiovascular surgery, or hip or knee resection. Autologous transfusions are also used to replace blood lost as a result of a traumatic injury, such as to the lungs, liver, chest wall, or heart.

Autologous transfusions provide immediately available blood and eliminate the risk of transfusion reactions and the spread of blood-borne pathogens. In addition, autologous blood has a greater oxygen-carrying capacity.

A patient receiving an autologous blood transfusion faces the potential for embolism, sepsis, coagulopathies, hemolysis, and citrate toxicity. Autologous transfusions are contraindicated in patients with malignant neoplasms, coagulopathies, excessive hemolysis, and active infections. They're also contraindicated in patients taking antibiotics and in those whose blood becomes contaminated by abdominal contents. In addition, patients who have recently lost weight because of illness or malnutrition shouldn't donate blood, to themselves or anyone else.

Perioperative donations

Autologous transfusions are frequently used for patients needing surgery and can occur before, during, or after the operation. Preoperative blood donation is often recommended for patients scheduled for orthopedic surgery, which can result in significant blood loss. Beginning 4 to 6 weeks before surgery, the patient donates a unit of blood as often as once a week, as needed, until 3 to 7 days before surgery.

Blood can be taken from patients during surgery or up to 12 hours afterward and reinfused. In addition, blood can be collected during the postoperative period from chest tubes, mediastinal drains, or wound drains, and then reinfused. In such cases, an autologous transfusion system, such as a Davol or Pleur-evac, is necessary to complete the autotransfusion. An anticoagulant, such as acid citrate dextrose or citrate phosphate dextrose, may be added to keep the blood from clotting. Reinfusion needs to be completed within 6 hours of the start of the collection process.

Acute normovolemic hemodilution
Acute normovolemic hemodilution is used primarily for patients undergoing open heart surgery. One or two units of blood are drawn immediately before or after anesthesia induction. The blood is replaced with a crystalloid or colloid solution so that the reduction in hemoglobin isn't accompanied by a resultant loss in volume, a condition referred to as *normovolemic anemia.*

The patient's blood is then reinfused immediately after surgery. The combination of reduced hemoglobin and the replacement solution causes the patient to lose fewer RBCs during surgery.

Banked blood products
Blood donated from someone other than the patient is always placed into a blood bank for storage. Types of banked blood products include whole blood, packed RBCs, leukocyte-poor RBCs, and plasma. WBCs; platelets; factors II, VII, VIII, IX, and X complex; antihemophilic factor, anti-inhibitor coagulant complex, human antithrombin III, and human $Rh_o(D)$ immune globulin intravenous are also available.

Whole blood
Whole blood, collected at the point of donation in an anticoagulated closed-collection system, requires no further processing after collection. Whole blood transfusions are rarely used except in instances of massive blood loss. Nearly always, the whole blood collected at donation sites is split later into the various blood components. Most often, leukocyte-poor RBCs, packed RBCs, and plasma are transfused.

Patients who receive a transfusion of whole blood have active bleeding, multiple trauma, hemorrhagic shock, or a combined need for increased oxygen-carrying capacity and expanded blood volume.

Leukocyte-poor RBCs
Patients who have had nonhemolytic febrile reactions to blood transfusions in the past may require a blood product without WBCs. Nonhemolytic febrile reactions occur in response to the WBCs present in a unit of PRBCs. Removing the WBCs can make the transfusion more comfortable and safer for patients with a history of these reactions. To remove the WBCs, some facilities use special leukocyte-removal filters during the transfusion. (See *Leukocyte-removal filters.*)

Leukocyte-removal filters

Leukocyte-removal filters protect against transfusion reactions by reducing the number of WBCs transfused in packed red blood cells. This photo shows two versions of a frequently used in-line filter. Similar filters are available (as separate units or preattached to blood tubing) to remove WBCs from platelet transfusions.

Photo courtesy of Pall Biomedical Products Corporation.

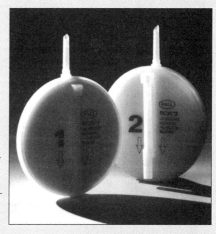

Packed RBCs

Packed cells, administered much more often than many other blood products, are prepared by separating the cellular portion of a unit of whole blood from the plasma. (See *Guide to commonly used blood components,* pages 196 to 200.) The shelf life of a unit of packed RBCs (PRBCs) is the same as a unit of whole blood. If an additive is mixed with the cells during separation, the shelf life of the unit is extended and can average 35 to 42 days.

Plasma

Plasma, also known as fresh frozen plasma and liquid plasma, is the anticoagulated, clear portion of the blood. Plasma is obtained by separating it from whole blood by centrifugation or sedimentation. Stable coagulation factors, such as fibrinogen and numerous clotting factors, are present in plasma.

Patients who might need a plasma transfusion include those with active bleeding and who have multiple factor deficiencies because of liver disease, and patients with disseminated intravascular coagulation, evidence of dilutional coagulopathy from large-volume

(Text continues on page 200.)

Guide to commonly used blood components

Administration procedures and other key considerations vary according to the type of blood component being transfused. Use this guide to commonly used blood components when administering them.

BLOOD COMPONENT	INDICATIONS
Packed red blood cells (PRBCs) Same RBC mass as whole blood with 80% of the plasma removed *Volume:* 250 ml	• To correct anemia due to chronic or malignant conditions • To restore or maintain oxygen-carrying capacity • To increase RBC mass
Leukocyte-poor RBCs Same as PRBCs except WBCs (70%) are removed *Volume:* 200 ml	• Same as PRBCs • To prevent frebrile reactions from WBC antibodies; recommended for patients with two or more febrile reactions • To treat immunosuppressed patients
WBCs Whole blood with all the RBCs and 80% of the supernatant plasma removed *Volume:* 150 ml	• To treat chronic or malignant conditions
Platelets Platelet sediment from RBCs or plasma *Volume:* 35 to 50 ml/unit; 1 unit of platelets = 7×10^7 platelets	• To treat thrombocytopenia caused by chronic or malignant conditions • To restore platelet count in a preoperative patient with a count of $100,000/mm^3$ or less
Fresh frozen plasma (FFP) Uncoagulated plasma separated from RBCs. FFP is rich in coagulation factors V, VIII, and IX. *Volume:* 200 to 250 ml	• To expand plasma volume • To treat postsurgical hemorrhage or shock • To correct an undetermined coagulation factor deficiency • To replace a specific factor when that factor alone is not available • To correct factor deficiencies resulting from hepatic disease
Albumin 5% (buffered saline); albumin 25% (salt-poor) A small plasma protein prepared by fractionation of pooled plasma *Volume:* 5% = 12.5 g/250 ml; 25% = 12.5 g/50 ml	• To treat chronic hypoproteinemia • To replace volume in treatment of shock from burns, trauma, surgery, or infections • To replace volume and prevent marked hemoconcentration

NURSING CONSIDERATIONS

- Cross-typing: Group A receives A or O; group B receives B or O; group AB receives AB, A, B, O; group O receives O.
- Use straight-line or Y-type IV set; infuse over 1½ to 4 hours.
- RBCs have the same oxygen-carrying capacity as whole blood without the hazards of volume overload.
- A microaggregate filter or leukocyte-removal filter may be used. WBC-removal filters may be used for patients with a history of febrile blood reactions.
- Posttransfusion hemoglobin and hematocrit is usually done the day after the transfusion.

- Cross-typing: Same as PRBCs; Rh match.
- Use straight-line or Y-type IV set. May require a leukocyte-removal filter for hard-spun, WBC-poor RBCs. Infuse over 1½ to 4 hours.
- Other considerations are same as for PRBCs.

- Cross-typing: Same as PRBCs; Rh match; preferably human leukocyte antigen (HLA)–compatible but not necessary unless patient is HLA sensitized from previous transfusions.
- Use straight-line set with standard in-line blood filter.
- May need to premedicate to prevent febrile reaction.
- WBC infusion induces fever and chills. Administer an antipyretic if fever occurs, but don't discontinue transfusion. Flow rate may be reduced for patient comfort. Notify the doctor.

- Cross-typing: ABO compatibility not necessary but preferable with repeated platelet infusions; Rh match preferred.
- Use a component administration set or a 170-micron blood set; infuse 100 ml over 15 minutes.
- A leukocyte-removal filter may be ordered.
- Usual dose is 6 to 8 units in adults or 1 or more units in children.
- A blood platelet count may be ordered 1 hour after platelet infusion to determine platelet transfusion increments.

- Cross-typing: Same as for platelets.
- Use straight-line set or Y-set and administer rapidly.
- Large-volume transfusions of FFP may require correction for hypocalcemia. Citric acid in FFP binds calcium.

- Cross-typing: Unnecessary.
- Use straight-line set at a rate and volume dependent on the patient's condition and response.
- A filtered set is often supplied by the manufacturer.
- Reactions to albumin (fever, chills, nausea) are rare.
- Shouldn't be mixed with protein hydrolysates and alcohol solutions.
- Often given as a volume expander until crossmatching for whole blood is complete.
- Contraindicated in severe anemia and administered cautiously in cardiac and pulmonary disease because of risk of heart failure from circulatory overload.
- Monitor blood pressure if given rapidly.

(continued)

Guide to commonly used blood components *(continued)*

BLOOD COMPONENT	INDICATIONS
Factor VIII (cryoprecipitate) Cold, insoluble portion of plasma recovered from FFP *Volume:* Approximately 30 ml (freeze-dried)	• To treat hemophilia A • To control bleeding associated with factor VIII deficiency • To replace fibrinogen or factor VIII
Factors II, VII, IX, X complex (prothrombin complex) *Volume:* Weight and situation dependent Lyophilized commercially prepared solution drawn from pooled plasma	• To treat a congenital factor V deficiency resulting from an acquired deficiency of factors II, VII, IX, and X
Antihemophilic factor (AHF, factor VIII) Sterile, lyophilized concentrate of factor VIII:C (coagulant portion of factor VIII complex) and small amounts of factor VIII:R (protein responsible for von Willebrand's factor activity) *Volume:* Dosage depends on patient's weight, severity of hemorrhage, and presence of inhibitors	• To provide hemostasis in factor VIII deficiency (hemophilia A) in the presence of mild, moderate, or severe bleeding, surgery, and bleeding near vital organs
Anti-inhibitor coagulant complex Prepared from pooled human plasma that has been tested for hepatitis and HIV and found to be negative; drug contains varying amounts of clotting factor precursors, activated clotting factors, and factors of the kinin-generating system; available as Autoplex T and Feiba VH Immuno *Volume:* Weight dependent	• To control hemorrhage in hemophilia A patients who have a factor VIII inhibitor level above 10 Bethesda U. • To treat joint, mucous membrane, soft tissue, and other severe hemorrhages
Antithrombin (AT) III, human Prepared from human plasma. Replaces AT-III in patients with hereditary AT-III deficiency, normalizing coagulation-inhibiting capability and inhibiting formation of thromboemboli *Volume:* Weight and situation dependent	• To treat patients with hereditary AT-III deficiency in connection with surgical or obstetric procedures or when suffering from thromboembolism

NURSING CONSIDERATIONS

- Cross-typing: ABO compatibility not necessary but preferable.
- Use the manufacturer-supplied administration set with a filter or a standard 170 micron blood set. Standard dosage recommended for treatment of acute bleeding episodes in hemophilia is 15 to 20 units/kg.
- Half-life of factor VIII (8 to 10 hours) necessitates repeat transfusions at these intervals to maintain normal levels.

- Cross-typing: No ABO/Rh matching.
- Use straight-line set.
- Hepatitis B and C are detectable about 90% of the time when all of the components are tested.
- Coagulation assays are performed before administration and at suitable intervals during treatment.
- Contraindicated when the patient has hepatic disease resulting in fibrinolysis.
- Contraindicated when the patient has intravascular coagulation and isn't undergoing heparin therapy.

- Cross-typing: Unnecessary
- Available in a kit, including single-dose vial with diluent, sterile needles for reconstitution and withdrawal, winged infusion set with microbore tubing, and alcohol swabs.
- Use within 3 hours of reconstitution.
- Administer by direct injection using a plastic syringe and the winged infusion set at a rate of 2 ml/minute.
- Intermittent and continuous infusions are not recommended.
- IV administration of 1 IU/kg increases circulating antihemophilic activity by about 2%.

- Cross-typing: Unnecessary
- To reconstitute, bring vials to room temperature and follow manufacturer's instructions.
- After reconstitution, do not refrigerate; use within 1 to 3 hours of reconstitution, depending on the specific product.
- Inject drug directly into vein: Autoplex T at 2 to 10 ml/minute, depending on patient tolerance, and Feiba VH Immuno no faster than 2 U/kg/minute.
- Feiba VH Immuno may be administered by intermittent infusion using a standard blood filter. Continuous infusion is not recommended.
- Stop administration if patient develops a headache, flushing, or change in pulse or blood pressure. Resume at a slower rate when symptoms disappear.
- Monitor patient for signs of intravascular coagulation (dyspnea, chest pain, cough, and pulse or blood pressure changes).

- Cross-typing: Unnecessary
- Reconstitute using 10 to 20 ml of sterile water for injection, 0.9% NaCl, or D_5W; if necessary, further dilute with same diluent solution.
- Bring solution to room temperature and administer within 3 hours of reconstitution.
- Dosage is individually calculated, but is usually 50 to 100 IU/minute IV, not to exceed 100 IU/minute.
- Administer by intermittent infusion over 10 to 20 minutes at an initial rate of 50 IU/minute (1 ml/minute).

(continued)

Guide to commonly used blood components (continued)

BLOOD COMPONENT	INDICATIONS
Rh₀(D) immune globulin intra-venous, human Immune serum that suppresses active antibody response and formation of anti-Rh₀ (D) antibodies in Rh₀ (D)-negative, Dᵘ-negative persons exposed to Rh-positive blood *Volume:* Weight and situation dependent	• To treat a patient after abortion, amniocentesis (after 34 weeks' gestation), or other manipulation late in pregnancy associated with increased risk of Rh isoimmunization • Indicated in pregnancy, transfusion accidents, and immune thrombocytopenic purpura in adults who are Rh₀ (D) antigen-positive

replacements, or congenital factor deficiencies. Plasma can also be given to patients requiring warfarin reversal.

Commercially prepared blood products

For situations that require transfusion therapy, several national regulatory organizations, including the American Red Cross and the American Association of Blood Banks, recommend that treatment with pharmaceutical and other commercially prepared products and solutions be considered instead of human blood products. Most experts agree that banked blood will be used less often in the future and that the use of autologous blood transfusions, intraoperative cell salvaging, and autotransfusions will increase. For now, commercial blood products such as Epogen can be used to boost the number of RBCs before and after surgery.

Compatibility testing

Compatibility testing is performed to make sure the recipient's plasma is compatible with the donor's RBCs. Only after testing is completed can transfusion therapy proceed as ordered.

Compatibility tests involve comparing ABO antigens. Located on the surface of RBCs, A, B, and O antigens determine the blood type of an individual. ABO antigens are genetically determined and together are the most important factor in determining compatibility. (See *Blood type compatibility,* page 202.)

The Rh system is also important in making that determination. A person whose RBCs have the D antigen is designated as Rh-

NURSING CONSIDERATIONS

- Cross-typing: Unnecessary
- Reconstitute drug with 0.9% NaCl only.
- Administer by direct injection into vein or free-flowing compatible IV solution over 3 to 5 minutes.
- Be sure epinephrine 1:1,000 is available in case of anaphylaxis.
- After delivery, if mother is Rh_o (D)-negative and D^u-negative and the infant is Rh_o (D)-positive or D^u-positive, administer drug as ordered.
- Minidose preparations are recommended for every patient undergoing miscarriage or abortion up to 12 weeks' gestation, if indicated.

positive. If the D antigen is absent, the person is considered Rh-negative. Blood grouping is performed on all donors and recipients to ensure that Rh-negative patients receive the correct component. Rh-positive recipients may receive either Rh-positive or Rh-negative blood. Rh-negative recipients must receive only Rh-negative blood; otherwise, they may form anti-D antibodies. A severe hemolytic reaction or, in newborns, hemolytic disease of the newborn may result from this antigen-antibody reaction.

In a crisis situation, when it may not be possible to wait for compatibility testing, the following products can be used until tested blood is available:

- type O, Rh-negative blood ("universal donor")
- plasma protein solution
- artificial plasma substitute
- dextran, normal saline, or lactated Ringer's solution.

Selecting blood administration devices

A number of administration devices are used when administering a blood transfusion, including IV administration sets, filters, and infusion delivery systems such as electronic infusion devices (EIDs).

Administration sets

Blood administration sets are available in various styles, including straight sets, multiple lead sets, or Y-type sets. Straight and Y-type administration sets are most commonly used. Most styles have a drip factor of 10 gtt/ml. Check the tubing package, which usually indicates the drip factor for that administration set.

Blood type compatibility

Precise typing and crossmatching of donor and recipient blood can avoid transfusions of incompatible blood, which can be fatal. RBCs are classified as type A, B, or AB, depending on the antigen detected on the cell, or type O, which has no detectable A or B antigens. Similarly, blood plasma has or lacks anti-A or anti-B antibodies.

A person with type O blood is a universal donor. Because his blood lacks A or B antigens, it can be transfused in an emergency in limited amounts to any patient regardless of blood type and with little risk of reaction. A person with AB blood is a universal recipient. Because his blood lacks A and B antibodies, he can receive types A, B, or O blood (given as packed RBCs). The chart below shows ABO compatibility at a glance.

BLOOD GROUP	ANTIBODIES IN PLASMA	COMPATIBLE RBCS	COMPATIBLE PLASMA
Recipient			
O	Anti-A and Anti-B	O	O, A, B, AB
A	Anti-B	A, O	A, AB
B	Anti-A	B, O	B, AB
AB	Neither Anti-A nor Anti-B	AB, A, B, O	AB
Donor			
O	Anti-A and Anti-B	O, A, B, AB	O
A	Anti-B	A, AB	A, O
B	Anti-A	B, AB	B, O
AB	Neither Anti-A nor Anti-B	AB	AB, A, B, O

Transfusions should be administered through a dedicated administration set and not piggy-backed into an existing infusion system. Use only normal saline solution when infusing blood products. Dextrose-containing solutions cause RBCs to agglutinate; hypotonic solutions cause fluid to enter the cells, resulting in hemolysis; and hypertonic solutions draw fluid from the cells, causing the cells to shrink.

Filters

Filters are used to remove particulate matter and debris, products of degradation from shelf-storage, and unwanted components such as WBCs. Generally, an 80- to 170-micron filter is appropriate for transfusing any blood product. The filter should be an integral part of the administration set; added-on filters pose an increased risk of microbial contamination.

Microaggregate filters, which have a pore size of 20 to 40 microns, are used primarily for autologous blood transfusions to remove contaminants (such as bone fragments and particles) and for blood exchange in a neonate.

Infusion delivery devices

A number of infusion delivery devices are available to assist in the administration of blood, from electronic infusion devices (EIDs) to pressure cuffs to blood warmers.

Electronic infusion device

EIDs are special rate-controlling devices that can deliver viscous fluids such as blood with a high degree of precision. These devices help reduce the risk of circulatory overload in pediatric, geriatric, and critically ill patients. An alarm sounds as soon an infusion is complete, which lets the nurse know that the blood tubing should be disconnected and the catheter flushed, according to facility policy. This feature is particularly useful when administering a blood transfusion through a central vein. Check your facility's policy and the manufacturer's recommendations for specific instructions on the use of an EID.

Pressure cuff

A pressure cuff can be used to ensure rapid administration of the transfusion. (See *Using a slip-on blood pump,* page 204.) The cuff consists of a sleeve, pressure gauge, and pressure bulb. To use the cuff, insert the blood bag into the sleeve, inflate the cuff, and begin the infusion. Continuously monitor the sleeve because the pressure decreases as the transfusion progresses and the cuff will need to be reinflated. You'll also need to monitor the insertion site carefully to detect infiltration.

Blood warmer

A blood warmer can be used for patients requiring a rapid infusion of large volumes of blood, neonates and children who receive blood for

EQUIPMENT EXPERTISE

Using a slip-on blood pump

When using a slip-on pump to administer a blood transfusion, follow these steps.

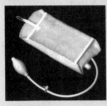

1. Insert the spike of the blood administration set into the blood bag and prime the tubing. Insert your hand into the pump envelope and pull the blood bag through the center opening. Grasp the pump envelope loops (used for hanging) and slip them through the blood bag loop, as shown below. Then hang the set on an IV pole.

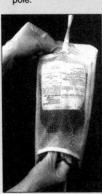

2. Turn the stopcock to the right (below).

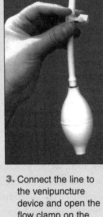

3. Connect the line to the venipuncture device and open the flow clamp on the administration set. Squeeze the bulb of the pump (below) until you've reached the desired flow rate.

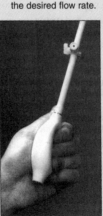

4. Don't let the pressure on the bag exceed 300 mm Hg. A pressure beyond that level may damage the blood cells, cause the line to disconnect, or rupture the bag. Turn the stopcock to the OFF position to maintain a constant pressure, as shown below.

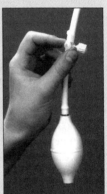

5. Repeat the procedure with each new blood bag. Remember that, as the bag empties, pressure decreases. Check the flow rate, and adjust the clamp as necessary. Observe the site carefully. If the vein is too small to accept blood under pressure, infiltration may result.

exchange transfusions, or patients needing delivery through a central venous catheter. In these situations, it may be necessary to warm the blood to normal body temperature to avoid the life-threatening cardiac arrhythmias that can result from the administration of chilled blood. In addition, they may be used for patients with a condition known as cold agglutinins. Cold agglutinins are antibodies that react at temperatures below 68° F (20° C) and cause RBC agglutination.

A blood warmer should maintain the transfusion temperature between 89.6° and 98.6° F (32° and 37° C) and provide infusion rates up to 150 ml/minute. Follow the manufacturer's recommendations for correct usage of the particular blood warmer used by your facility.

Administering a blood product

To administer a transfusion, you'll need to gather the equipment, prepare the patient and the blood product to be administered, and then infuse it correctly and safely.

Gathering the equipment
Gather the following items to administer a transfusion:
• gloves
• IV pole
• 100- to 250-ml container of normal saline solution
• the specific blood product to be transfused
• appropriate filter, if indicated
• other infusion delivery devices, as needed.

Preparing the patient
Prior to the transfusion, make sure to explain the procedure to the patient and obtain his consent (according to your facility's policy). (See *Commonly asked questions about blood transfusions,* page 206.) Check the compatibility of the blood to be administered. Obtain a preliminary set of vital signs and notify the doctor if the patient has a temperature elevation. Fever can mask adverse reactions to the transfusion. Also report other changes in vital signs.

If the patient has a history of allergic reactions to transfusions, diphenhydramine and acetaminophen may be administered to reduce the symptoms associated with these reactions.

Commonly asked questions about blood transfusions

A patient receiving a blood transfusion may ask questions about the transfusion and its aftermath. This chart lists commonly asked questions about transfusions and their answers.

QUESTION	ANSWER
Why am I being given a transfusion?	• The transfusion replaces blood lost from heavy bleeding. Or you may be receiving a transfusion to help treat anemia or another blood disorder.
What will happen before the transfusion?	• A blood sample is taken to determine your blood type. • If you have a history of blood transfusion reactions, the nurse will give you medications. • Your vital signs are checked just before the transfusion starts.
What will happen during the transfusion?	• Depending on the severity of your condition, transfusions are performed in the hospital or in an outpatient setting. • The blood is delivered into your veins through special tubing. • Commonly, saline solution is used to keep the vein open if the transfusion must be stopped or delayed.
What are the possible complications?	• Blood transfusions carry the risk of serious complications, including an acute hemolytic reaction (in which red blood cells are destroyed) or an allergic reaction. • Reactions can occur during, immediately after, or up to 10 days after a blood transfusion but most often occur immediately after the transfusion begins or within an hour after it's completed. • Another serious complication is the transmission of infectious diseases, such as hepatitis C, cytomegalovirus, and AIDS. Because of current techniques for testing donor blood for these diseases, such transmission is uncommon. However, because of these risks, many people elect to donate their own blood so that it can be used subsequently—for example, during a planned surgery. • Certain complications—such as hypothermia and bleeding tendencies—may result from multiple or massive transfusions.

Commonly asked questions about blood transfusions *(continued)*

QUESTION	ANSWER
What will happen after the transfusion?	• If the transfusion is being given on an outpatient basis, you'll be observed for at least 2 hours before discharge. • If you're receiving platelets, don't use aspirin. It interferes with platelet function. Use Tylenol or another product that contains acetaminophen for pain relief or fever. • You and your caregiver need to watch for the symptoms of a delayed transfusion reaction and of hepatitis: fever, headache, loss of appetite, nausea, vomiting, and abdominal pain. These symptoms most often occur 3 to 10 days after the transfusion and must be reported to your doctor immediately.

Before administering a blood product, make sure two nurses have identified the unit of blood as being the correct unit for that patient. Next, positively identify the patient. If the patient is alert and responsive, ask him to state his full name, and always check it against the name and hospital number on his identification wristband or bracelet. When a patient has had a blood sample taken before a transfusion, a wristband or bracelet is placed on his wrist. This identification band lists the patient's full name, medical record number, date and time the sample was drawn, the number of the blood component compatibility tag, and the name of the person who performed the blood collection.

After confirming the patient's identity, two nurses should examine the compatibility tag attached to the unit and the information printed on the bag. Make sure that the ABO group, Rh type, and unit number match. Report discrepancies immediately to the blood bank, and delay the transfusion until those discrepancies are resolved.

You'll also need to make sure the patient has an 18G or 20G venous access catheter in place; smaller catheters may inhibit flow rates. In patients with poor venous access, however, it may be necessary to use 22G or 24G catheters. Don't force blood through small cannulae with a pressure cuff or EID; cell damage may result.

If the patient's existing venipuncture site or infusion don't appear infected or otherwise compromised, proceed with the transfusion.

Preparing the blood product

Make sure the blood product to be transfused is obtained from the blood bank not more than 30 minutes before the expected start time. Administer only one blood product at a given time, unless the patient has experienced sudden, severe blood loss requiring emergency treatment. Administering one transfusion at a time allows you to detect signs of a transfusion reaction earlier and identify the cause of the reaction.

Check the expiration date on the blood bag, and observe the bag's contents for clumping, gas bubbles, and other extraneous materials that may indicate bacterial contamination. If the blood appears contaminated in any way, return the unit to the blood bank immediately.

Initiating the transfusion

To start a transfusion, first put on gloves. Open the package with the transfusion administration set and remove the tubing. If a Y-type set is being used, close all clamps and inspect the set for defects.

Check your facility's policy about priming the administration set; some facilities allow priming of the infusion set with a small amount of normal saline solution before connecting the set to the blood product. (See *Tips for administering blood products.*) If the patient's condition allows for an infusion of a small amount of normal saline solution, remove the protective wrapper from the infusate container and insert the tubing spike into the container.

Next, remove the cap from the spike on the administration set. Pull back the protective tab on the blood product container to expose the access port. Insert the administration set spike into the port. Hang the entire Y-type set on an IV pole.

With the clamp on the blood line closed, open the clamp to the normal saline solution. Squeeze the drip chamber until the saline completely covers the filter. Blood cells can be damaged if they drop directly onto a filter. Open the main tubing clamp, purging the entire line with normal saline solution. Close both clamps.

Open the blood line clamp. Squeeze the drip chamber until the blood completely covers the filter. Attach the blood administration set to the patient's catheter hub, and begin the tranfusion slowly. Check the integrity of the access device and venipuncture site. Adjust the administration set to deliver the infusion at the prescribed initial rate.

Remain with the patient, observing for signs of a transfusion reaction. If a reaction occurs, stop the transfusion immediately and notify

CLINICAL
PEARLS

Tips for administering blood products

Administering a blood transfusion requires extreme care. Review the following tips on what you should and shouldn't do during a transfusion.

Do

- Write the number of the blood bag on the intake-and-output sheet so you'll have a backup if the sticker falls off.
- Record vital signs before the transfusion, 15 minutes later, and after the transfusion (per facility policy). Most acute hemolytic reactions occur during the first 50 ml of the transfusion, so watch your patient carefully for the first 30 minutes.
- Act promptly if the patient develops wheezing and bronchospasm. These reactions may indicate an allergic reaction or anaphylaxis. If, after a few milliliters of blood are transfused, a patient becomes dyspneic and shows generalized flushing and chest pain, he could be having an anaphylactic reaction. Stop the blood and change the tubing. Start a slow infusion of normal saline solution. Administer oxygen, and call the doctor. Monitor the patient's vital signs, and keep the head of the bed elevated. Tell the patient what's happening.
- Send the blood bag and its tubing to the blood bank, collect a urine specimen, and call the laboratory to request a repeat crossmatching if the patient shows signs worse than a rash or slight fever. Only laboratory tests can determine whether a severe reaction is hemolytic, pyrogenic, allergic, or anaphylactic.
- Watch elderly and cardiac patients for signs of circulatory overload and heart failure. Slow the transfusion to a keep-vein-open rate, raise the head of the bed, and administer oxygen. Then notify the doctor.

Don't

- Don't add medications to the blood bag.
- Never give blood or blood products without checking the order against the blood bag label. Most life-threatening reactions result when this step is omitted.
- Don't piggyback blood into an existing line. Most solutions are incompatible with blood. Administer blood with normal saline solution only.
- When you can't give the blood as planned, don't put blood bags in the unit refrigerator. The refrigerator's temperature isn't controlled, and the blood might be damaged. Return the blood to the blood bank and get it when you're ready to hang it.
- Don't expect to discontinue the transfusion if the patient develops an itchy rash or hives. Most likely, these signs indicate an allergic reaction. If the patient isn't dyspneic, interrupt the transfusion and call the doctor. The transfusion will most likely be resumed after the patient receives antihistamines and his symptoms dissipate.
- Don't hesitate to stop the transfusion if your patient shows vital sign changes, is dyspneic or restless, or if he develops chills, hematuria, or pain in the flank, chest, or back. He could go into shock, so don't remove the IV line. Instead, keep it open with a slow infusion of 0.9% NaCl solution while you call the doctor and the laboratory.
- Never transfuse blood that's been unrefrigerated for more than 4 hours. The risk of sepsis or bacterial contamination would be too high.

CLINICAL
PEARLS

What to do if a transfusion stops

If the transfusion stops or becomes sluggish, run the following checks to pin-point the problem.

• Check that the IV container is at least 3 ft (1 m) above the IV site.
• Verify that the flow clamp is open.
• Ensure the blood in the blood bag completely covers the filter. If it doesn't, squeeze the drip chamber (as shown in the illustration at right) until it does.
• Gently rock the blood bag, agitating any blood cells that may have settled on the bottom.
• For a straight-line set, flush the line with sterile normal saline solution (NSS) and restart the infusion.
• For a Y-type set, close the clamp to the patient and lower the blood bag. Open the clamp to the NSS and allow 50 to 100 ml to flow into the bag. Rehang the bag, open the clamp to the patient and restart the flow rate.

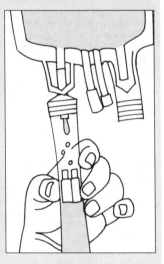

the doctor and other emergency personnel, as appropriate. Take the patient's vital signs at once. Change the IV set to a new, blood-free administration set primed with normal saline solution. Infuse this solution slowly while awaiting the arrival of the doctor and emergency personnel.

If no signs of a reaction appear within the first 15 minutes, continue with the infusion. Adjust the flow rate as prescribed or according to facility policy. A unit of PRBCs, for instance, may be infused over a period of 1½ to 4 hours. Monitor the transfusion frequently, being especially alert for transfusion reactions or a sluggish infusion. (See *What to do if a transfusion stops.*)

After the transfusion is complete, put on gloves and flush the filter and tubing with normal saline solution until the tubing is fairly clear. Disconnect the transfusion administration set. If your facility doesn't require sending the empty blood bag to the blood bank, discard the bag and tubing according to standard precautions.

Make sure to obtain and record the patient's vital signs at the completion of the transfusion.

Complications

Many transfusion-related complications occur immediately; others may occur 96 hours or more after completion of the transfusion. Complications are categorized as transfusion reactions or metabolic complications. Transfusion-related complications typically result from blood incompatibility, contamination of the transfusion system, or a too-rapid infusion.

Transfusion complications

Transfusion reactions can occur after either single-unit infusions or massive or multiple transfusions. The reactions include allergic reaction, hemolytic reaction, nonhemolytic febrile reaction, and plasma protein incompatibility.

ALLERGIC REACTION. Allergic reactions to blood products are common and probably the result of the presence of a foreign substance in the blood. For example, a patient might have an allergic reaction if he receives blood from a donor who's allergic to a particular drug. In that case, the donor's body would have developed antibodies to the drug. The antibodies would then be infused with the donated blood and cause an allergic reaction in the recipient, who might never have taken the drug.

Symptoms of allergic reaction include fever, nausea, vomiting, mild localized itching, hives, and urticaria. The reaction may progress to a full anaphylactic reaction, complete with laryngeal edema, bronchospasm, dyspnea, and wheezing. Allergic reactions can occur immediately or within 1 hour of the transfusion.

If a reaction occurs, the transfusion should be stopped. If the reaction is mild, the transfusion may be continued after the administration of antihistamines and after signs and symptoms of the reaction dissipate. Severe reactions can usually be treated successfully with epinephrine or corticosteroids.

To prevent an allergic reaction, determine if the patient has a history of allergic reactions. Administer antihistamines before the transfusion, as ordered. Patients with a history of allergic reactions may be transfused with washed or deglycerolized RBCs.

HEMOLYTIC REACTION. Caused by an ABO or Rh incompatibility or by improper storage of the blood, a hemolytic reaction is considered serious and potentially life-threatening. Signs and symptoms include shaking, chills, fever, chest pain, dyspnea, hypotension, oliguria, hemoglobinuria, flank pain, and abnormal bleeding.

If these signs and symptoms occur, stop the transfusion immediately. Keep the IV access open with a secondary line of normal saline solution. Be prepared to treat the patient's shock by administering oxygen, fluids, and epinephrine, as ordered. In addition, mannitol, dopamine, and furosemide or other diuretics may be administered.

Collect blood and urine samples for laboratory testing, as necessary. If a hemolytic reaction has occurred, blood tests will indicate hemolysis and urine tests will confirm the presence of hemoglobin. Record fluid intake and output, observing for diuresis or oliguria. Notify the doctor if either occurs.

To prevent a hemolytic reaction, ensure that the blood being transfused is compatible with the patient's blood type. Always double-check the patient's identification before initiating the transfusion, and begin the transfusion slowly, monitoring for signs of reaction for at least the first 15 minutes.

NONHEMOLYTIC FEBRILE REACTION. Nonhemolytic febrile reactions usually occur because the recipient's anti–human leukocyte antigen antibodies react with antigens on the donor's WBCs or platelets. Febrile reactions occur in only 1% of transfusions. Repeat reactions seldom occur. The reaction can appear immediately or within 2 hours of completion of the transfusion.

Symptoms include a temperature elevation of 1.8° F (1° C) or more noted in association with the transfusion, chills (including severe shaking chills called rigors), palpitations, chest tightness, lower back pain, and headache. Treatment involves the administration of antipyretics and antihistamines. Severe cases are treated the same way a hemolytic reaction is treated. Nonhemolytic febrile reactions can be avoided or their severity reduced by using leukocyte-poor blood products or leukocyte-removal filters.

PLASMA PROTEIN INCOMPATIBILITY. Caused by immunoglobulin A (IgA) incompatibility, plasma protein incompatibility is a rare but serious reaction. The patient may experience flushing, abdominal pain, diarrhea, chills, fever, dyspnea, and hypotension. Symptoms may progress to shock, requiring oxygen, fluids, epinephrine, and corticosteroids. Only IgA-deficient blood products should be infused to prevent this reaction.

Metabolic complications

Metabolic complications can occur when a patient receives a large amount of blood over a short period of time and include circulatory overload, hypothermia, hypocalcemia, hyperkalemia, and microbial contamination.

CIRCULATORY OVERLOAD. Circulatory overload is a common and easily avoidable reaction. Overload occurs when blood is infused rapidly or in excessive amounts over a short period of time. Signs and symptoms include dyspnea, enlarged or engorged neck veins, chest or back pain, and hypertension.

Treatment includes discontinuing the transfusion, notifying the doctor, elevating the patient's head to facilitate respiratory exchange, and administering diuretics, as ordered. Prevention is directed toward minimizing the risk of overload by using PRBCs, infusing components more slowly, and administering a diuretic at the start of the transfusion in high-risk patients.

HYPOTHERMIA. Hypothermia is the result of a rapid infusion of large amounts of chilled blood or the infusion of chilled blood through a central venous catheter. The patient may experience shaking chills, hypotension, and possibly cardiac arrhythmias. If untreated, hypothermia may progress to cardiac arrest.

To treat hypothermia, stop the transfusion and wrap the patient with blankets. Obtain an ECG to monitor cardiac activity. Prevention of hypothermia involves use of a blood warmer during transfusion.

HYPOCALCEMIA. Hypocalcemia, a rare complication, results from multiple transfusions. Also known as citrate toxicity, hypocalcemia occurs when citrate-treated blood is infused too rapidly. Citrate combines with calcium and results in calcium deficiency. Normal citrate metabolism may be affected by liver disease. The liver may be unable to metabolize large quantities of citrate circulating in the blood during or after a transfusion.

Signs and symptoms of hypocalcemia included tingling in the extremities, muscle cramps, nausea, vomiting, hypotension, cardiac arrhythmias, and possibly seizures. If symptoms of hypocalcemia occur, slow or stop the transfusion, depending on the severity of the symptoms. The condition should eventually correct itself. If symptoms persist, however, replacement therapy with an oral calcium supplement or IV calcium gluconate may be required.

HYPERKALEMIA. As cells in stored plasma disintegrate, the level of potassium within the blood climbs. Hyperkalemia, a potentially serious complication, may result. The longer blood is stored, the higher the extracellular level of potassium. Symptoms vary depending on the number of units given and their storage age as well as the potassium level of the patient prior to transfusion. If hyperkalemia occurs, obtain an ECG and administer Kayexalate, glucose 50% and insulin, bicarbonate, or calcium, as ordered.

MICROBIAL CONTAMINATION. Bacterial contamination is a rare but serious event. Caused by cold-growing, gram-negative bacteria, such as *Pseudomonas*, *Staphylococcus*, coliform, or *Achromobacter* bacteria, contaminated blood may cause chills, fever, vomiting, abdominal cramping, diarrhea, shock, and signs of renal failure.

Contamination of a donated unit can occur in many ways, including bacterial infection of the donor and contamination during phlebotomy or the processing phase of the donation.

Blood products can also be contaminated with other microorganisms, including *Treponema pallidum*, the spirochete that causes syphilis. Once considered a blood-borne pathogen (as well as a sexually transmitted disease), syphilis is now rarely found in stored blood products. All donated units are serologically tested. In addition, *T. pallidum* can't survive temperatures of $39.2°$ to $42.8°$ F ($4°$ to $6°$ C) for more than 72 hours. Blood components stored at room temperature, however, may carry some risk.

Treatment of microbial contamination includes high doses of antibiotics and therapies to combat shock, including steroids and vasopressors. Always examine blood to be transfused for evidence of gas, clots, or changes in color. Blood storage is strictly controlled; therefore, never hang blood that has been out of the refrigerator for longer than 30 minutes.

To help prevent contamination, use strict aseptic technique when infusing the blood, change the administration infusion set every 4 hours or every 2 units, and discard used tubing and containers according to standard precautions.

Administering transfusions in the home

To give a transfusion in a patient's home, follow these guidelines:

1. Transport the blood product in a container with the appropriate coolant for the product. The proper temperature for transporting blood is between 33.8° and 50° F (1° and 10° C); for platelets, it's between 68° and 75° F (20° and 24° C).

2. Encourage the patient to void before beginning the transfusion because the procedure may take up to 2 hours.

3. Set up and transfuse the product according to facility policy.

4. After the transfusion, keep the IV line open and stay with the patient for at least 30 minutes to watch for delayed reaction to the transfusion.

5. If no reactions occur within 30 minutes, remove the IV line and give the patient or caregiver posttransfusion instructions.

6. Place all equipment, including the containers and infusion devices, in a bag labeled "Biohazard" and then into the transport container. Return the container to the blood bank for proper disposal.

7. If a transfusion reaction occurs, notify the transfusion service and the patient's doctor immediately.

Teaching the patient

Explain the transfusion procedure to the patient and family before starting it. Reassure the patient that the blood product being transfused has been tested for impurities and communicable diseases. Explain that during the transfusion, the patient's vital signs will be monitored and continually assessed and that the entire transfusion will be completed in 2 to 4 hours. Instruct the patient to report discomfort, including chest pain, shortness of breath, itching, chills, or pain at the IV site.

If the transfusion is being administered at home, explain that quality control practices ensure the same safety for home transfusions as for those in an acute care setting. (See *Administering transfusions in the home.*) Make sure emergency services are available in the patient's community and that you or the patient has access to those services. Check that electricity and running water are available. In addition, make sure an emergency anaphylaxis kit is on hand and that you have emergency corrective orders from the prescribing doctor.

Give the patient a list of signs and symptoms to report, the doctor's or facility's 24-hour telephone number, and telephone numbers for the ambulance and other health care personnel, as indicated.

Documentation

Make sure each step of a transfusion is thoroughly documented. If your facility's policy requires it, documentation may be placed in a separate blood administration record. In any case, make sure you document:

• names of the nurses who identified the blood product and the patient

• type of blood product administered and its identification number and expiration date

• patient's vital signs before, during, and after the transfusion

• date and time that the transfusion was started and completed

• total volume transfused

• other IV solutions used

• patient teaching done

• patient's response to the transfusion, including signs and symptoms of transfusion reactions

• actions taken to prevent or reverse transfusion reactions.

CHAPTER

Administering parenteral nutrition

The term *parenteral nutrition* refers to IV administration of nutritional support. Prescribed when a patient's nutritional needs can't be met orally or through enteral feedings, parenteral nutrition may be administered for a wide variety of conditions, including debilitating illness lasting 2 weeks or more, weight loss of over 10% of the patient's weight prior to illness, serum albumin level below 3.5 g/dl, chronic vomiting or diarrhea, continued weight loss despite adequate oral or enteral intake, a disorder that severely reduces or prevents GI absorption, excessive nitrogen loss from wound infections, hyperemesis gravidarum, fistulas, abscesses, or renal or hepatic failure if accompanied by GI tract failure.

Parenteral nutrition can also be used for patients with Crohn's disease, ulcerative colitis, radiation enteritis, short-bowel syndrome, bowel fistulas, severe acute pancreatitis, peritonitis, or severe burns.

This chapter examines peripheral and total parenteral nutrition and lipid emulsions, as well as total nutrient admixture and protein-sparing therapy.

Parenteral nutrition solutions

Selecting the right parenteral solution for each patient is critical for successful treatment. This chart outlines the type and composition of parenteral nutrition solutions and the uses and special considerations for each.

TYPE AND COMPONENTS	USES
Total parenteral nutrition (TPN) Composed of dextrose 15% to 25% in water (1 L of dextrose 25% contains 850 nonprotein calories) and crystalline amino acids 2.5% to 8.5%. Contains electrolytes, minerals, vitamins, and trace elements. Lipid emulsion 10% or 20% is given as a separate solution.	Given for 2 weeks or longer. Can provide 2,000 to 4,000 calories/day. Helps restore nitrogen balance and replaces electrolytes, minerals, vitamins, and trace elements. Also promotes tissue synthesis, wound healing, and normal metabolic function; allows the bowel to rest and heal; reduces activity in the gallbladder, pancreas, and small intestine; and improves the patient's tolerance for surgery.
Peripheral parenteral nutrition Composed of dextrose 5% to 10% in water, crystalline amino acids 2.5% to 5%, electrolytes, minerals, vitamins, and trace elements. Lipid emulsion 10% or 20% is given as a separate solution. Heparin or hydrocortisone is administered as ordered.	Given for 2 weeks or less. Can provide up to 2,000 calories/day. Used to maintain nutritional status in patients who can tolerate relatively high fluid volumes, who will resume oral feedings after a few days, and who are susceptible to CV catheter infections.
Total nutrient admixture Also called 3-in-1 solution; combines lipid emulsion with other parenteral nutrition components. A 3-L bag contains a 1-day supply of nutrients.	Given for 2 weeks or longer. Typically administered to patients who are relatively stable because solution components can only be adjusted once daily. Other uses are the same as those for TPN.
Protein-sparing therapy Contains crystalline amino acids (in the same amount as in TPN), electrolytes, vitamins, minerals, and trace elements.	Given for 2 weeks or less. Used to augment oral or tube feedings. May preserve body protein in a stable patient.

Advantages and disadvantages

The type of solution used for parenteral nutrition varies according to the specific needs of each patient, the expected duration of therapy, and other factors. (See *Parenteral nutrition solutions.*)

Parenteral nutrition shouldn't be used for well-nourished patients with a functioning GI tract or a nonfunctioning GI tract expected to resume function within 10 days. The potential risks of mechanical, infectious, and metabolic complications from parenteral nutrition therapy may outweigh the benefits.

SPECIAL CONSIDERATIONS

Must be administered through a central venous (CV) catheter. The *basic solution* is nutritionally complete, highly hypertonic, and may cause metabolic complications (such as glucose intolerance, electrolyte imbalances, and acid/base disturbances). The *lipid emulsion* may be ineffective in severely stressed patients, such as those with burns. It may interfere with immune mechanisms and, in patients suffering respiratory compromise, it reduces carbon dioxide buildup.

The *parenteral solution* is nutritionally complete for short-term use. Because the site must be rotated every 72 hours, the patient must have accessible veins. Although the solution is less hypertonic than TPN given through a CV catheter, it can't exceed 900 mOsm/L. May cause phlebitis, and increases risk of metabolic complications. Contraindicated in nutritionally depleted patients and volume-restricted patients. Does not cause weight gain. The *lipid emulsion* is as effective a calorie source as dextrose. If infused with the nutrient solution, the patient's risk for phlebitis decreases.

Because the bag is hung only once a day, the risk of contamination decreases. Allows for increased patient mobility and is easier to use in a home setting. The solution and tubing require changing every 24 hours. Use is limited because not all types and amounts of components are compatible. The solution precludes the use of certain infusion pumps (because many can't accurately deliver large volumes), as well as standard IV tubing filters (because 0.22-micron filters block lipid molecules).

Nutritionally complete solution requires little mixing. May be started and stopped at any time during the patient's stay. Other IV fluids, medications, and blood by-products may be administered through the same line. Carries a lower risk of phlebitis but is expensive and has limited benefits.

To take full advantage of the type of parenteral nutrition to be used, make sure pertinent patient-focused goals have been identified. These goals may include providing all essential nutrients in the amounts required to sustain nutrition balance, preserving or restoring the body's protein metabolism to regain or maintain the anabolic state, maintaining or increasing body weight, slowing weight-loss progression, or promoting tissue healing and repairing nutritional deficits.

When to use a peripheral versus a central vein

Parenteral nutrition therapy can be given through a peripheral or central venous access device. This chart lists criteria to follow when determining whether a patient should receive peripheral or central parenteral nutrition.

Peripheral vein
- Interrupted enteral intake, but patient can resume enteral feedings in 5 to 7 days
- Mild-to-moderate malnutrition for which supplements are needed for enteral feedings
- Normal or mildly elevated metabolic rate
- Absence of fluid restrictions
- Availability of suitable peripheral veins

Central vein
- Inability to tolerate enteral intake for more than 7 days
- Moderate-to-severe malnutrition that can't be corrected with enteral feedings
- Restricted fluid intake
- Poor or inaccessible peripheral veins
- Readily accessible central vein.

Selecting a patient

Depending on need, a patient may benefit most from peripheral parenteral nutrition (PPN) or total parenteral nutrition (TPN). TPN must be given through a central vein; PPN may be infused through a peripheral vein. Patients who are well-nourished or have mild malnutrition with no fluid restrictions may benefit most from PPN. Malnourished patients with fluid restrictions might benefit most from TPN. (See *When to use a peripheral versus a central vein.*)

When a higher caloric value is required than can be delivered peripherally, 10% or 20% lipid solutions may be added and can, together with PPN, increase the calorie content to as much as 2,000 calories a day. With or without lipid administration, a patient receiving PPN must be able to tolerate large volumes of fluid. In addition, PPN can't satisfy a patient's nutritional demands for long; typically, it's used for no more than 2 weeks. TPN, in contrast, may be more beneficial for patients who can't tolerate large fluid volumes or who need nutritional support for longer than 2 weeks.

Selecting a solution or additive

When selecting a solution or additive for a patient, consideration should be given to the caloric and other nutritional needs of the patient to determine which solutions or additives—and how much of each—can best meet those needs.

Peripheral parenteral nutrition
PPN solutions contain nutrients in lesser concentrations than in TPN solutions, so they can be infused through a peripheral vein with less risk of damaging the vein lining. Keep in mind that because peripheral veins are used for PPN infusions, the final concentration of parenteral solution shouldn't exceed 900 mOsm/L and the total dextrose content shouldn't exceed 10%.

Total parenteral nutrition
TPN solutions contain the complete nutritional requirements of the patient. Because TPN solutions are highly concentrated (up to approximately 2,400 mOsm/L) and can damage the intima of a peripheral vein, TPN must be given in the central circulation, where a greater hemodilution helps protect the lining of the veins.

Usually providing more than 2,000 calories daily, TPN may be given continuously or in cycles. Continuous TPN is more commonly used in acute care settings; cyclic therapy is reserved for patients who need TPN for months to years, such as home care patients who receive TPN at night but are disconnected from it during the day.

Lipid emulsion
With more than twice the calories per gram as dextrose or amino acids, lipid emulsion is a major source of energy and helps to provide calories, typically 20% to 40% of the total caloric intake. These solutions also prevent essential fatty acid deficiency.

Lipid emulsion may be used in children and infants but its use is limited by the child's ability to metabolize fats. These solutions may be given as part of a parenteral nutrition solution, piggybacked into a parenteral nutrition line at the lowest Y-port, or administered separately through a central or peripheral vein.

Additives
Certain agents—from drugs such as insulin and heparin to vitamins and trace elements—may be added to PPN or TPN solutions to enhance the effectiveness of the solutions or avoid complications. Insulin, for example, may be added in small quantities to control hyperglycemic reactions to the dextrose in the TPN solutions. Separate insulin therapy, however, has been proved more effective in controlling blood sugar and is more cost-effective.

CLINICAL
◊◊◊◊◊◊◊◊◊◊
PEARLS

Calculating calories for total parenteral nutrition

Computation of the number of calories contained in a total parenteral nutrition (TPN) formulation can be critical. Here's an easy way to calculate calories for each administration of a TPN solution.

To calculate the calories in 1 L of TPN solution, you need to know the final concentration of the carbohydrate, protein, and fat additives. Remember that each percent of that concentration equals 1 g/100 ml.

Next, know the calories in each gram of dextrose, protein, and fat.
• 1 g of dextrose = 3.4 kcal
• 1 g of amino acid (protein) = 4 kcal
• 1 g of lipid emulsion (fat) = 9 kcal*

For example, an order reads, "1,000 ml TPN to contain 30% dextrose and 20% amino acids every 12 hours. Add 500 ml 20% lipid emulsion on Tuesdays and Saturdays." To calculate the calories for the dextrose component, remember that 30% dextrose means there's 30 g in each 100 ml. Because you need 1,000 ml, multiply 30 g by 10 (10 x 100 = 1,000 ml),

which equals 300 g dextrose per liter. Then multiply 300 g by the number of kcal/g to get 1,020 kcal/L. Use the same method to calculate the kcal of protein (800 kcal) in a liter of 20% amino acids.

The 800 protein calories and the 1,020 dextrose (carbohydrate) calories amount to 1,820 calories every 12 hours, or 3,640 calories/24 hours (1,820 calories x 2 L).

On Tuesdays and Saturdays, an additional 500 ml of 20% lipids are added. This calculates as 20% = 20 g/100 ml x 5 (500 ml) = 100 g x 9 kcal/g = 900 calories.

When the 900 fat calories are added to the 3,640 calories in the TPN, the patient receives 4,540 calories on Tuesdays and Saturdays.

*The Intravenous Nurses Society (INS) says a 10% lipid emulsion contains 1.1 kcal/ml; a 20% emulsion contains 2 kcal/ml. Therefore, according to INS guidelines, 500 ml of 20% lipid emulsion would contain 1,000 kcal, not 900 kcal as noted in the above formula. Use whichever calculation your facility recommends.

From *Plumer's Principles & Practice of Intravenous Therapy,* 5th edition. Reprinted with permission of Lippincott-Raven Publishers.

Heparin may be added to decrease the risk of phlebitis and fibrin formation on the venous access catheter. Ranitidine, cimetidine, or famotidine may be added to inhibit gastric acid secretion and lower the risk of stress ulcers. Albumin may also be added to TPN solutions to normalize plasma oncotic pressure during therapy. Care must be taken to avoid vascular overload, however. In addition, albumin has been associated with an increased risk of solution contamination.

Dextrose supplies most of the calories (3.4 kcal/g) in a TPN solution and has a significant nitrogen-sparing effect. (See *Calculating calories for total parenteral nutrition.*) The number of nonprotein calories needed to gain or maintain a positive nitrogen balance depends on the patient's diagnosis and severity of disease.

Amino acids supply protein (4 kcal/g) to replace essential amino acids and maintain protein stores, which prevents amino acid loss from muscle mass. Various amino acid formulations have been developed. Selections of a formulation for a specific patient are based on the patient's age, condition, and other factors.

The amount and type of electrolytes added to the parenteral nutrition solution are based on current electrolyte losses. Common electrolytes added to PPN and TPN solutions include sodium, potassium, calcium, chloride, phosphate, and magnesium. These additions are added in a specific order at a specific temperature to prevent precipitation. Additions should never be made after the formula is mixed.

Water- and fat-soluble vitamins are frequently added to a PPN or TPN solution in varying amounts, depending on the patient's specific needs. (See *Vitamins and trace elements in TPN therapy,* pages 224 and 225.) Vitamin K is not routinely added because some patients may also be receiving anticoagulant therapy and vitamin K might interfere with that therapy. If needed, vitamin K is usually given in a weekly parenteral (IM or SC) injection.

Micronutrients, also called trace elements, promote normal metabolism by increasing the efficient use of nutrients for energy production and protein synthesis. Commonly added micronutrients include zinc, chromium, copper, manganese, iodine, and selenium. Iron is added only if it's absolutely essential; its safety in parenteral nutrition therapy has not been established. If iron is necessary, it may be added in the form of iron dextran.

Water requirements vary widely, from 35 ml/kg/day for adults up to 150 ml/kg/day for infants. Fluid needs may be dramatically increased during the treatment of starvation, injury, sepsis, or burns. The amount of water added to the parenteral nutrition solution depends on the patient's current condition and may change daily.

Administration of parenteral nutrition

The administration of parenteral nutrition involves performing a full nutritional assessment, determining the type of solution to be used, and initiating the infusion.

(Text continues on page 226.)

Vitamins and trace elements in TPN therapy

Total parenteral nutrition (TPN) solutions can contain a variety of vitamins and trace elements. This chart describes the functions of these components and signs and symptoms of deficiencies related to them.

COMPONENT	FUNCTION	SIGNS AND SYMPTOMS OF DEFICIENCY
Water-soluble		
Vitamin B_1 (thiamine)	Aids absorption of carbohydrates and protein	Beriberi, fatigue, muscle atrophy, tenderness, peripheral neuropathy
Vitamin B_2 (riboflavin)	Aids absorption of carbohydrates and protein	Chapping and fissuring of lips, dermatitis, corneal inflammation, dryness, redness of eye
Vitamin B_3 (niacin)	Coenzyme for cell respiration; aids in synthesis of fat and glucolysis and in the absorption of carbohydrates and protein	Pellagra, weakness, anorexia, glossitis, dermatitis, emotional instability or irritability
Vitamin B_5 (pantothenic acid)	Coenzyme A	Malaise, headache, nausea and vomiting
Vitamin B_6	Coenzyme for amino acid metabolism; essential for enzyme formation; aids in glycogen breakdown	Personality changes, irritability, depression
Vitamin B_9 (folic acid)	Coenzyme in the synthesis of amino acids	Glossitis
Vitamin B_{12}	Assists with movement of folate into the cells; needed for metabolism	Glossitis, mental slowness or poor memory and confusion, peripheral paresthesia, pernicious anemia
Vitamin C	Needed for the formation of collagen; helps in the regulation of cholesterol metabolism	Gingivitis, petechiae, scurvy (anemia, joint pain, bleeding gums), delayed wound healing
Fat-soluble		
Vitamin A	Retinal function; prevents night blindness; development and repair of epithelial tissues; aids in bone metabolism	Night blindness, conjunctivae dryness, decrease in ability to taste and smell, reproductive problems
Vitamin D	Calcium and phosphate absorption; mobilization of calcium and phosphate from bones	Rickets, low serum calcium and phosphate, tetany, osteomalacia (softening of the bones)

Vitamins and trace elements in TPN therapy (continued)

COMPONENT	FUNCTION	SIGNS AND SYMPTOMS OF DEFICIENCY
Fat-soluble (continued)		
Vitamin E	Protects cellular membranes; prevents oxidation of vitamins A and C	Deficiency may contribute to hemolytic anemia and liver necrosis or decrease in RBC survival time; skeletal muscle lesions; increased platelet aggregation
Vitamin K (given separately intra-muscularly)	Prothrombin formation	Prolonged clotting and bleeding time
Trace elements		
Chromium	Glucose use	Decreased glycogen reserves or impaired glucose tolerance and insulin resistance, growth retardation, weight loss
Copper	Aids in hemoglobin synthesis; aids in connective tissue integrity; necessary for amino acid metabolism	Anemia associated with neutropenia, delayed wound healing, osteoporosis
Iodine	Thyroid function and the regulation of body metabolism	Hypothyroidism or enlarged thyroid, delayed growth, decreased metabolic rate or fatigue
Iron	Necessary in the production of hemoglobin or oxygen transport; necessary in the function of some essential metabolic enzymes	Anemia
Manganese	Cofactor for many enzymes	Slow growth, weight loss, CNS dysfunction, hair color changes
Molybdenum	Component of enzyme formation	Growth retardation
Selenium	Essential component of several enzymes	Cardiomyopathy, muscle weakness, myalgia
Zinc	Cofactor of many enzymes; essential for mobilization of vitamin A; aids in metabolism of lipids, proteins, and carbohydrates	Alopecia, diminished taste or smell, diarrhea, depression, growth retardation or gonadal dysfunction, poor wound healing or rash

Assessing nutritional needs

A full assessment of the patient's nutritional needs must be completed before parenteral nutrition therapy begins. The nutritional assessment will allow the doctor and other members of the health care team to customize the parenteral solution, including setting the number of calories in the solution and the type and amount of vitamins, minerals, and other nutrients.

The nutritional assessment should include a full physical assessment as well as a dietary history and laboratory analysis to determine the patient's current nutritional status. Obtain measurements of the patient's height, weight, and percent of body fat and lean muscle mass. Measurements of nitrogen balance help to determine if, in general, the patient is in an anabolic (muscle-building) state with a positive nitrogen balance or a catabolic (muscle-breakdown) state with a negative nitrogen balance. In a severe, long-term catabolic state, the body has depleted its supply of skeletal muscle protein and turns instead to breaking down proteins in internal organs for energy. This breakdown process can lead to organ failure and requires immediate treatment.

In addition to tests for electrolyte levels, plasma protein and albumin levels can be used to evaluate the patient's current and recent past nutritional status. Levels of albumin, which has a long half-life of 20 days, may be helpful in the initial screening process to determine past protein intake. Serum transferrin has a shorter half-life (8 to 10 days) and is more sensitive to recent events. The most sensitive serum protein is prealbumin, with a half-life of 2 to 3 days. Although expensive, a prealbumin test offers a more accurate picture of current visceral protein status.

Initiating parenteral nutrition

Administering PPN, TPN, or lipid emulsions requires that you gather the appropriate equipment, prepare the patient for the infusion, properly prepare the solution, and initiate the infusion. (See *Tips for administering parenteral nutrition.*)

Gathering the equipment

Before proceeding with a PPN or TPN infusion, you'll need to obtain this equipment:
- clean gloves
- 70% alcohol swabs
- container of parenteral solution
- suitable administration set

Tips for administering parenteral nutrition

Infusions of parenteral nutrition must be done with care. Here are some expert tips to help you manage parenteral nutrition therapy more efficiently.

- Don't play "catch up" with flow rates. Speeding up and slowing down a parenteral nutrition solution causes changes in the patient's blood sugar levels.
- Don't allow the total parenteral nutrition (TPN) solutions to hang for more than 24 hours.
- Change the TPN tubing and filter every 24 hours.
- If the solution container is damaged and an immediate replacement isn't available, hang a container of dextrose 10% at the same rate as prescribed for the parenteral nutrition. This will prevent an extreme hypoglycemic reaction. Monitor the patient; the blood sugar may still change significantly.
- Don't use the lumen dedicated to parenteral nutrition for other functions, including infusion of blood products, bolus injections, simultaneous IV solutions, blood draws for laboratory analysis, or measurement of central venous pressure. If a multiple-lumen catheter is used, label one lumen as "TPN only." The remaining lumens may be used for other needs. If a single-lumen catheter is being used, another access will be required for other therapies.
- Inform the patient who can't use the oral route that frequent oral care will provide comfort and prevent sores.
- Provide emotional support because a patient who has lost the ability to eat and enjoy the social and emotional pleasures attached to eating may go through a grieving process.

- needleless connector (for lipid emulsions)
- tape (if administration tubing lacks luer-lock connectors)
- filter, as needed
- infusion pump.

Preparing the patient
Explain the procedure to the patient before initiating the infusion. Make sure to check the name on the solution container against the patient's wrist identification band to ensure that you're giving the correct solution to the correct patient.

Preparing parenteral nutrition solutions
Preparation of the solution depends on the solution being used, whether it's a PPN or TPN solution or a lipid emulsion.

Preparing PPN or TPN solutions
PPN and TPN solutions are prepared in the pharmacy under a laminar flow hood and using strict aseptic technique. The solutions are then refrigerated until ready for use. Although a pharmacist pre-

pares the actual solution, you may be involved in determining the components of a particular patient's solution. A basic TPN solution consists of varying amounts of dextrose, amino acids, electrolytes, and other components.

Whatever the composition, the parenteral nutrition solution should be removed from the refrigerator at least 1 hour before administration to allow it to warm to room temperature. Check the solution and label against the doctor's order for correct formula components. Also check the patient's identification and the solution's expiration date.

Check the container for holes or cracks and the solution for turbidity, precipitates, and cloudiness. If lipids have been added to a solution, also look for separation or a brown discoloration. Return the solution to the pharmacy if these findings exist.

Obtain an appropriate filter. Filters are used to remove particulate matter and bacteria from the solution before they reach the patient. Filters may be part of the administration set (called in-line filters) or added to the administration set during setup.

A 0.22-micron filter is recommended for solutions without fat emulsion. For a lipid-containing solution (known as a total nutrient admixture or a 3-in-1 solution), a 1.2-micron filter is used because the lipids in solution are too large to pass through a 0.22-micron filter.

To prepare the solution for infusion, connect in this sequence the infusion pump tubing, filter (unless the tubing has an in-line filter), and reflux valve. Place the filter as close to the catheter insertion site as possible.

If the tubing doesn't have luer-lock connections, tape all connections to prevent accidental separation. Hang the unopened solution container on the IV pole. Squeeze the IV drip chamber and, holding the drip chamber upright, insert the tubing spike into the solution container. Release the drip chamber. Squeezing the drip chamber before spiking the container prevents accidental leakage of the solution during spiking.

Prime the tubing slowly, gently tapping it to dislodge air bubbles trapped in the Y-ports and filter. Load the administration set into the infusion pump according to the manufacturer's instructions, and program the prescribed rate and volume.

Attach a time tape to the container so you can check the accuracy of the infusion pump. Label the container and tubing with the date and time and your initials.

Preparing lipid emulsions

Fats are supplied in lipid emulsions and, at 9 kcal/g, are a concentrated source of energy. They help meet calorie needs and prevent or correct fatty-acid deficiencies. Lipids are available in concentrations of 10% or 20%. Lipid emulsions may be given separately, piggybacked into the parenteral nutrition tubing at the lowest additive site, or sometimes mixed into the parenteral nutrition in a total nutrient admixture (TNA) or 3-in-1 solution.

Inspect the lipid emulsion for color and texture. If the emulsion looks frothy, oily, has brownish discoloration, appears to have separated, or if there is any question regarding the solution's stability or sterility, return the emulsion to the pharmacy.

Verify the order, identify the patient, and make sure the correct lipid emulsion is being used. To prevent aggregation of fat globules, avoid shaking the container. Don't freeze the emulsion or add anything to it.

To prepare the solution for infusion, connect the IV tubing to the needleless connector. If the tubing doesn't contain luer-lock connections, tape all connections securely to prevent accidental separation, which can lead to exsanguination, air embolism, or sepsis. Close the flow clamp on the IV tubing. Using aseptic technique, remove the protective cap from the lipid emulsion bottle and clean the rubber stopper with an alcohol sponge. Hang the bottle on the IV pole, and insert the vented spike through the inner circle of the rubber stopper.

Squeeze the drip chamber until it fills to the indicated level. Open the flow clamp slowly, and prime the tubing. Gently tap the tubing to dislodge air bubbles trapped in the Y-ports and filter, if used. Attach a time tape to the container to allow accurate measurement of flow rate. Label the container and tubing with the date and time and your initials.

Infusing parenteral nutrition solutions

Infusion procedures for parenteral nutrition solutions vary with the type of solution being infused—PPN, TPN, or lipid emulsions—and the route of administration.

Infusing PPN or TPN solutions

If you're initiating the infusion, place the patient in the supine position, clean the catheter injection cap with an alcohol sponge, and allow the solution to dry. Flush the catheter with normal saline solution, according to your facility's policy.

Central venous infusion of parenteral nutrition

Total parenteral nutrition (TPN) therapy is always given through a central venous catheter, as shown here. Because of its gentle arch, the left subclavian vein is commonly used for central venous infusion.

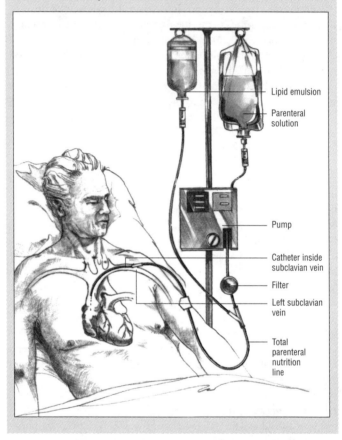

Lipid emulsion

Parenteral solution

Pump

Catheter inside subclavian vein

Filter

Left subclavian vein

Total parenteral nutrition line

If you're replacing a completed infusion, you'll need to change the tubing. Clamp the catheter before disconnecting the tubing from the catheter, to prevent air from entering the catheter. (See *Central venous infusion of parenteral nutrition.*) If a clamp isn't available, ask the patient to perform Valsalva's maneuver as the tubing is being changed. If the patient is being mechanically ventilated, change the IV tubing immediately after the machine delivers a breath at peak inspiration. These techniques increase intrathoracic pressure and prevent air embolism.

For either TPN or PPN infusions, use aseptic technique to re-move the injection cap or old tubing and attach the new IV line. Once the new tubing is connected, unclamp the catheter.

Make sure that the catheter junction is secure. Check the pump to make sure it's set at the correct rate. Then start the infusion. If it's the first infusion, start with incremental rate increases, as or-dered. An incrementally increased infusion rate (a process called ramping) allows the beta cells in the pancreas time to increase their output of insulin in response to the high glucose load in the solu-tion. Initial rates range from 40 to 50 ml/hour. Increase this rate in 20 to 25 ml/hour increments every 6 to 8 hours until the desired rate is achieved. If the patient is extremely sensitive to the dextrose, increase the rate more slowly, in increments of 20 ml/hour every 24 hours. If a patient's blood glucose levels change dramatically over several hours, the entire TPN bottle may need to be discarded.

When initiating therapy, check the infusion pump's volume and time tape every 30 minutes. Once you know how the patient's blood glucose levels react from the infusion, begin monitoring as appropriate for each patient.

At the start of therapy, check vital signs, including temperature, every 4 hours. An increased temperature is one of the earliest signs of catheter-related sepsis. Because many patients require supple-mental insulin during parenteral nutrition therapy, most facilities re-quire finger-stick blood glucose testing every 6 hours and treatment with sliding-scale insulin based on the blood glucose readings.

Perform a complete physical assessment daily, noting heart func-tion, lung sounds, blood pressure, pulse, and presence of edema. Weigh the patient at the same time each morning, after voiding, in similar clothing, and using the same scale. Suspect fluid imbalance if the patient gains 1 lb (0.5 kg) or more in a day.

Assess the patient's response to therapy and laboratory test results, watching for early signs of metabolic or mechanical complications. Notify the doctor if a problem arises.

When TPN therapy is to be discontinued, reverse the slow rate adjustment done during the initial infusion. PPN has a much lower dextrose concentration and can usually be initiated at the ordered rate and discontinued without ramping.

Infusing lipid emulsions

For a patient's first lipid infusion, administer a 30-minute test dose of 1 ml/minute for 10% lipids or 0.5 ml/minute for 20%. Monitor the patient's vital signs, and watch closely for signs and symptoms of adverse reactions, such as fever, chills, flushing, sweating, muscle pain, chest or back pain, urticaria, nausea, vomiting, headache, or a pressure sensation over the eyes. Allergic reactions may be more common among patients allergic to eggs because of the addition of certain egg products during emulsification.

If the test dose causes no adverse reactions, infuse the lipid emulsion at the prescribed rate. The maximum rate for infusing a lipid emulsion is 125 ml/hour for a 10% emulsion and 60 ml/hour for a 20% emulsion, although most emulsions are infused more slowly.

As with other IV procedures, strict aseptic technique is essential. Change the IV tubing and lipid container every 24 hours. Because lipid emulsion is an excellent medium for bacterial and fungal growth, never hang a partially empty container of emulsion, and always remove the container promptly after the infusion is complete.

Monitor the patient closely for reactions to the lipid emulsion. Note that some patients experience an unpleasant metallic taste during the infusion and that most patients say they feel satiated after completion of the infusion. You'll also need to monitor laboratory tests to detect early signs of complications. Tests include liver function studies, platelet counts, prothrombin times, and serum triglyceride levels. To avoid falsely elevated triglyceride levels, draw blood at least 6 hours after the infusion has been completed.

Cloudy plasma in a centrifuged sample of citrated blood may signal that the rate or amount of the lipid infusion should be decreased. Lipid emulsion can clear from the blood faster in patients with multiple trauma, full thickness burns, and other conditions affecting metabolic balance.

Complications

Complications of parenteral nutrition therapy vary with the type of therapy—PPN, TPN, or lipid emulsions.

PPN– or TPN–related complications

Complications of PPN or TPN therapy include catheter-related sepsis, phlebitis, air embolism, glucose imbalances, hepatic dysfunction, hypercapnia, hyperosmolarity, hypocalcemia, hypokalemia, hypo-

magnesemia, hypophosphatemia, metabolic acidosis, metabolic alkalosis, a clotted IV catheter, cracked or broken tubing, a dislodged
catheter, and a too-rapid infusion.

CATHETER-RELATED SEPSIS. Catheter-related sepsis is one of the most
serious complications of parenteral nutrition therapy. The most
common cause is skin contamination at the entry site. Many
instances stem from microbes present on the hands of health care
workers. The need for frequent, rigorous hand washing and strict
aseptic technique when performing all catheter-related procedures
cannot be overemphasized.

To detect site infection or other kinds of related infections,
monitor the patient's temperature closely. The frequency should be
based on your facility's policy and depends on the patient's underlying disease. If a normally afebrile patient has an unexpected temperature elevation during a TPN infusion, the entire IV system should
be changed and cultured immediately, to rule out solution contamination. A new TPN container and tubing should be started.

Next, a complete workup for fever will be done. The doctor may
remove the catheter, depending on the patient's condition, culture
results, and nature of the infecting organisms. Infections (except for
fungemia) related to long-term implanted vascular access devices
may be treated with antibiotics.

PHLEBITIS. Phlebitis is a common complication of TPN or PPN
therapy. Signs and symptoms include pain, tenderness, redness, and
warmth at the insertion site. For phlebitis, apply gentle heat to the
area and elevate the site, if possible.

AIR EMBOLISM. Air embolism is always a risk when a central venous
catheter is in place. Air can enter the central venous system when
the administration set is being changed or during accidental
disconnection of tubing junctions. A crack at any point can provide
access for air. Air may also enter through the tract left when a
central catheter is removed.

To prevent air embolism, use luer-lock connections on the tubing or tape the connections carefully. Assess the tubing and catheter
for signs of cracking, and always apply pressure to the tract and then
an occlusive dressing after removing a central venous catheter.

GLUCOSE IMBALANCES. The most common metabolic complications
are related to glucose imbalances. Glucose levels may also be

adversely affected by sepsis, stress, shock, starvation, renal or hepatic failure, pancreatic disease, and certain medications. Because many patients receiving PPN or TPN have one or more of these conditions, you'll need to remain extra vigilant for alterations in glucose metabolism. Patients may become hyperglycemic or hypoglycemic.

A patient with hyperglycemia may appear fatigued, restless, confused, anxious, or weak. You may note polyuria, dehydration, elevated serum glucose levels, delirium, or coma. The rate of infusion or dextrose concentration should be decreased. Calories should be replaced with lipid emulsion. Insulin therapy should be initiated.

Sweating, shaking, and irritability after the infusion has stopped are common signs of hypoglycemia in a patient receiving TPN. For this patient, the dextrose intake should be increased or the exogenous insulin intake decreased.

HEPATIC DYSFUNCTION. Signs and symptoms of hepatic dysfunction include elevated AST, alkaline phosphatase, and serum bilirubin levels. The patient's total caloric and dextrose intakes should be reduced. Lost calories should be replaced with lipid emulsion. In addition, a cyclical infusion schedule should be used. Keep in mind that specific hepatic formulations should be used only for patients with encephalopathy.

HYPERCAPNIA. With hypercapnia, you'll see increased oxygen consumption and carbon dioxide production and a measured respiratory quotient of 1 or more. For a patient with hypercapnia, the total caloric and dextrose intake should be reduced. Intake of dextrose and fat calories should be balanced.

HYPEROSMOLARITY. Confusion, lethargy, seizures, hyperosmolar non-ketotic syndrome, hyperglycemia, dehydration, and glycosuria are signs and symptoms of hyperosmolarity. Dextrose infusions should be stopped. Insulin should be administered along with 0.45% NaCl solution with 10 to 20 mEq/L of potassium, for rehydration.

HYPOCALCEMIA. A patient with hypocalcemia may exhibit polyuria, dehydration, and elevated blood and urine glucose levels. Calcium supplements should be increased.

HYPOKALEMIA. Muscle weakness, paralysis, paresthesia, and arrhythmias are common signs and symptoms of hypokalemia. Potassium supplements should be given.

HYPOMAGNESEMIA. A patient with hypomagnesemia may feel tingling around the mouth or paresthesia in the fingers. You may note mental changes or hyperreflexia. For this patient, magnesium supplementation should be increased.

HYPOPHOSPHATEMIA. Signs and symptoms of this TPN-related condition include irritability, weakness, paresthesia, coma, and respiratory arrest. Phosphate supplementation should be increased.

METABOLIC ACIDOSIS. With metabolic acidosis, you'll note an elevated serum chloride level and a decreased serum bicarbonate level. For a patient with this condition, the amount of acetate in the TPN solution should be increased and the chloride decreased.

METABOLIC ALKALOSIS. A patient with metabolic alkalosis will have a diminished serum chloride level and an elevated serum bicarbonate level. The amount of acetate in the TPN solution should be decreased in this case, and the chloride increased.

CLOTTED IV CATHETER. If a patient's IV catheter becomes clotted, you'll note an interrupted flow rate and resistance when flushing or withdrawing blood. Attempt to aspirate the clot. If you're unsuccessful, urokinase may be instilled to clear the catheter lumen.

CRACKED OR BROKEN TUBING. You'll see fluid leaking from the tubing if it's cracked or broken. Apply a padded hemostat between the break and the patient to prevent air from entering the system and causing an air embolism. Replace the tubing.

DISLODGED CATHETER. If a catheter being used to deliver TPN comes out of the vein, apply pressure to the site with a sterile gauze pad. Then alert the doctor.

TOO-RAPID INFUSION. If a TPN infusion is flowing too rapidly, the patient may complain of nausea or headache or appear lethargic. Adjust the rate and, if applicable, check the infusion pump for accuracy.

Lipid emulsion–related complications

Complications related to the administration of lipid emulsions can occur early in therapy or be delayed.

EARLY COMPLICATIONS. Early adverse reactions to lipid emulsion therapy occur in fewer than 1% of patients. These reactions can include fever, dyspnea, cyanosis, nausea, vomiting, flushing, diaphoresis, headache, lethargy, syncope, chest or back pain, and pressure over the eyes. Insertion site irritation, hyperlipidemia, and thrombocytopenia may also occur. Treatment may be aimed at alleviating the symptoms or, in severe reactions, halting therapy.

DELAYED COMPLICATIONS. Delayed complications associated with prolonged administration of lipid emulsion are rare and may include hepatomegaly, splenomegaly, jaundice secondary to central lobular cholestasis, and blood dyscrasias, such as thrombocytopenia and leukopenia. Transient increases in liver function test results may also occur. Abnormal liver function test results aren't limited to lipid administration; they also occur in long-term TPN therapy.

Thrombocytopenia has been reported in infants receiving a 20% lipid emulsion. In premature or low-birth-weight infants, PPN with lipid emulsion may cause lipids to accumulate in the lungs.

Treatment of delayed complications varies with the specific type of complication and may involve discontinuation of lipid therapy.

Teaching the patient

Patients receiving parenteral nutrition in any form need to understand the treatment, its goals, risks, and benefits. Assess the patient's ability and willingness to learn and participate in his care prior to instruction. Include caregivers in this process whenever possible, especially if parenteral nutrition will be administered at home. (See *Using parenteral nutrition at home.*)

For patients who'll be receiving parenteral nutrition, explain the purpose and use of aseptic techniques. Demonstrate each step of each procedure, explaining why proper technique is essential. Allow the patient to practice each procedure until his knowledge and techniques are perfected.

Explain the signs and symptoms to watch for, what to do if a complication occurs, and when to report complications. With cyclic feedings, the patient normally will infuse solution for 12 hours, usu-

CLINICAL PEARLS

Using parenteral nutrition at home

Patients often receive parenteral nutrition at home. You may be asked to assess a patient's suitability for home therapy and to teach the patient how to administer the therapy.

Assessing the patient

To determine a patient's suitability for home therapy, consider the patient's motivation, his mental aptitude, and his job or other daily activities. Assess his relationships with family or other household members: Can they assist him with parenteral nutrition therapy?

Also consider the accessibility of hospitals, home nursing services, and other health care support systems. If a patient's psychological state or home environment interferes with his safety, he shouldn't receive parenteral nutrition at home. Home parenteral nutrition is also contraindicated if the patient's primary disease is untreatable or if other medical problems require in-patient care.

Teaching the patient

If the patient is scheduled to receive parenteral nutrition at home, provide careful teaching before discharge. (Include a family member or caregiver if possible.) Conduct your teaching sessions in a quiet area where you and the patient will be undisturbed.

Teach the patient to change the catheter site dressing as ordered (usually every 2 to 3 days) or whenever it becomes soiled or nonocclusive. Also emphasize the importance of changing the IV tubing as scheduled.

Instruct the patient to take only sponge baths, and to wash gently around the catheter site. Tell him he may be allowed to remove his dressing and bathe or shower after the implanted catheter has been in place for 1 month or longer.

Tell the patient to protect his catheter against contact with granular or lint-producing surfaces. Explain that airborne particles and surface contaminants could cause a local tissue reaction.

Work with the patient to devise a suitable parenteral nutrition schedule, considering both his nutritional needs and his lifestyle. Suggest that he wear a medical identification bracelet or subscribe to a medical alert service. Reassure him that a nurse from the home health care team will always be available in case of an emergency.

Because the financial burden of long-term or permanent home parenteral nutrition can be overwhelming, even if the patient has health insurance, make a social services referral. Tell the elderly patient that Medicare may assume the cost of supplies and medications if he meets eligibility requirements.

Providing emotional support

Many patients receiving home parenteral nutrition experience depression related to a change in body image, a loss of ability to eat normally, a change in family structure, financial strain, and a change in activity level. Encourage the patient and his family to verbalize their concerns and to join a support group of other persons receiving home parenteral nutrition. Also encourage the patient to resume his normal activities as soon as possible.

ally at night. Teach the patient to ramp up slowly for the first 1 or 2 hours to reach the prescribed rate, and then to keep the infusion at that rate until 1 or 2 hours before discontinuing. In the last 2 hours, the infusion is ramped down slowly to avoid hypoglycemia. Some pumps have this feature built-in.

Remind the patient and caregiver that TPN bags should be refrigerated until 1 hour before use and hang for not more than 24 hours. Teach them how to check each container for precipitate, leaks, turbidity, or, if a 3-in-1 solution is used, separation or discoloration.

Teach the patient how to obtain accurate weight and body temperature measurements. Instruct them to check blood glucose levels. If this isn't possible or feasible, they can check urine glucose and ketones routinely. Help them set up a chart to graph temperatures, weights, and blood glucose levels, which will serve to remind them when to perform these functions and will show gradual changes that could be reported to the doctor.

Explain how to order supplies and to properly dispose of used material. Always give them a list of emergency phone numbers and personnel they can call if they have a question or problem.

Documentation

Documentation for any form of parenteral nutrition involves recording information about the infusion and the patient's response to it. Record:
• date, time, type and amount of solution, and the infusion rate
• equipment used for rate regulation
• dressing changes
• observations of the site and catheter patency before, during, and after the infusion
• weight, intake and output, and blood glucose measurements
• signs of complications or complaints of discomfort, the intervention taken, and the outcome of each intervention
• date, time, and all supplies used when an administration set is changed
• patient education done
• difficulties the patient had learning concepts or procedures and the steps taken to correct these problems
• patient's response to the procedures.

Administering chemotherapy

Chemotherapeutic agents, also called antineoplastic agents, are used to treat cancer. Chemotherapeutic agents may be used alone or in combination with other treatments, including surgery, radiation therapy, and biotherapy. This chapter examines how to select and administer a chemotherapeutic agent. It also explains complications of chemotherapy, patient teaching, and documentation.

Selecting a chemotherapeutic agent

Selecting a suitable chemotherapeutic agent for a patient with a particular cancer depends in large measure on an understanding of the cell cycle and how each chemotherapeutic agent affects that cycle.

Understanding the cell cycle
Normal and abnormal cells alike progress through five phases of development, identified as G_0, G_1, S, G_2, and M, and collectively known as the cell cycle. (See *Phases of the cell cycle,* page 240.) In the G_0 (or resting) phase, the cells are temporarily out of cycle and not

239

Phases of the cell cycle

Chemotherapeutic agents may be categorized as cell cycle–specific or cell cycle–nonspecific. Cell cycle–specific agents such as methotrexate act at one or more cell cycle phases, shown in this illustration. Cell cycle–nonspecific agents such as busulfan can act on replicating and resting cells. (Agents listed in this diagram are examples of cell cycle–specific agents.)

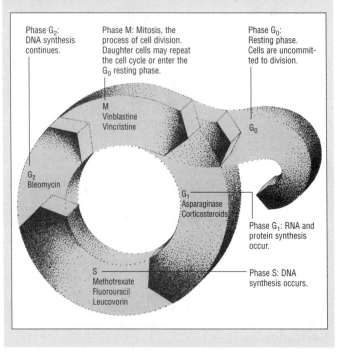

Phase G_2: DNA synthesis continues.

Phase M: Mitosis, the process of cell division. Daughter cells may repeat the cell cycle or enter the G_0 resting phase.

Phase G_0: Resting phase. Cells are uncommitted to division.

M
Vinblastine
Vincristine

G_0

G_2
Bleomycin

G_1
Asparaginase
Corticosteroids

Phase G_1: RNA and protein synthesis occur.

S
Methotrexate
Fluorouracil
Leucovorin

Phase S: DNA synthesis occurs.

currently dividing. The length of time a cell remains in this phase depends on the type of cell. Skin cells, for instance, spend little time in the resting phase; neurons spend much more time in the G_0 phase. A cell can stay in the G_0 phase from 8 to 48 hours.

During the G_1 phase, the cell makes RNA and proteins. Cells remain in this phase from hours to days, depending on the cell type. After the G_1 phase, the cell enters the S phase, which lasts approximately 10 to 30 hours. During this phase, the cell synthesizes DNA in preparation for dividing.

When DNA synthesis is complete, the cell moves into the G_2 phase, which lasts about 2 hours. The cell makes more RNA and protein. It also produces the mitotic spindle apparatus.

Cell cycle–specific and cell cycle–nonspecific agents

Use of a particular agent depends on the phase of the cell cycle affected by that agent. This chart lists commonly used chemotherapeutic agents according to the cell cycle phase affected.

CELL CYCLE–SPECIFIC AGENTS		CELL CYCLE–NONSPECIFIC AGENTS	
G₁ phase	**G₂ phase**	**Alkylating agents**	**Nitrosoureas**
Asparaginase	Bleomycin	Busulfan	Carmustine
Prednisone	Etoposide	Carboplatin	Lomustine
	Teniposide	Chlorambucil	Streptozocin
S phase		Cisplatin	
Clodribine	**M phase**	Cyclophosphamide	**Miscellaneous**
Cytarabine	Paclitaxel	Ifosfamide	Dacarbazine
Fludarabine	Vinblastine	Mechlorethamine	Procarbazine
5-Fluorouracil	Vincristine	Melphalan	
Hydroxyurea	Vindesine		
Mercaptopurine	Vinorelbine	**Antibiotics**	
Methotrexate		Dactinomycin	
Pentostatin		Daunorubicin	
Thioguanine		Doxorubicin	
		Idarubicin	
		Mitomycin	

During the M phase, the final phase of the cell cycle, cell division occurs, usually in about 1 hour. When the division occurs (called mitosis in nonsex cells and meiosis in sex cells), two daughter cells are formed, each of which contains the same complement of genetic material. The two daughter cells mature and either enter the G_1 phase to repeat the cell cycle or remain in G_0 phase until triggered to begin dividing.

Agents that alter the cell cycle

Depending on the specific agent used, an antineoplastic agent alters a particular phase or all phases of the cell cycle. (See *Cell cycle–specific and cell cycle–nonspecific agents.*) Agents designed to disrupt a specific phase of the cell cycle are called cell cycle–specific agents. These agents work best on rapidly dividing tumors and are usually given in divided doses or by continuous infusion.

Chemotherapeutic agents that act in all phases of the cell cycle are called cell cycle–nonspecific agents. These agents have a prolonged action independent of the cell cycle, so they produce cell damage throughout the entire cell cycle. Cell cycle–nonspecific agents are most effective if given in large single doses because the more agent given, the greater the number of tumor cells killed.

The response of the cancer to the chemotherapeutic agents is influenced directly by the size of the tumor and the degree of metastasis. These agents are most effective when the cancer is small and when the tumor hasn't spread.

The condition of the patient should also be considered when choosing a chemotherapeutic agent. The better the patient's condition before chemotherapy, the more likely the agents will be well tolerated and the outcome successful.

The dosage required to effect a desired response plays a role in selection of the most suitable chemotherapeutic agent. Higher doses of these agents are more likely to destroy cancerous cells, but the patient is also more likely to experience toxic effects. Generally, chemotherapeutic agents are administered in cycles; first, a cycle of chemotherapy, and then a rest period for the patient, to allow for normal cells to repair and the immune system to recover. This intermittent therapy allows repeated treatments using high doses of chemotherapy.

Not all cancers can be treated with high-dose chemotherapy, however. The drug-free interval needed after high-dose chemotherapy could provide sufficient time for cancer cells in the G_0 phase at the time to begin reproducing. If these cells reproduce more quickly than the recovery time needed by normal cells, frequent low-dose chemotherapy or high doses of combination chemotherapy may be used. Frequent low-dose chemotherapy generally continues until the patient shows signs of toxicity. Combination therapy is usually well tolerated by patients and may minimize immunosuppression.

Another important factor to consider when selecting chemotherapeutic agents relates to the destruction of cells occurring at a constant fractional rate. If a chemotherapeutic agent kills 90% of cancer cells after the first dose, the second dose will kill 90% of the remaining cancer cells. The third administration would kill 90% of those, and so forth. To destroy the entire tumor would require either continued administration of the chemotherapy agent in increasing dosages or the administration of the agent when the tumor is small enough to allow cell destruction at a tolerable dose.

Chemotherapeutic agents can also be given in combination. The formulation of combination therapy depends on each drug's effectiveness, action within the cell cycle, and toxicity. Selections of agents used in combination are driven by four main principles of combination therapy: Each chemotherapeutic agent should be effective when administered alone; each agent should have a different mechanism of action in the cell cycle, all agents should be able to

Irritant, vesicant, and nonvesicant agents

Chemotherapeutic agents may be inadvertently administered into surrounding tissues. To administer these agents safely, you need to know whether an agent is an irritant (capable of producing undue sensitivity), a vesicant (capable of producing blisters and other tissue damage), or a nonvesicant agent.

IRRITANT AGENTS	VESICANT AGENTS	NONVESICANT AGENTS
Bleomycin	Cisplatin	Asparaginase
Carmustine	Dactinomycin	Carboplatin
Cisplatin	Daunorubicin	Cyclophosphamide
Dacarbazine	Doxorubicin	Cytarabine
Etoposide	Mitomycin	Floxuridine
5-Fluorouracil	Nitrogen mustards	Ifosfamide
Mitoxantrone	Paclitaxel	
Streptozocin	Plicamycin	
Teniposide	Vinblastine	
	Vincristine	
	Vindesine	
	Vinorelbine	

work together and not inhibit each other's action in the cell cycle, and each agent should produce toxicities at different times and in different organ systems.

Selecting a route

Chemotherapeutic agents can be administered by several routes. The selection of the most appropriate route varies with the optimal effect of the agent, the patient's ability to tolerate the agent, and the agent's effects on normal and malignant cells.

Chemotherapy, whether an irritant, vesicant, or nonvesicant agent is used, is most commonly administered IV. (See *Irritant, vesicant, and nonvesicant agents.*) It may be given by IV push directly into the catheter or through the Y-site of a free-flowing IV line.

The oral route may be used when the agent can be absorbed through the GI system and the patient can swallow and has an obstruction-free GI tract. The IM and SC routes are rarely chosen.

Chemotherapeutic agents may be administered by the intrathecal route, used when the blood-brain barrier prevents the agent from reaching its intended target in the brain. Agents delivered by this method are administered through a lumbar puncture when

Using an Ommaya reservoir

Not all drugs cross the blood-brain barrier. For those that don't cross the barrier to reach their intended target in the brain, an Ommaya reservoir may be used. To insert an Ommaya reservoir, the doctor drills a burr hole and inserts the device's catheter through the patient's nondominant frontal lobe into the lateral ventricle. The reservoir, which has a self-sealing silicone injection dome, rests over the burr hole under a scalp flap. This creates a slight, soft bulge on the scalp, about the size of a quarter. Drugs are injected into the dome with a syringe, as shown in this illustration.

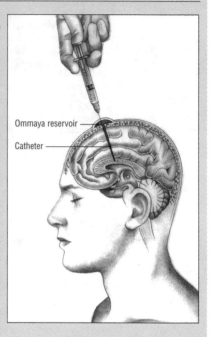

short-term therapy is anticipated or through a ventricular reservoir for long-term therapy. (See *Using an Ommaya reservoir.*) Complications associated with intrathecal administration include infection, bleeding, and leakage of cerebrospinal fluid.

Selecting a device

Many patients with cancer face an increased risk for extravasation; their veins are often fragile, they're subjected to repeated venipunctures, and many exhibit a tendency toward lymphedema. For those patients, therapy through a central venous access device may be essential.

Central venous access devices allow for long-term therapy (from weeks to years) and the ability to infuse more caustic chemotherapeutic agents. Central venous access may also prove helpful for patients receiving IV therapy at home or those requiring frequent venipuncture for blood tests or the administration of blood products. Refer to earlier chapters for a description of each type of vascular access device including implantable ports.

Administration of a chemotherapeutic agent

The administration of a chemotherapeutic agent carries with it a great deal of responsibility for the nurse, perhaps more than what most other agents carry. Errors in administration of a chemotherapeutic agent can cause severe toxic effects. To properly and safely administer a chemotherapeutic agent, you'll need to prepare the patient and the agent and follow rigid administration guidelines.

Preparing the patient
In preparation for administering a chemotherapeutic agent, make sure the doctor has obtained the patient's consent for the therapy. The patient should be given a description of the therapy, an explanation of its risks and benefits, and information about alternatives to the proposed therapy including an explanation of their risks and benefits. Explain the procedure to the patient and the need for whatever special precautions are necessary in the handling of that patient's particular chemotherapeutic agents.

Preparing the chemotherapeutic agent
Preparation for the administration of chemotherapy actually starts long before the patient reaches the health care facility. Safe and effective preparation and administration of these agents require specialized knowledge and skills. Nurses who administer chemotherapeutic agents receive special training in the handling and administration of these agents.

Some chemotherapeutic agents need to be administered through IV tubing designed especially for use with these agents. Some need to be protected from light or administered before or after another agent. In addition, some chemotherapeutic agents, when administered to patients also receiving radiation, may cause more severe adverse effects than usual because the patient is receiving two kinds of antineoplastic treatment at once. You'll need to be familiar with all of these aspects of drug therapy—and more—to administer chemotherapy properly.

You'll also need to check the accuracy of the prescribed dosage. Dosages of chemotherapy agents may be standardized according to established protocols or calculated based on the patient's weight or body surface area (BSA). Most often, dosages are calculated according to the patient's BSA. To calculate the BSA, use a body surface nomogram or this formula:

$$BSA(m^2) = \frac{\text{Height (cm) x weight (kg)}}{3600}$$

$$BSA(m^2) = \frac{\text{Height (inches) x weight (lb)}}{3131}$$

Handling chemotherapeutic agents themselves carries significant risks for the nurse. Most of these agents can cause cancer, genetic mutations, or fetal defects. Moreover, several of the agents cause local irritation if they come into contact with the skin, eyes, or mucous membranes. They can also cause tissue ulceration and necrosis. However, these risks can be minimized by following certain guidelines. All chemotherapeutic agents should be prepared in a well-ventilated area and within a class II, type A or B laminar flow biological safety cabinet. The cabinet helps to prevent accidental inhalation of aerosolized agents.

A chemotherapy spill kit should be readily available wherever chemotherapeutic agents are prepared or given, and all health care providers should be instructed in its proper use. The kit should contain the following items:
- latex, powder-free gloves
- impermeable long-sleeved gown with cuffs
- shoe covers
- goggles and mask
- disposable dust pan and scraper (for broken glass)
- absorbent towels and a container of desiccant powder or granules (to absorb wet content)
- disposable sponges
- leak-proof container labeled "Biohazard"
- container of 70% alcohol (for cleaning the spill area).

Depending on the agent being used, chemotherapeutic agents may be mixed by pharmacists, pharmacy technicians, or nurses. To prepare an agent for administration, wipe the surface top of the safety cabinet with 70% alcohol and a disposable towel before and after mixing. Wash your hands before and after preparation and before administration. Wear protective equipment—goggles, face shield, impermeable gown with long sleeves and cuffs, and latex gloves—when mixing the agents. Also wear appropriate gown and gloves during administration.

When drawing up agents from a vial, use a needle with a filter to avoid the inadvertent administration of particulate matter from the vial. Label all syringes or solution containers with the name of the patient and name and dose of the medication. Once the medication has been drawn up, discard needles intact in a sharps container suitable for chemotherapy waste and dispose of protective attire in a chemotherapy waste container. If a chemotherapeutic agent comes in contact with skin, wash the area with soap and water. If the agent comes in contact with an eye, flood the eye with water for at least 5 minutes while holding the eyelid open.

Administering an IV chemotherapeutic agent

Before administering an IV chemotherapeutic agent, carefully check the patient's CBC results and chemotherapy order. Make sure the patient has a patent venous access device. Avoid using a peripheral IV catheter distal to the site of a recent (within the past 24 hours) venipuncture. Infusing a chemotherapeutic agent through a catheter in that vein could result in leakage of the agent through the venipuncture site and subsequent tissue damage.

Also avoid extremities with compromised circulation as a result of lymphedema, phlebitis, fractures, or other conditions. Avoid using veins in the antecubital fossa, wrist, and hands; extravasation in these areas can destroy nerves and tendons, affecting the patient's function and mobility.

Once a patent line has been established, wash your hands and put on latex gloves and a nonpermeable long-sleeved gown with cuffs. Then administer the chemotherapeutic agent. Some nonvesicant agents may be given by the two-syringe method. This method involves saline flushes before and after administration of the chemotherapeutic agent. To employ the two-syringe method, flush the venous access device with normal saline solution in a syringe. Remove the saline syringe, attach the syringe with the chemotherapeutic agent, and administer the agent at the prescribed rate. At the completion of the push, reattach the saline syringe and flush the device again.

When administering a vesicant chemotherapeutic agent by IV push, do so through a compatible, running IV line and check for a blood return every 2 to 3 ml. An absence of subcutaneous swelling, pain, or burning in the area and the presence of a blood return indicate catheter patency.

When administering a vesicant agent by a short-term (15 to 30 minutes) piggyback infusion, check for a blood return at the beginning and end of the infusion. For a continuous infusion of a vesicant agent, check for a blood return before starting therapy and then again every hour.

Continuous infusions of vesicant chemotherapeutic agents are generally administered through a central venous access device to reduce the risk of extravasation. When given in combination with other agents, vesicants may be administered first or last, depending on facility policy. After the chemotherapy has been administered, dispose of used supplies in a chemotherapy waste container, according to your facility's policy. Caregivers who administer chemotherapeutic agents in the home also need to follow rigid guidelines for the safe handling and disposal of the drug, supplies, and linens contaminated with an agent or the patient's body fluids, which may also contain the chemotherapeutic agent.

Complications

In addition to monitoring for and trying to prevent numerous drug-specific complications of chemotherapy, you'll need to pay particular attention to preventing extravasation and watching for hypersensitivity reactions. (See *Preventing adverse reactions of chemotherapy*.)

EXTRAVASATION. Vesicant and nonvesicant agents may infiltrate into surrounding tissues. If a nonvesicant agent infiltrates, stop the infusion (or bolus injection). The venous access device may need to be removed. Monitor the area for edema, changes in color, or other signs of local tissue damage.

If a vesicant agent infiltrates, it may destroy tissue or cause tissue necrosis. When a vesicant extravasation occurs, stop the agent immediately. If extravasation occurs, prompt treatment and careful follow-up for several weeks are critical. (See *Preventing and managing extravasation,* pages 251 and 252.)

HYPERSENSITIVITY REACTIONS. Hypersensitivity reactions represent serious and potentially life-threatening adverse effects of chemotherapy. A hypersensitivity reaction occurs in response to an exposure to a chemotherapeutic agent identified by the immune system as an antigen. That exposure, in turn, triggers antibody production and subsequent allergic response. Symptoms include urticaria, redness, pruritus, shortness of breath, wheezing, stridor, facial swelling, hypotension, cyanosis, and loss of consciousness.

CLINICAL PEARLS

Preventing adverse reactions of chemotherapy

Chemotherapeutic agents can be highly toxic and cause numerous adverse reactions. This chart explains how the patient can prevent common adverse reactions of chemotherapy and nursing interventions for those reactions.

ADVERSE REACTION	PREVENTIVE MEASURES	NURSING INTERVENTIONS
Alopecia May occur suddenly, 10 to 21 days after start of therapy	Patient should: • avoid using scalp tourniquets if disease originates with or metastasizes to the scalp. • keep head covered to prevent heat loss in the winter and sunburn in the summer.	• Inform the patient that alopecia may affect the scalp, eyebrows, eyelashes, and body hair and that hair will regrow when chemotherapy ends.
Anemia Dizziness, fatigue, pallor and shortness of breath after minimal exertion; may develop slowly over several courses of treatment	Patient should: • rest more frequently and increase dietary intake of iron-rich foods. • take a multivitamin with iron as prescribed.	• Monitor patient's hematocrit, hemoglobin level, RBC count. Remember, dehydration from nausea, vomiting, or anorexia may cause false-normal hematocrit readings. • Be prepared to administer a blood transfusion to a symptomatic patient. • Plan patient teaching to include bone marrow suppression, blood counts, potential sites of infection, and personal hygiene.
Leukopenia Low granulocyte count, especially below 1,000/mm^3	Patient should: • observe good hygiene. • learn signs and symptoms of infection: fever, cough, sore throat, burning sensation on urination. • avoid crowds and people with colds or flu during blood count nadir (usually 7 to 14 days after drug administration). • avoid fresh fruit, fresh flowers, and plants. • learn to take own temperature regularly.	• Watch for blood count nadir, the point of greatest risk. • Plan patient teaching to include bone marrow suppression, blood counts, potential sites of infection, and good hygiene. • As ordered, carry out risk-reduction treatment with colony-stimulating factors.

(continued)

Preventing adverse reactions of chemotherapy
(continued)

ADVERSE REACTION	PREVENTIVE MEASURES	NURSING INTERVENTIONS
Nausea and vomiting Occurrence and severity varying with the agent and the patient	Patient should: • avoid fatty and greasy foods. • eat small frequent meals. • avoid unpleasant sights, tastes, and odors. • consider music therapy.	• Watch for electrolyte imbalance. • Offer clear liquid diet if vomiting is severe. • Plan on use of an antiemetic for 3 to 5 days.
Stomatitis Most commonly on oral mucosa; symptoms may be mild or severe and debilitating	Patient should: • begin preventive mouth care before chemotherapy, as taught, to provide comfort and decrease symptom severity.	• Provide therapeutic mouth care, including topical antibiotics if prescribed.
Thrombocytopenia Bleeding gums, increased bruising or petechiae, hypermenorrhea, tarry stools, hematuria, and coffee ground–like vomitus	Patient should: • report sudden headaches. • avoid cuts and bruises, and use a pediatric toothbrush and an electric razor. • use a stool softener to prevent colonic irritation or bleeding. • avoid using rectal thermometer or receiving IM injections.	• Watch platelet count: below 50,000/mm³, the patient risks excessive bleeding; below 20,000/mm³, he's at severe risk for excessive bleeding and may need a platelet transfusion. • Plan patient teaching to include bone marrow suppression, blood counts, potential sites of infection, and personal hygiene.

Chemotherapeutic agents known to cause hypersensitivity reactions include L-asparaginase, cisplatin, procarbazine, bleomycin, paclitaxel, teniposide, melphalan, and anthracycline antibiotics, such as doxorubicin and daunorubicin. Discontinue administration at the first sign of symptoms, and notify the doctor. Don't leave the patient alone; symptoms can progress quickly.

Emergency measures may need to be instituted. Assess the patient continuously, and reassure the patient and family. If the offending chemotherapeutic agent is essential for treatment, consideration should be given to substituting a similar agent, increasing the dilution of the agent, administering the agent over a longer period of time, giving the patient an antihistamine or corticosteroid before administration of the chemotherapeutic agent, or desensitizing the patient to the agent.

CLINICAL PEARLS

Preventing and managing extravasation

Extravasation—the infiltration of a vesicant drug into the surrounding tissue—can result from a punctured vein or from leakage around a venipuncture site. If vesicant drugs or fluids extravasate, severe local tissue damage may result. This may cause prolonged healing, infection, cosmetic disfigurement, and loss of function, and may necessitate multiple debridements and possibly amputation.

Preventing extravasation
To avoid extravasation when giving vesicants, adhere strictly to proper administration techniques and follow these guidelines:
• Don't use an existing IV line unless its patency is assured. Perform a new venipuncture to ensure correct needle placement and vein patency.
• Select the site carefully. Use a distal vein that allows successive proximal venipunctures. To avoid tendon and nerve damage through possible extravasation, avoid using the dorsum of the hand. Also avoid the wrist and digits (they're hard to immobilize) and areas previously damaged or with compromised circulation.
• If you need to probe for a vein, you may cause trauma. Stop and begin again at another site.
• Start the infusion with D_5W or 0.9% NaCl solution.
• Use a transparent film dressing to allow inspection.
• Check for extravasation before starting the infusion. Apply a tourniquet above the needle to occlude the vein and see if the flow continues. If the flow stops, the solution isn't infiltrating. Another method is to lower the IV container and watch for blood backflow. This is less reliable because the needle may have punc-

tured the opposite vein wall yet still rests partially in the vein. Flush the needle to ensure patency. If swelling occurs at the IV site, the solution is infiltrating.
• Give by slow IV push through a free-flowing IV line or by small-volume infusion (50 to 100 ml).
• During administration, observe the infusion site for erythema or infiltration. Tell the patient to report burning, stinging, pruritus, or temperature changes.
• After drug administration, instill several milliliters of 0.9% NaCl solution to flush the drug from the vein and to preclude drug leakage when the needle is removed.
• Give vesicants after the IV is tested with saline and before manipulations dislodge the needle.
• Avoid using an infusion pump to administer vesicants. A pump infuses even if infiltration occurs.

Treating extravasation
Extravasation of vesicant drugs requires emergency treatment. Follow your facility's protocol. Essential steps include:
• Stop the IV flow, aspirate the remaining drug in the catheter, and remove the IV line, unless you need the needle to infiltrate the antidote.
• Estimate the amount of extravasated solution and notify the doctor.
• Instill the appropriate antidote according to facility protocol.
• Elevate the extremity.
• Record the extravasation site, the patient's symptoms, the estimated amount of infiltrated solution, and the treatment. Include the time you notified the doctor and the doctor's name. Continue documenting the appearance of the site and associated symptoms.

(continued)

Preventing and managing extravasation *(continued)*

- Follow facility protocol, and apply either ice packs or warm compresses to the affected area. Ice is applied to all extravasated areas for 15 to 20 minutes every 4 to 6 hours for about 3 days. However, for etoposide and vinca alkaloids, heat is applied.
- If skin breakdown occurs, apply dressings, as ordered.
- If severe tissue damage occurs, plastic surgery and physical therapy may be needed.

Teaching the patient

The patient needs to be kept well informed about the risks and benefits of treatment. Explain adverse effects of each agent and how those effects might be prevented or treated. Anticipating that the patient's blood cell count will decrease during therapy, teach the patient how to avoid infection, recognize early signs and symptoms of infection, and report them immediately.

Because chemotherapy often leads to lowered platelet counts, the patient may be at increased risk for bleeding. Review the patient's daily activities, and encourage appropriate lifestyle adjustments that might reduce the risk of bleeding while also helping to maintain the patient's independence. Tell the patient that infection and bleeding may still occur despite compliance with these precautions.

Caregivers should be involved in all education efforts. However, the patient has the right to withhold information about any aspect of his disease from them. A patient may have difficulty if a caregiver becomes overinvolved. If a caregiver experiences difficulty in coping, refer the person to the appropriate support groups.

Documentation

Documentation of chemotherapy should include all aspects of the treatment, including these points:
- pretreatment vital signs, allergies, general condition, and mental status
- pertinent laboratory values
- learning needs and patient teaching done
- aspects of care related to age or cultural factors
- names and dosages of the agents

- type and gauge of the catheter
- sequence of administration for combination therapy
- IV solution coadministered with the chemotherapy
- presence of a blood return during administration
- appearance and location of the site and the patient's response to treatment after the IV has been discontinued
- complications that occurred and what you did about them
- issues discussed by the patient or caregiver that require nursing intervention.

IV

INTRAVENOUS DRUGS AND SOLUTIONS

abciximab

ReoPro

Pregnancy Risk Category: C

INDICATIONS & DOSAGES

Adjunct to percutaneous translumi-nal coronary angioplasty (PTCA) or atherectomy for the prevention of acute cardiac ischemic complications in patients at high risk for abrupt clo-sure of the treated coronary vessel—
Adults: 0.25 mg/kg as an IV bolus administered 10 to 60 minutes be-fore start of PTCA or atherectomy, followed by a continuous IV infu-sion of 10 mcg/minute for 12 hours.

Note: Abciximab should be used with heparin and aspirin.

PREPARATION & STORAGE

Supplied in 5-ml vials at a concentra-tion of 2 mg/ml.

Withdraw 4.5 ml of abciximab for continuous IV infusion through a sterile, nonpyrogenic, low protein-binding 0.2- or 0.22-micron filter. Mix with 250 ml of sterile 0.9% NaCl solution or D_5W.

Inspect solution for particulate matter before administration and discard if visible opaque particles are found. Do not freeze or shake. Store drug at 36° to 46°F (2° to 8°C).

Incompatibility
None reported; however, no other medication should be added to the infusion solution.

ADMINISTRATION

Direct injection: Withdraw the neces-sary amount through a sterile, non-pyrogenic, low protein-binding 0.2- or 0.22-micron filter into syringe.
Continuous infusion: Infuse at a rate of 10 mcg/minute for 12 hours via a continuous infusion pump equipped with an in-line filter. Discard unused portion at the end of the 12-hour in-fusion.

Administer drug in a separate IV line; no other medication should be added to the infusion solution.

CONTRAINDICATIONS & CAUTIONS

• Contraindicated in patients with hypersensitivity to any component of drug or to murine proteins; in those with active internal bleeding, recent GI or GU bleeding of clinical signifi-cance, history of CVA within past 2 years or CVA with significant resid-ual neurologic deficit, bleeding diathesis, thrombocytopenia (less than 100,000/mm^3), recent (within 6 weeks) major surgery or trauma, intracranial neoplasm, arteriovenous malformation or aneurysm, severe uncontrolled hypertension, or histo-ry of vasculitis.
• Contraindicated when oral antico-agulants have been administered within past 7 days unless PT is 1.2 times control or less.
• Contraindicated with use of IV dextran before PTCA or intent to use it during PTCA.
• Use cautiously in patients at in-creased risk for bleeding, including those who weigh below 165 lb (75 kg), are over age 65, or are re-ceiving thrombolytic agents. Condi-tions that also increase the patient's risk of bleeding include PTCA with-in 12 hours of onset of symptoms for acute MI, prolonged PTCA (last-ing more than 70 minutes), or failed PTCA.

SPECIAL CONSIDERATIONS

• Avoid noncompressible IV sites.
• Institute bleeding precautions. Maintain patient on bed rest for 6 to 8 hours following sheath removal or discontinuation of drug infusion, whichever is later. Minimize or avoid, if possible, arterial and venous punctures; IM injections; use of uri-nary catheters, nasogastric tubes, or automatic blood pressure cuffs; and nasotracheal intubation.
• Consider saline or heparin locks for blood drawing.
• Provide gentle care when remov-ing dressings.

• Document and monitor vascular puncture sites.
• Before infusion, measure platelet count, PT, and APTT. Monitor platelet count, activated clotting time, and APTT during and following treatment.

acetazolamide sodium

Diamox♦

Pregnancy Risk Category: C

INDICATIONS & DOSAGES
To rapidly lower intraocular pressure or when patient is unable to take drug orally—
Adults: 500 mg IV May repeat IV dose in 2 to 4 hours, if necessary. Therapy is usually continued with 125 to 250 mg PO q 4 to 6 hours, based on patient's response.
Acute glaucoma—
Children: 5 to 10 mg/kg IV q 6 hours.
As a diuretic—
Adults: 5 mg/kg IV p.r.n.
Children: 5 mg/kg or 150 mg/m² IV once daily in morning for 1 or 2 days alternated with a drug-free day.

PREPARATION & STORAGE
Available as a powder in a 500-mg vial. Reconstitute with 5 ml of sterile water for injection to provide a solution containing no more than 100 mg/ml, preferably before use. Alternatively, refrigerate reconstituted drug and use within 24 hours.

Incompatibility
Incompatible with multivitamins.

ADMINISTRATION
Direct injection: Using a 21G or 23G needle, inject 100 to 500 mg/ minute into a large vein.

CONTRAINDICATIONS & CAUTIONS
• Contraindicated in patients with hepatic or renal disease or dysfunction; hyponatremia, hypokalemia, or hyperchloremic acidosis; or adrenal

gland failure and in those with long-term therapy for chronic noncongestive angle-closure glaucoma.
• Use cautiously in patients with sulfonamide sensitivity.
• Use cautiously in patients with respiratory acidosis, emphysema, or chronic pulmonary disease because of increased risk of respiratory acidosis.
• Give cautiously in patients with diabetes mellitus because glucose levels may become elevated and in those with gout and renal calculi because drug may exacerbate these conditions.

SPECIAL CONSIDERATIONS
• Give drug under continuous medical supervision. IV administration reduces intraocular pressure rapidly.
• Carefully monitor intake and output and serum electrolytes, especially potassium.
• Weigh patient daily. Elderly patients are especially susceptible to excessive diuresis.
• Monitor arterial blood gases of patients with COPD for respiratory acidosis.

acyclovir sodium (acycloguanosine)

Avirax◇, Zovirax♦

Pregnancy Risk Category: C

INDICATIONS & DOSAGES
Mucocutaneous herpes simplex virus (HSV)-I and HSV-II infections in immunocompromised patients with normal renal function—
Adults: 5 mg/kg q 8 hours for 7 days.
Infants and children under age 12: 250 mg/m² q 8 hours for 7 days.
Initial herpes genitalis in nonimmunocompromised patients with normal renal function—
Adults: 5 mg/kg q 8 hours for 5 days.

Children under age 12:
250 mg/m^2 q 8 hours for 5 days.
Herpes simplex encephalitis—
Adults: 10 mg/kg q 8 hours for 10 days.
Children ages 6 months to 12 years: 500 mg/m^2 q 8 hours for 10 days.
Varicella zoster in immunocompromised patients—
Adults: 10 mg/kg q 8 hours for 7 days (with normal renal function).
Children under age 12:
500 mg/m^2 q 8 hours for 7 days.
   Note: Dosage in renal failure is based on creatinine clearance. For adults, give 50% of dose q 24 hours if clearance is less than 10 ml/minute; 100% of dose q 24 hours if it is 10 to 25 ml/minute; 100% of dose q 12 hours if it is 25 to 50 ml/minute; and 100% of dose q 8 hours if clearance exceeds 50 ml/minute.

PREPARATION & STORAGE
Available as a powder supplied in 10- and 20-ml sterile vials (equivalent to 500 and 1,000 mg of acyclovir, respectively). Store at 59° to 77° F (15° to 25° C). To reconstitute, add 10 ml of sterile water for injection to the 10-ml vial and 20 ml to the 20-ml vial to yield a concentration of 50 mg/ml.
   If refrigerated, reconstituted solution may form a precipitate that dissolves when warmed to room temperature. Once reconstituted, drug should be used within 12 hours.
   For intermittent infusion, dilute reconstituted drug with commercially available electrolyte and glucose solutions and use within 24 hours. Dilute with at least 70 ml for a concentration of 7 mg/ml or less. Greater concentrations can cause phlebitis.

Incompatibility
Drug may precipitate when combined with parabens. Also incompatible with biological or colloidal solutions and idarubicin hydrochloride.

ADMINISTRATION
Intermittent infusion: Administer over at least 1 hour using an intermittent infusion device or an IV line containing a free-flowing, compatible solution. Shorter infusion time risks nephrotoxicity.

CONTRAINDICATIONS & CAUTIONS
• Contraindicated in acyclovir hypersensitivity.
• Use cautiously in patients with previous CNS reaction to cytotoxic drugs or with neurologic abnormalities.
• Also use cautiously in renal impairment or dehydration.
• Use cautiously in serious hepatic disease, electrolyte imbalances, or significant hypoxia.

SPECIAL CONSIDERATIONS
• Use drug for infusion only. Avoid rapid infusion or bolus IV injection.
• To treat drug overdose, maintain sufficient urine flow to prevent precipitation in renal tubules. Recommended urine output is 500 ml/g or more of drug infused. Acyclovir can be removed by hemodialysis.
• Carefully monitor intake and output. Because maximum drug concentration occurs in kidneys during first 2 hours of infusion, ensure that adequate hydration and urine output is maintained during this period.
• Concentrated solutions (10 mg/ml or more) may be associated with a higher incidence of phlebitis.
• Notify doctor if serum creatinine level does not return to normal within a few days. He may increase hydration, adjust dose, or stop therapy.

adenosine

Adenocard

Pregnancy Risk Category: C

INDICATIONS & DOSAGES
Conversion of paroxysmal supraventricular tachycardia (PSVT) to sinus rhythm—

Adults: 6 mg IV by rapid bolus injection (over 1 to 2 seconds). If PSVT is not eliminated in 1 to 2 minutes, give 12 mg by rapid IV push. Repeat 12-mg dose once if necessary.

Note: Adenosine is useful for treating PSVT associated with accessory bypass tracts (Wolff-Parkinson-White syndrome).

PREPARATION & STORAGE
Supplied in vials containing 6 mg/2 ml. Store at controlled room temperature (59° to 86° F [15° to 30° C]). Do not refrigerate.

Observe solution for crystals, which may appear if solution has been refrigerated. If crystals are visible, gently warm solution to room temperature. Do not use solutions that are not clear. Discard unused drug because it lacks preservatives.

Incompatibility
Do not mix with other drugs.

ADMINISTRATION
Direct injection: Rapid IV injection is necessary for drug action. Administer over 1 to 2 seconds directly into a peripheral vein if possible; if using an IV line, use the most proximal port and follow the injection with a rapid saline flush to hasten drug delivery to systemic circulation.

CONTRAINDICATIONS & CAUTIONS
• Contraindicated in patients with known hypersensitivity to drug.
• Avoid use in known or suspected bronchoconstrictive or bronchospastic lung disease such as asthma. Use with caution in obstructive lung disease without bronchoconstriction such as emphysema.
• Also contraindicated in patients with atrial flutter, atrial fibrillation, and ventricular tachycardia because drug is ineffective in the treatment of these arrhythmias.
• Adenosine may briefly induce a first-, second-, or third-degree heart block. Thus, it is contraindicated in patients with second- or third-degree

heart block or sick sinus syndrome, unless the patient has an artificial pacemaker. Patients in whom significant block develops after a dose of adenosine should not receive additional doses.

SPECIAL CONSIDERATIONS
• Single doses over 12 mg are not recommended.
• Bolus dosages of 6 or 12 mg usually do not elicit systemic hemodynamic effects.
• Drug must reach the systemic circulation in sufficient quantity to provide an adequate therapeutic effect. Therefore, rapid IV bolus injection is necessary.
• Adverse effects usually resolve quickly when injection is discontinued.
• Give drug only under medical supervision with continuous ECG monitoring. Be alert for arrhythmias.

aldesleukin (interleukin-2, IL-2)

Proleukin
Pregnancy Risk Category: C

INDICATIONS & DOSAGES
Metastatic renal cell carcinoma—
Adults age 18 and over:
600,000 IU/kg (0.037 mg/kg) infused over 15 minutes q 8 hours for 5 days (total of 14 doses). After a 9-day rest, repeat sequence for another 14 doses. Repeat courses may be administered after a rest period of at least 7 weeks from hospital discharge. Or investigationally, 18 million IU (1.1 mg)/m^2 of body surface area by 24-hour continuous infusion for 5 days; repeat in 1 week.

PREPARATION & STORAGE
Available as a powder for injection containing 22 million IU (1.3 mg)/vial. Reconstitute by adding 1.2 ml of sterile water for injection; the resultant solution contains 18 million

IU (1.1 mg)/ml. To avoid excessive foaming, direct water diluent toward side of vial and swirl gently; do not shake. The reconstituted drug should be particle-free and colorless to slightly yellow.

To dilute, add the ordered dose of reconstituted drug to 50 ml of 5% dextrose injection, preferably in a plastic container for more consistent drug delivery. Store powder for injection and reconstituted solutions in the refrigerator. After reconstitution and dilution, drug must be administered within 48 hours. Discard unused drug. Return solution to room temperature before administration.

Incompatibility
Incompatible with albumin, bacteriostatic water for injection, and 0.9% NaCl solution. Avoid mixing with other drugs.

ADMINISTRATION
Intermittent infusion: Infuse diluted dose over 15 minutes. Use of an in-line filter is not recommended.
Continuous infusion: Give diluted solution over 24 hours (investigational).

CONTRAINDICATIONS & CAUTIONS
• Contraindicated in hypersensitivity to drug or components of the formulation.
• Contraindicated in patients with abnormal results from thallium stress test or pulmonary function tests or in those with organ allografts.
• Retreatment is contraindicated in patients who experience the following toxicities: pericardial tamponade, disturbances in cardiac rhythm that are uncontrolled or unresponsive to intervention; sustained ventricular tachycardia (five consecutive beats or more); chest pain accompanied by ECG changes consistent with MI or angina; renal dysfunction requiring dialysis for more than 72 hours; coma or toxic psychosis lasting more than 48 hours; seizures that are repetitive or difficult to control; is-

chemia or perforation of the bowel; or GI bleeding requiring surgery.
• *Use with extreme caution* in patients with history of seizure disorders or cardiac or pulmonary disease.
• Drug should be used only in a hospital setting under the direction of a doctor experienced in the use of chemotherapeutic agents. An intensive care facility and intensive care or cardiopulmonary specialists must be available.
• Because fluid management or administration of pressor agents may be essential to treat capillary leak syndrome (CLS), use cautiously in patients who require large volumes of fluid (such as hypercalcemic patients).

SPECIAL CONSIDERATIONS
• Be prepared to adjust dosage of other drugs patient may be taking to compensate for aldesleukin-induced renal and hepatic impairment.
• Patients should be neurologically stable with a negative computed tomography scan for CNS metastases.
• Severe anemia or thrombocytopenia may occur. Administer packed RBCs or platelets, as ordered.
• In cases of overdose, treat continuing symptoms supportively. Life-threatening toxicities have been ameliorated with IV dexamethasone, which may result in loss of therapeutic effect from aldesleukin.
• Withhold dose and notify doctor if moderate to severe lethargy or somnolence develops because continued administration can result in coma.
• Drug has been associated with CLS, a condition that results from the loss of vascular tone in which plasma proteins and fluids escape into the extravascular space. Mean arterial blood pressure begins to drop within 2 to 12 hours of treatment; edema and effusions may be severe, and death can result from hypoperfusion of major organs.
• Treat CLS with careful monitoring of fluid status, pulse, mental status, urine output, and organ perfusion.

Central venous pressure monitoring is necessary.

alteplase, recombinant alteplase, tissue plasminogen activator (t-PA)

Activase, Activase rt-PA◇

Pregnancy Risk Category: C

INDICATIONS & DOSAGES

Destruction of coronary artery thrombi in acute MI (3-hour infusion)—
Adults weighing 143 lb (65 kg) and over: 100 mg over 3 hours, with 60 mg given in first hour (6 to 10 mg in first 1 to 2 minutes), 20 mg in second hour, and 20 mg in third hour. Do not exceed dosage; doses above 100 mg have been linked with intracranial bleeding.
Adults weighing below 143 lb: 1.25 mg/kg over 3 hours, with 60% of dose given in first hour (10% in first 1 to 2 minutes) and rest over next 2 hours.
Accelerated dosing for acute MI—
Adults weighing more than 148 lb (67 kg): total dosage of 100 mg given as follows: 15 mg by rapid IV bolus over 1 to 2 minutes, then 50 mg IV over the next 30 minutes, followed by remaining 35 mg IV over 1 hour.
Adults weighing 148 lb or less: initially, 15 mg by rapid IV bolus over 1 to 2 minutes; followed by 0.75 mg/kg (not to exceed 50 mg) over the next 30 minutes; then 0.5 mg/kg (not to exceed 35 mg) over the next hour.
Acute ischemic stroke within 3 hours of symptom onset—
Adults: 0.9 mg/kg (maximum, 90 mg) IV infusion over 1 hour, with 10% of the dose given initially as an IV bolus over 1 minute.
Lysis of acute pulmonary emboli—
Adults: 100 mg over 2 hours.

PREPARATION & STORAGE
Available as lyophilized powder in 20-, 50-, and 100-mg vials. Store at room temperature or refrigerate. Reconstitute just before injection. Using an 18G needle, reconstitute to 1 mg/ml by adding 50 ml or 100 ml of preservative-free, sterile water for injection, provided by manufacturer. (Do not use bacteriostatic water for injection.) Aim diluent at lyophilized cake and expect slight foaming. Let vial stand for several minutes.
    If necessary, dilute drug to 0.5 mg/ml in glass bottles or polyvinyl chloride bag. For 50-ml vial, add 50 ml of 0.9% NaCl or D₅W; for 100-ml vial, add 100 ml. Avoid undue agitation. Diluted solution remains stable for 8 hours at room temperature.

Incompatibility
Do not mix with other drugs.

ADMINISTRATION
Direct injection: Bolus doses can be administered over 1 to 2 minutes.
Continuous infusion: Infuse diluted solution at recommended rate.

CONTRAINDICATIONS & CAUTIONS
• Contraindicated in patients with evidence of intracranial hemorrhage, suspicion of subarachnoid hemorrhage, seizure at onset of stroke, internal bleeding, aneurysm, arteriovenous malformation, bleeding diathesis, history of CVA, brain tumor, CNS surgery or trauma in previous 2 months, or systolic blood pressure above 179 mm Hg or diastolic blood pressure above 109 mm Hg.
• Use cautiously in patients with acute pericarditis, cerebrovascular disease, diabetic hemorrhagic retinopathy, significant hepatic disease, risk of left-sided heart thrombus, marked hypertension, subacute bacterial endocarditis, septic thrombophlebitis, or an occluded arteriovenous cannula at an infected site.
• Also use cautiously in patients over age 75; within 10 days after GI or GU bleeding, major surgery, or trau-

ma; and during oral anticoagulant therapy.
• Safety and efficacy in children have not been established.

SPECIAL CONSIDERATIONS
• Recanalization of occluded coronary arteries and improvement of heart function are time-dependent phenomena and require initiation of treatment within 6 to 12 hours after onset of symptoms.
• To prevent new clot formation, give heparin during or after alteplase infusion, if ordered. Do not give heparin when treating acute ischemic stroke with t-PA.
• Avoid IM injections because of high risk of bleeding into muscle. Also avoid turning and moving the patient excessively during infusion.
• Treatment of acute ischemic stroke must be initiated within 3 hours of symptom onset.
• If possible, obtain coagulation studies (PT, PTT, INR, fibrin split products) before starting therapy.
• Have antiarrhythmic agents readily available, and carefully monitor ECG.
• If unable to stop severe bleeding with local pressure, discontinue alteplase and heparin infusions.
• Avoid venipuncture and arterial puncture during therapy because of increased risk of bleeding. If arterial puncture is necessary, select a site on an arm and apply pressure for 30 minutes afterward. Also use pressure dressings, sandbags, or ice packs on recent puncture sites to prevent bleeding.

amifostine

Ethyol

Pregnancy Risk Category: C

INDICATIONS & DOSAGES
Reduction of the cumulative renal toxicity associated with repeated administration of cisplatin in patients
with advanced ovarian cancer or non-small-cell lung cancer—
Adults: 910 mg/m^2/day as a 15-minute IV infusion, starting 30 minutes before chemotherapy. If hypotension occurs and blood pressure does not return to normal within 5 minutes after treatment is stopped, subsequent cycles should use a dose of 740 mg/m^2.

PREPARATION & STORAGE
Supplied as a sterile lyophilized powder mixture in 10-ml single-use vials requiring reconstitution for IV infusion. Each single-use vial contains 500 mg of amifostine (anhydrous basis) and 500 mg of mannitol. Reconstitute with 9.7 ml of normal saline; reconstituted solution is stable for up to 5 hours at room temperature (about 77° F [25°C]) or up to 24 hours if refrigerated (35° to 46° F [1.5° to 8° C]).
    Do not use solution if cloudiness or precipitate is observed.

Incompatibility
Do not mix with other solutions. Compatibilities with solutions other than 0.9% NaCl for injection are unknown.

ADMINISTRATION
Intermittent infusion: Infuse over 15 minutes.

CONTRAINDICATIONS & CAUTIONS
• Contraindicated in patients hypersensitive to aminothiol compounds or mannitol.
• Do not use drug in patients receiving chemotherapy for potentially curable malignancies, except for those involved in clinical studies.
• Contraindicated in hypotensive or dehydrated patients.
• Contraindicated in patients receiving antihypertensive drugs that cannot be stopped during the 24 hours preceding amifostine administration.
• Use cautiously in elderly patients, in those with preexisting CV or cerebrovascular conditions, and when nausea, vomiting, or hypotension

may be more likely to have serious consequences.
• Safety and effectiveness in children have not been established.

SPECIAL CONSIDERATIONS
• Do not infuse for more than 15 minutes; a longer infusion has been associated with a higher incidence of adverse reactions.
• Patient should be adequately hydrated before administration.
• Keep patient in a supine position during infusion.
• Administer antiemetic medications before and in conjunction with amifostine administration.
• The most common symptom of overdosage is hypotension, which should be treated with supportive measures.
• Monitor blood pressure every 5 minutes during infusion.
• Monitor serum calcium levels in patients at risk for hypocalcemia such as those with nephrotic syndrome.

amikacin sulfate

Amikin◆

Pregnancy Risk Category: D

INDICATIONS & DOSAGES
Septicemia, peritonitis, and severe burn, bone, joint, respiratory tract, skin, and soft-tissue infections caused by susceptible organisms—
Adults and children with normal renal function: 15 mg/kg/day in equally divided doses at 8- or 12-hour intervals for 7 to 10 days, not to exceed 1.5 g/day.
Adults and children with renal impairment: loading dose, 7.5 mg/kg. Subsequent dosage based on serum levels and degree of impairment.
Neonates with normal renal function: initially, 10 mg/kg, then 7.5 mg/kg q 12 hours.

PREPARATION & STORAGE
Supplied as a 50-mg/ml concentration in 2-ml vials or as a 250 mg/ml concentration in 2- and 4-ml vials.
    For infusion, add 500 mg of amikacin to 100 to 200 ml of 0.9% NaCl or D₅W. All solutions remain stable for 24 hours at room temperature. Yellowing of solution does not indicate loss of potency.

Incompatibility
Incompatible with amphotericin B, bacitracin, cisplatin, vancomycin, cephalothin, cephapirin, heparin, phenytoin, thiopental, and vitamin B complex with C. Manufacturer recommends that amikacin not be mixed with other drugs.

ADMINISTRATION
Intermittent infusion: Using a 21G to 23G needle, infuse diluted drug over 30 to 60 minutes in children and adults and over 1 to 2 hours in infants.

CONTRAINDICATIONS & CAUTIONS
• Contraindicated in aminoglycoside hypersensitivity.
• Give cautiously in dehydration and renal impairment because of increased risk of toxicity, in eighth cranial nerve damage because of risk of ototoxicity, and in myasthenia gravis or Parkinson's disease because drug can cause neuromuscular blockade.
• Give cautiously to premature infants, neonates, and the elderly because of increased risk of toxicity.

SPECIAL CONSIDERATIONS
• Obtain periodic peak and trough levels, and adjust dosage as ordered.
• Drug may contain sulfites.
• To treat drug overdose, use hemodialysis or peritoneal dialysis to remove drug, if ordered. Exchange transfusions may be considered for neonates.
• Evaluate patient's hearing before and during treatment.
• Be alert to loss of balance in ambulatory patients if therapy is prolonged (over 2 weeks).

• Keep patient well hydrated to reduce risk of nephrotoxicity; measure intake and output. Monitor urine for decreased specific gravity.

aminocaproic acid

Amicar◆

Pregnancy Risk Category: C

INDICATIONS & DOSAGES

Life-threatening hemorrhage caused by systemic hyperfibrinolysis associated with complications of cardiac surgery and portacaval shunt; cancer of the lung, prostate, cervix, or stomach; abruptio placentae; hematologic disorders such as aplastic anemia; and urinary fibrinolysis associated with severe trauma, shock, and anoxia—
Adults: initially, 4 to 5 g infused over 1 hour, then 1 to 1.25 g hourly. Alternatively, continuous infusion of 1 g/hour for about 8 hours to maintain plasma level of 130 mcg/ml. Maximum dosage, 30 g/day.
Children: 100 mg/kg or 3 g/m^2 body surface area during first hour, then continuous infusion of 33 mg/kg/hour or 1 g/m^2/hour. Maximum dosage, 18 g/m^2/day.

PREPARATION & STORAGE

Available in 250 mg/ml solutions containing 5 g (20 ml) or 24 g (96 ml) with benzyl alcohol. Further dilute with 0.9% NaCl, D$_5$W, lactated Ringer's solution, or sterile water for injection. (Do not use sterile water for injection when patient has subarachnoid hemorrhage.) Store at 59° to 86° F (15° to 30° C); avoid freezing.

Incompatibility
Incompatible with fructose solution.

ADMINISTRATION

Continuous infusion: Slowly infuse 4 to 5 g of diluted drug during first hour. Then infuse 1 g/hour to maintain serum level of 130 mcg/ml.

CONTRAINDICATIONS & CAUTIONS

• Contraindicated in active intravascular clotting associated with possible fibrinolysis and bleeding as a primary disorder.
• Also contraindicated in DIC unless used with heparin. Otherwise, drug could cause potentially fatal thrombi.
• Use cautiously in cardiac disorders because of possible hypotension and bradycardia, in renal disorders, in hepatic disease, and in patients predisposed to thrombosis.
• Also use cautiously in upper urinary tract bleeding because glomerular capillary thrombosis or clots in the renal pelvis and ureter could cause intrarenal obstruction.

SPECIAL CONSIDERATIONS

• Rapid infusion may induce hypotension and bradycardia.
• Drug has been used as antidote for alteplase, anistreplase, streptokinase, or urokinase; not beneficial in treating thrombocytopenia.
• Monitor coagulation studies, heart rhythm, and blood pressure. Notify doctor of change immediately.
• Guard against thrombophlebitis by using proper technique for needle insertion and positioning

aminophylline

Aminophyllin Injection◆
Pregnancy Risk Category: C

INDICATIONS & DOSAGES

Acute bronchial asthma and reversible bronchospasm associated with chronic bronchitis and emphysema—
Adults not currently receiving theophylline: initially, 6 mg/kg, followed by maintenance doses; for nonsmoking adults, 0.7 mg/kg/hour for first 12 hours, then 0.5 mg/kg/hour for next 12 hours; for elderly patients and those with cor pulmonale, 0.6 mg/kg/hour for first 12 hours, then 0.3 mg/kg/hour for next 12 hours; for patients with heart failure or liver failure,

0.5 mg/kg/hour for first 12 hours, then 0.1 to 0.2 mg/kg/hour for next 12 hours.
Children not currently receiving theophylline: initially, 6 mg/kg, followed by maintenance doses; for children ages 6 months to 9 years, 1.2 mg/kg/hour for first 12 hours, then 1 mg/kg/hour for next 12 hours; for children ages 9 to 16, 1 mg/kg/hour for first 12 hours, then 0.8 mg/kg/hour for next 12 hours.
Adults and children currently receiving theophylline: dosage form, amount, time, and administration rate of last theophylline dose determine initial dose. Ideally, initial dose deferred until serum theophylline level is obtained. When there is sufficient respiratory distress, a loading dose of 2.5 mg/kg may be given.

PREPARATION & STORAGE
Available as a 25 mg/ml solution in 10-ml (250 mg) and 20-ml (500 mg) ampules.
   Store containers at room temperature and protect from freezing and light. Inspect for precipitate and discoloration before use.

Incompatibility
Incompatible with amikacin sulfate, amiodarone, ascorbic acid, bleomycin sulfate, cephalothin sodium, cephapirin sodium, chlorpromazine hydrochloride, ciprofloxacin, clindamycin phosphate, codeine phosphate, corticotropin, dimenhydrinate hydrochloride, dobutamine hydrochloride, doxapram hydrochloride, doxorubicin hydrochloride, epinephrine hydrochloride, erythromycin gluceptate, fat emulsion 10%, fructose 10% in 0.9% NaCl, hydralazine hydrochloride, hydroxyzine hydrochloride, insulin (regular), invert sugar 10% in 0.9% NaCl injection, invert sugar 10% in water, levorphanol bitartrate, meperidine hydrochloride, methadone hydrochloride, methylprednisolone sodium succinate, morphine sulfate, naf-

cillin sodium, norepinephrine bitartrate, ondansetron hydrochloride, papaverine hydrochloride, penicillin G potassium, pentazocine lactate, phenobarbital sodium, phenytoin sodium, procaine hydrochloride, prochlorperazine edisylate, promazine hydrochloride, promethazine hydrochloride, vancomycin hydrochloride, verapamil hydrochloride, and vitamin B complex with C.

ADMINISTRATION
Direct injection: Give undiluted loading dose (25 mg/ml) slowly, not exceeding 25 mg/minute. Do not give through a central venous catheter. Rapid injection can be fatal.
Continuous infusion: For maintenance therapy, administer desired dose in a large volume (500 to 1,000 ml) of compatible solution. Adjust infusion rate to deliver prescribed amount each hour.

CONTRAINDICATIONS & CAUTIONS
• Contraindicated in hypersensitivity to theophylline, caffeine, theobromine, and other xanthine compounds.
• Use cautiously in severe cardiac disease, severe hypoxemia, hypertension, hyperthyroidism, peptic ulcer, diabetes mellitus, acute MI, and heart failure because drug may exacerbate symptoms.
• Use cautiously in neonates, elderly patients, and those with liver disease due to increased risk of toxicity.
• In prostatic enlargement, give cautiously because of increased risk of urine retention.
• Also give cautiously in cor pulmonale, prolonged fever, and febrile viral respiratory infections because of prolonged half-life of theophylline.

SPECIAL CONSIDERATIONS
• IV administration can cause vein irritation and burning. Dilute with compatible solution if necessary.
• In cases of overdose, stop drug immediately and provide supportive and symptomatic treatment. Avoid giving sympathomimetic drugs.

• Base dosage on lean body weight and serum theophylline level. Monitor serum trough level to manage regimen; monitor serum peak levels to assess for toxicity. Optimum therapeutic levels, 10 to 20 mcg/ml.
• Warn elderly patient that dizziness, a common adverse reaction, may occur at the start of therapy.

amiodarone hydrochloride

Cordarone◆

Pregnancy Risk Category: C

INDICATIONS & DOSAGES
Initiation of treatment and prophylaxis of frequently recurring ventricular fibrillation (VF) and hemodynamically unstable ventricular tachycardia (VT) in patients refractory to other therapy; in patients with VF or VT for whom oral amiodarone is indicated but who are unable to take oral medication—
Adults: initially, rapid loading infusion of 150 mg administered over first 10 minutes (15 mg/minute), then a slow loading phase of 1 mg/minute over 6 hours for a total of 360 mg, followed by a maintenance phase of 0.5 mg/minute for 18 hours for a total of 540 mg. After the first 24 hours, the maintenance infusion of 0.5 mg/minute should be continued (this may be increased to control arrhythmia). There is limited experience using IV amiodarone for more than 3 weeks.

PREPARATION & STORAGE
Available in 3-ml ampules at a concentration of 50 mg/ml. Store at room temperature and protect from light.
    IV amiodarone must be diluted before use. For rapid loading dose, dilute 150 mg of drug in 100 ml D_5W; for maintenance infusion, final concentrations can range from 1 to 6 mg/ml.

Incompatibility
Incompatible with quinidine gluconate, aminophylline, cefamandole nafate, cefazolin sodium, mezlocillin sodium, heparin sodium, and sodium bicarbonate.

ADMINISTRATION
Direct injection: Give initial bolus over 10 minutes (must be diluted in 100 ml of D_5W).
Continuous infusion: Must be administered by a volumetric infusion pump. Use central venous catheter when possible. An in-line filter should be used.

CONTRAINDICATIONS & CAUTIONS
• Pediatric dosage is not established.
• Contraindicated in amiodarone hypersensitivity, severe sinus bradycardia, and second- and third-degree AV block.
• Use cautiously in preexisting pulmonary disease and in the elderly because of possibly fatal cardiopulmonary effects.
• Monitor patient closely during loading phase.

SPECIAL CONSIDERATIONS
• In cases of overdose, provide symptomatic and supportive care. Monitor ECG and blood pressure. If needed, give an IV beta-adrenergic antagonist (such as isoproterenol) or assist with transvenous pacemaker insertion to treat bradycardia. Infuse IV fluids and place in the Trendelenburg position to correct hypotension. Also give an IV vasopressor or inotropic drugs (such as norepinephrine or dopamine) to improve tissue perfusion. Hemodialysis and peritoneal dialysis are *not* helpful.
• Monitor for dry eyes, halo vision, and photophobia. Recommend a sunscreen or sunglasses.
• Assess respiratory system for pulmonary toxicity.
• Monitor ECG status continuously for AV block, bradycardia, paradoxical arrhythmias, and prolonged QT segments.

ammonium chloride

Pregnancy Risk Category: B

INDICATIONS & DOSAGES
Metabolic alkalosis caused by chloride loss from vomiting, gastric suction, pyloric stenosis, or gastric fistula drainage; diuretic-induced chloride depletion—
Adults: dosage reflects severity of alkalosis and patient tolerance. It is calculated by amount of chloride deficit and estimated in milliequivalents. First, establish patient's estimated fluid volume by multiplying 20% of body weight in kilograms by serum chloride level. For example, in a patient weighing 154 lb (70 kg) with a chloride level of 94 mEq/ml, multiply 14 by 94 for a dosage of 1,316 mEq. One liter of 2.14% solution provides 400 mEq of ammonium and chloride ions.

PREPARATION & STORAGE
Prepare diluted solution by adding one or two vials (100 or 200 mEq) of aqueous ammonium chloride to 500 or 1,000 ml of 0.9% NaCl for injection. Also available as prepared solution in a 500-ml bottle containing 2.14 g/dl (0.4 mEq/ml).
    Solution may crystallize if stored at low temperature. Crystals will dissolve when solution is placed in warm water.

Incompatibility
Incompatible with alkalis and their carbonates, strong oxidizing agents such as potassium chloride, and dimenhydrinate, levorphanol tartrate, and methadone.

ADMINISTRATION
Continuous infusion: Infuse diluted solution at no more than 5 ml/minute to avoid pain, toxic effects, and local irritation. Infuse the 2.14% solution at 0.9 to 1.3 ml/minute (but always under 2 ml/minute). Start infusion at half the calculated rate to determine patient tolerance.

CONTRAINDICATIONS & CAUTIONS
• Contraindicated in hypersensitivity to drug, severe hepatic disease, and hepatic coma.
• Also contraindicated in primary respiratory acidosis because of risk of developing systemic acidosis.
• Use cautiously in pulmonary insufficiency and edema.

SPECIAL CONSIDERATIONS
• To treat drug overdose, stop drug and give potassium chloride IV or sodium bicarbonate IV for acidosis. Signs of overdose include arrhythmias, asterixis, bradycardia, coma, Kussmaul's respirations, pallor, local or generalized twitching, sweating, tonic seizures, and vomiting.
• Assess for pain at infusion site and adjust rate if necessary.
• To prevent acidosis, determine serum electrolyte levels during therapy.
• Monitor input and output, edema, weight, and urine pH during therapy. Expect diuresis for the first 2 days.
• Assess respiratory pattern frequently.

amobarbital sodium

Amytal Sodium◆

Controlled Substance Schedule II

Pregnancy Risk Category: B

INDICATIONS & DOSAGES
Agitation in psychoses, insomnia, seizures, and status epilepticus—
Adults and children over age 6 when used as sedative or anticonvulsant: 65 to 500 mg, not to exceed 1 g. IV route typically used only in emergencies; dosage varies by patient.

PREPARATION & STORAGE
To prepare the standard 100-mg/ml (10%) injection, dissolve 250 or 500 mg of sterile powder in 2.5 or 5 ml, respectively, of sterile water for injection. Rotate the ampule to facilitate mixing; do not shake. If solution becomes cloudy after 5 minutes, discard; drug breaks down in solution or on exposure to air. Drug also precipitates if diluent pH is 9.2 or less. Give within 30 minutes of reconstitution.

Incompatibility
Incompatible with cefazolin, cephaloridine, cephalothin, chlorpromazine, cimetidine, clindamycin, droperidol, isoproterenol, metaraminol bitartrate, methyldopa, norepinephrine bitartrate, penicillin G, pentazocine lactate, propiomazine, succinylcholine, and thiamine.

ADMINISTRATION
Direct injection: Do not exceed rate of 100 mg/minute for adults or 60 mg/m^2/minute for children. Avoid extravasation, which can cause necrosis.

CONTRAINDICATIONS & CAUTIONS
• Contraindicated in liver impairment from cirrhosis, drug or alcohol abuse, or lengthy exposure to hepatic carcinogens.
• Also contraindicated in patients with history of acute intermittent or variegate porphyria.
• Use especially cautiously in patients with history of drug abuse.
• Also use cautiously in elderly or debilitated patients; in renal impairment, uremia, or shock because of prolonged or intensified hypnotic effects; in cardiac disease; in pulmonary disease; in asthma; in hyperthyroidism or hyperkinesis; in borderline hyperadrenalism; in acute or chronic pain; and in hypertension because drug may cause hypotension.

SPECIAL CONSIDERATIONS
• Give drug only to hospitalized patients under close observation and respiratory monitoring. Keep resuscitation equipment available.
• Barbiturates potentiate narcotic effect. If given during labor, reduce narcotic dose to lessen risk of neonatal respiratory depression.
• Do not give drug within 24 hours of liver function tests.
• Signs of drug overdose include clammy skin, coma, cyanosis, hypotension, and pupillary constriction. If overdose occurs, maintain airway and, if needed, provide ventilatory support. Monitor vital signs and fluid balance. For shock, give fluids and follow standard care measures; for hypotension, give vasopressors, as ordered. In normal renal function, forced diuresis may help remove drug; hemodialysis or hemoperfusion may enhance removal.
• Monitor PT carefully when patient starts or ends anticoagulant therapy. Anticoagulant dose may need adjustment.

amphotericin B

Abelcet, Amphocin, Fungizone♦

Pregnancy Risk Category: B

INDICATIONS & DOSAGES
Systemic fungal infections (aspergillosis, blastomycosis, candidiasis, coccidioidomycosis, cryptococcosis, histoplasmosis, and phycomycosis)—
Adults and children: initially, 0.25 mg/kg infused over 6 hours (if tolerated, may be infused over 3 to 4 hours). A test dose of 1 mg in 20 ml of D$_5$W is infused over 20 to 30 minutes. Monitor patient's vital signs q 30 minutes for 4 hours. Dosage is increased gradually, depending on patient tolerance and severity of infection, to a maximum of 1 mg/kg/day. Dosage must never exceed 1.5 mg/kg/day. If discontinued for 1 week or more, therapy resumes

with initial dose and gradually increases as described. Therapy may last for months.

PREPARATION & STORAGE
For 50-mg vial, reconstitute with 10 ml of sterile (not bacteriostatic) water for injection. Shake until solution clears. Further dilute in 500 ml of D_5W with a pH above 4.2. Final concentration will be 0.1 mg/ml.

Store concentrate at room temperature for 24 hours or refrigerate for 1 week. When diluted, use drug promptly. Protect from light until ready to hang.

Incompatibility
Incompatible with amikacin, calcium chloride, calcium gluceptate, chlorpromazine, cimetidine, diphenhydramine, edetate calcium disodium, gentamicin, kanamycin, melphalan hydrochloride, metaraminol, methyldopate, paclitaxel, penicillin G potassium, penicillin g sodium, polymyxin B, potassium chloride, prochlorperazine mesylate, lactated Ringer's solution, 0.9% NaCl, streptomycin, and verapamil.

ADMINISTRATION
Continuous infusion: Administer 500 ml of diluted solution over 3 to 6 hours. In-line filter should have a pore diameter exceeding 1 micron. Because of severe adverse reactions, remain with home care patient during entire infusion.

CONTRAINDICATIONS & CAUTIONS
• Contraindicated in patients with known hypersensitivity unless infection is life-threatening and susceptible only to this drug.
• Use only in patients (under close supervision) with confirmed diagnosis of potentially fatal fungal infection. Use cautiously in renal impairment.

SPECIAL CONSIDERATIONS
• Adding a small amount of heparin (1,200 to 1,600 U) to solution may lessen risk of thrombophlebitis.

• Giving small doses IV of an adrenal corticosteroid just before or during administration of drug may reduce febrile reaction.
• Antihistamines, antipyretics, corticosteroids, and antiemetics may be ordered to prevent adverse reactions.
• Do not dilute with diluent that contains bacteriostatic agent, which can cause drug to precipitate.
• In cases of overdose, stop therapy, monitor patient's clinical status, and administer supportive therapy. Amphotericin B cannot be removed by dialysis.
• Monitor vital signs every 30 minutes for 4 hours during initial therapy. Fever may appear 1 to 2 hours after start of infusion; it should subside within 4 hours after stopping drug.
• Monitor intake and output.
• Monitor serum potassium and magnesium levels. Monitor hemoglobin and hematocrit.

amphotericin B cholesteryl sulfate

Amphotec

Pregnancy Risk Category: B

INDICATIONS & DOSAGES
Invasive aspergillosis in patients in whom renal impairment or unacceptable toxicity precludes use of amphotericin B deoxycholate in effective doses and in those with invasive aspergillosis in whom prior amphotericin B deoxycholate therapy has failed—
Adults and children: 3 to 4 mg/kg/day; can increase to 6 mg/kg/day if no improvement occurs or if fungal infection has progressed.

Dilute in D_5W and administer by continuous infusion at 1 mg/kg/hour. A test dose is advised when commencing new courses of treatment; infuse a small amount of drug (10 ml of final preparation containing 1.6 to 8.3 mg of drug) over 15 to 30 minutes and monitor for next

30 minutes. Infusion time can be shortened to 2 hours or lengthened based on tolerance.

PREPARATION & STORAGE
Available in preservative-free 50- and 100-mg lyophilized powder vials. Store vials at room temperature. Reconstitute 50-mg vial with rapid addition of 10 ml of sterile water for injection, and 100-mg vial with rapid addition of 20 ml sterile water with a sterile syringe and 20G needle. Shake vial gently. Do not use any diluent other than sterile water for injection.

Reconstituted drug is clear or opalescent liquid and is stable for 24 hours refrigerated. Discard partially used vials.

Dilute to a final concentration of approximately 0.6 mg/ml (range, 0.16 to 0.83 mg/ml) with D_5W only. Final product is stable for 24 hours refrigerated when diluted with D_5W. Do not administer undiluted. Do not filter or use an in-line filter and do not freeze.

Incompatibility
Incompatible with saline, electrolyte solutions, and bacteriostatic agents.

ADMINISTRATION
Intermittent infusion: Infuse over at least 2 hours. Do not mix with other drugs. If administered through an existing IV line, flush line with D_5W before infusion or use a separate line.

CONTRAINDICATIONS & CAUTIONS
• Contraindicated in patients with documented hypersensitivity to any component of drug, unless doctor believes that the benefits outweigh the risk of hypersensitivity.
• It is unknown whether drug is excreted in breast milk. Use in pregnancy only if anticipated benefits outweigh potential risks to the fetus.

SPECIAL CONSIDERATIONS
• Pretreatment with antihistamines and corticosteroids or reducing the rate of infusion (or both) and

prompt administration of antihistamines and corticosteroids may reduce the acute infusion-related reactions.
• Drug cannot be removed by dialysis. Amphotericin B deoxycholate overdose has been reported to result in cardiopulmonary arrest. If overdose is suspected, discontinue therapy, monitor clinical status, and administer supportive therapy.
• Monitor vital signs every 30 minutes during initial therapy.
• Monitor intake and output.
• Monitor renal and hepatic function tests, serum electrolytes (especially potassium, magnesium, and calcium), CBC, and PT.

ampicillin sodium

Ampicin◇, Omnipen-N, Penbritin◇, Polycillin-N, Totacillin-N

Pregnancy Risk Category: B

INDICATIONS & DOSAGES
Systemic, respiratory tract, skin, GI, and acute urinary tract infections—
Adults: 250 to 500 mg q 6 hours; in more severe infections, 500 mg q 6 hours. **Children:** 25 to 50 mg/kg q 6 hours.
Bacterial meningitis—
Adults: 1 to 2.5 g q 3 to 4 hours for 3 days, then given IM
Children: 12.5 to 50 mg/kg q 3 to 4 hours for 3 days, then given IM
   Note: Adjust dosage in renal failure. In adult patients with a creatinine clearance of 10 ml/minute or less, increase dosage interval to q 12 hours.

PREPARATION & STORAGE
Supplied in vials containing 125 mg, 250 mg, 500 mg, 1 g, and 2 g. Reconstitute by adding 5 ml of sterile water for injection to the 125-, 250-, or 500-mg vial; 7.5 ml to 1-g vial; or 10 ml to 2-g vial. Dilute for infusion

with 50 or 100 ml 0.9% NaCl, D_5W, dextrose 5% and 0.45% NaCl, invert sugar 10% and water, 1/6 M sodium lactate, lactated Ringer's solution, or sterile water for injection. Concentration of the drug should not exceed 30 mg/ml. Solution remains stable for 2 to 4 hours in dextrose solutions and for up to 8 hours in other solutions when refrigerated.

When frozen, drug is stable for 30 days. Allow solution to thaw for 8 hours before administration.

Incompatibility
Incompatible with amikacin, amino acid solutions, chlorpromazine, dextran solutions, dopamine, erythromycin lactobionate, 10% fat emulsions, fructose, gentamicin, heparin sodium, hetastarch, hydrocortisone sodium succinate, hydromorphone hydrochloride, kanamycin, lidocaine hydrochloride, lincomycin, polymyxin B, prochlorperazine edisylate, sodium bicarbonate, and streptomycin.

ADMINISTRATION
Direct injection: Inject reconstituted drug into a large vein or cannula over 10 to 15 minutes. After injection, flush cannula with 0.9% NaCl.
Intermittent infusion: Give diluted solution through IV piggyback or cannula over 30 to 60 minutes.

CONTRAINDICATIONS & CAUTIONS
• Contraindicated in penicillin hypersensitivity and infectious mononucleosis.
• Use cautiously in the elderly and in patients with cephalosporin hypersensitivity or renal impairment.

SPECIAL CONSIDERATIONS
• Obtain specimens for culture and sensitivity testing before giving first dose. Therapy may start before results are available.
• Intermittent infusion reduces risk of vein irritation.
• Discontinue drug if acute interstitial nephritis, bone marrow depres-

sion, or pseudomembranous colitis develops.
• Monitor hematologic and renal function studies during therapy.
• Monitor for signs of bacterial or fungal superinfection.

ampicillin sodium/ sulbactam sodium

Unasyn
Pregnancy Risk Category: B

INDICATIONS & DOSAGES
Peritonitis and gynecologic, skin, and skin structure infections caused by susceptible organisms—
Adults: 1.5 (1 g ampicillin, 0.5 g sulbactam) to 3 g (2 g ampicillin, 1 g sulbactam) q 6 hours, not to exceed 4 g/day of sulbactam.

Note: Dosage in renal failure is based on creatinine clearance. In adult patients, give 1.5 to 3 g q 6 to 8 hours if creatinine clearance exceeds 29 ml/minute; 1.5 to 3 g q 12 hours if it is 15 to 29 ml/minute; or 1.5 to 3 g q 24 hours if it is 5 to 14 ml/minute.

PREPARATION & STORAGE
Available in 1.5- and 3-g vials and in piggyback vials. Reconstitute with sterile water for injection to yield a concentration of 375 mg/ml. For infusion, immediately dilute reconstituted solution with compatible diluent to yield 3 to 45 mg/ml.

Storage times reflect diluent and concentration. Using sterile water for injection or 0.9% NaCl injection, a 45-mg/ml solution remains stable for 8 hours at 77° F (25° C) and for 48 hours at 39° F (4° C); a 30-mg/ml solution remains stable for 72 hours at 39° F.

Using D_5W, a 30-mg/ml solution is stable for 2 hours at 77° F and for 24 hours at 39° F.

Using lactated Ringer's solution, a 45-mg/ml solution remains stable for 8 hours at 77° F and for 24 hours at 39° F.

Other compatible diluents include dextrose 5% and 0.45% NaCl or 10% invert sugar.

Incompatibility
Incompatible with amikacin, amino acid solutions, chlorpromazine, dextran solutions, dopamine, erythromycin lactobionate, 10% fat emulsions, fructose, gentamicin, heparin sodium, hetastarch, hydrocortisone sodium succinate, kanamycin, lidocaine hydrochloride, lincomycin, netilmicin, polymyxin B, prochlorperazine edisylate, sodium bicarbonate, streptomycin, or tobramycin.

ADMINISTRATION
Direct injection: Inject reconstituted drug into large vein or cannula over at least 10 to 15 minutes. Then flush with 0.9% NaCl.
Intermittent infusion: After diluting reconstituted drug (usually in 100 ml of solution), infuse over 15 to 30 minutes.

CONTRAINDICATIONS & CAUTIONS
• Contraindicated in penicillin or sulbactam hypersensitivity; also in mononucleosis.
• Use cautiously in the elderly and in patients with cephalosporin hypersensitivity or renal impairment.
• Safety and efficacy in children have not been established.

SPECIAL CONSIDERATIONS
• Obtain specimens for culture and sensitivity testing before administering first dose. Therapy may start before results of tests are known.
• Discontinue drug if acute interstitial nephritis, bone marrow depression, or pseudomembranous colitis develops.
• Give ampicillin sulbactam at least 1 hour before bacteriostatic antibiotics.
• In cases of overdose, hemodialysis may be used to remove ampicillin and probably sulbactam.

• Observe patient for fungal and bacterial superinfection with large doses or prolonged use.
• Monitor patients with renal impairment for signs of toxicity.

amrinone lactate

Inocor♦

Pregnancy Risk Category: C

INDICATIONS & DOSAGES
Short-term management of heart failure (primarily in patients unresponsive to cardiac glycosides, diuretics, and vasodilators)—
Adults: initially, 0.75 mg/kg given over 2 to 3 minutes, followed by 200 mg in 100 ml of 0.9% NaCl given at 5 to 10 mcg/kg/minute. If needed, additional bolus of 0.75 mg/kg can be given 30 minutes after therapy starts. Dosages should be individualized based on patient response. Maximum daily dosage is 10 mg/kg. Steady-state plasma level should be maintained at 3 mcg/ml.

PREPARATION & STORAGE
Available in 20-ml ampules of clear yellow solution containing 5 mg/ml. Protect ampules from light and store at room temperature. Do not use if solution is discolored or has precipitates. Administer undiluted or dilute in 0.45% or 0.9% NaCl. Concentrations of 1 to 3 mg/ml remain stable for 24 hours.

Incompatibility
Incompatible with furosemide, glucose, bicarbonate, and dextrose-containing solutions.

ADMINISTRATION
Direct injection: Over 2 to 3 minutes, inject diluted or undiluted drug into vein or IV tubing containing a free-flowing, compatible solution. Avoid extravasation. After injection, flush with 0.9% NaCl.

Continuous infusion: Dilute only with NaCl solution to 1 to 3 mg/ml. May be piggybacked into line close to insertion site containing D$_5$W. Infusion rate is usually controlled by pump at 5 to 10 mcg/kg/minute.

CONTRAINDICATIONS & CAUTIONS
• Contraindicated in hypersensitivity to amrinone and sulfites.
• Contraindicated in acute MI or ischemic coronary artery disease *without heart failure*; in severe aortic or pulmonary valve disease (surgery is required to relieve the obstruction); and in hypertrophic cardiomyopathy.

SPECIAL CONSIDERATIONS
• Because amrinone may increase ventricular response rate, patients with atrial fibrillation or flutter may require concomitant therapy with cardiac glycosides.
• In cases of overdose, reduce infusion rate and treat hypotension symptomatically.
• Carefully monitor fluid and electrolyte levels, hepatic and renal function, and platelet count. Expect to decrease dosage if platelet count drops below 150,000/mm³.
• During infusion, check vital signs every 5 to 15 minutes. If blood pressure drops, slow or stop infusion and notify doctor.

anistreplase (anisoylated plasminogen-streptokinase activator complex; APSAC)

Eminase♦
Pregnancy Risk Category: C

INDICATIONS & DOSAGES
Lysis of coronary artery thrombi following acute MI—
Adults: 30 U IV over 2 to 5 minutes. Administer by direct injection.

PREPARATION & STORAGE
Available in vials containing 30 U. Refrigerate drug at 36° to 46° F (2° to 8° C). Reconstitute drug by slowly adding 5 ml of sterile water for injection. Direct the stream against the side of the vial, not at the drug itself. Gently roll the vial to mix the dry powder and water. To avoid excessive foaming, do not shake the vial. Reconstituted solution should be colorless to pale yellow. Inspect for precipitate. Do not dilute reconstituted solution.
   If drug is not administered within 30 minutes of reconstituting, discard the vial.

Incompatibility
Do not mix with other drugs.

ADMINISTRATION
Direct injection: Inject drug over 2 to 5 minutes into an IV line or vein.

CONTRAINDICATIONS & CAUTIONS
• Contraindicated in patients with active internal bleeding, history of CVA, recent (within the past 2 months) intraspinal or intracranial surgery or trauma, aneurysm, arteriovenous malformation, intracranial neoplasm, or known bleeding diathesis.
• Use cautiously in patients for 10 days following major surgery, trauma (including CPR), or GI or GU bleeding.
• Administer cautiously in patients with cerebrovascular disease or hypertension (systolic, 180 mm Hg; diastolic, 110 mm Hg), in mitral stenosis or atrial fibrillation or other condition that may lead to left-sided heart thrombosis, in acute pericarditis or subacute bacterial endocarditis, in septic thrombophlebitis, in patients age 75 and older, in diabetic hemorrhagic retinopathy, and in those receiving anticoagulants.

SPECIAL CONSIDERATIONS
• Drug must be given within 6 hours after onset of symptoms.

• Avoid IM injections because of high risk of bleeding into muscle. Also avoid turning and moving the patient excessively.
• Monitor for reperfusion arrhythmias, including sinus bradycardia, accelerated idioventricular rhythm, ventricular tachycardia, or PVCs. Have emergency treatment readily available.
• If arterial puncture is necessary, select a compressible site (such as an arm) and apply pressure for 30 minutes afterward. Also use pressure dressings, sandbags, or ice packs on recent puncture sites to prevent bleeding.

aprotinin

Trasylol◆

Pregnancy Risk Category: B

INDICATIONS & DOSAGES
Reduction of excessive blood loss and blood transfusions during cardiopulmonary bypass—
Adults: 1-ml (1.4 mg or 10,000 U) test dose 10 minutes before scheduled administration time, followed by a loading dose of 200 ml (280 mg or 2 million U) given over 20 to 30 minutes after induction of anesthesia. Patient should be in a supine position. A 200-ml pump-priming dose is provided for the bypass machine before the bypass is begun. During surgery, a constant infusion of 50 ml/hour (70 mg/hour or 500,000 U/hour) of aprotinin is given until the incision is closed. Once closed, the infusion is stopped.
Children: dosage has not been established.

PREPARATION & STORAGE
Available as 100- and 200-ml vials containing 1.4 mg/ml (10,000 U) aprotinin. Store at room temperature. May dilute with D_5W or 0.9% NaCl before infusion.

Incompatibility
Incompatible with corticosteroids, heparin, tetracycline, and nutrient solutions containing amino acids or fat emulsions. If aprotinin is given concurrently with other drugs, each drug should be administered separately through different venous lines or catheters.

ADMINISTRATION
Direct injection: By slow IV injection over at least 4 minutes.
Intermittent infusion: By slow IV infusion at a rate of 200 ml over 20 to 30 minutes.
Continuous infusion: During surgery at a rate of 50 ml/hour until incision is closed.

CONTRAINDICATIONS & CAUTIONS
• Contraindicated in hypersensitivity to aprotinin or its components or to bovine products.
• Contraindicated in patients with thromboembolic disease requiring anticoagulant therapy.
• Use cautiously in patients with renal impairment.
• Also use cautiously in patients receiving aprotinin for the second, third, or fourth time because significant adverse reactions have occurred. Patient may experience anaphylaxis after the full therapeutic dose even if he remains asymptomatic after the test dose.

SPECIAL CONSIDERATIONS
• A test dose is recommended before infusion because allergic reactions, including anaphylaxis, have occurred.
• Administer drug through a central line.
• Make sure patient is supine when giving test dose to avoid hypotension.
• Watch for increased serum creatinine, signaling nephrotoxicity.

asparaginase (colaspase, L-asparaginase)

Elspar, Kidrolase◇

Pregnancy Risk Category: C

INDICATIONS & DOSAGES

Induction phase of acute lymphocytic leukemia (in combination therapy)—
Adults and children:
1,000 IU/kg/day for 10 days.
Note: Asparaginase has been used in many combination regimens. Consultation of current medical literature is recommended to determine the most appropriate dosage.
Induction phase of acute lymphocytic leukemia (as sole agent)—
Adults and children:
200 IU/kg/day for 28 days.
Note: Dosage varies with protocol.

PREPARATION & STORAGE

Use extreme caution when preparing or giving drug to avoid mutagenic, teratogenic, and carcinogenic risks. Use a biological containment cabinet and avoid contact with skin. Wear mask and gloves. If solution comes in contact with skin or mucosa, immediately wash thoroughly with soap and water. Correctly dispose of needles, syringes, vials, and unused drug.

Asparaginase is available in 10,000-IU vials, which are stable for 2 years at room temperature, 4 years if refrigerated. Reconstitute drug with 2 to 5 ml of 0.9% NaCl (without a preservative) or sterile water for injection. Drug may be clear or slightly cloudy. Dilute in D_5W or 0.9% NaCl within 8 hours after reconstitution.

Incompatibility
None reported.

ADMINISTRATION

Intermittent infusion: Start new IV site in distal vein to allow for successive venipunctures, if necessary, using a 23G or 25G butterfly needle. Give drug through side port of rapidly infusing D_5W or 0.9% NaCl solution and administer over at least 30 minutes.

CONTRAINDICATIONS & CAUTIONS

• Contraindicated in asparaginase hypersensitivity and in patients with past or current pancreatitis.
• Also contraindicated in chickenpox, herpes, or recent exposure to these viral illnesses.
• Use with caution in diabetes mellitus, in gout or history of urate stones, in hepatic impairment, and in infection.

SPECIAL CONSIDERATIONS

• Skin testing and desensitization are mandatory before first dose or if more than 1 week has elapsed between treatments. Life-threatening hypersensitivity occurs in 20% to 35% of patients. For skin test, inject 2 IU intradermally at least 1 week before first asparaginase dose and observe injection site for at least 1 hour for flare or wheal. If skin test is positive or if patient was previously treated with asparaginase, desensitize by gradually increasing IV doses until reaching ordered daily dose (provided no allergic reaction occurs). A negative skin test does not rule out future allergic reactions. Keep emergency equipment nearby during therapy.
• Adequate hydration, alkalinization of urine, and possibly allopurinol administration reduce risk of uric acid nephropathy.
• Loss of potency has been observed with use of 0.2-micron filter.
• Observe patient for signs of CNS toxicity or thromboembolism. Be especially alert for dyspnea and chest pain, which may indicate pulmonary embolism.
• Teach patient to recognize signs of hepatic impairment (jaundice, dark

orange urine, and clay-colored stools).

atenolol

Tenormin

Pregnancy Risk Category: D

INDICATIONS & DOSAGES
To reduce CV mortality and risk of reinfarction in hemodynamically stable patients who have survived the acute phase of an MI—
Adults: 5 mg IV, followed by another 5 mg IV 10 minutes later. Initiate oral therapy 10 minutes after the final IV dose in patient who can tolerate the full IV dose. Give 50 mg PO, followed by another 50 mg PO q 12 hours later. Then give 50 mg PO b.i.d. or 100 mg PO once daily for at least 6 to 9 days, or until patient is discharged from the hospital. If not contraindicated, therapy may sometimes be continued for 1 to 3 years.

PREPARATION & STORAGE
Available in 10-ml ampules containing 5 mg atenolol. Store drug at room temperature (59° to 86° F [15° to 30° C]) and protect from light. Dilute with 0.9% NaCl, D_5W, or NaCl and dextrose injection. Dilutions are stable for 48 hours.

Incompatibility
Do not mix with other drugs.

ADMINISTRATION
Direct injection: Administer over at least 5 minutes into a large vein.

CONTRAINDICATIONS & CAUTIONS
• Contraindicated in patients with sinus bradycardia, heart block greater than first degree, cardiogenic shock, hypotension, and overt cardiac failure. Also contraindicated in patients with acute MI accompanied by cardiac failure that is not effectively and promptly controlled.
• Use cautiously in patients with history of bronchospastic disease.

• Also use cautiously in diabetic patients.
• Use cautiously in patients with heart failure controlled by cardiac glycosides or diuretics. Intrinsic sympathetic stimulation is necessary to support circulatory function in heart failure, and excessive beta blockade may exacerbate heart failure.

SPECIAL CONSIDERATIONS
• Administration of IV atenolol should be restricted to a critical care area such as the cardiac care unit (CCU).
• During the acute phase of MI, beta-adrenergic blocker therapy should supplement standard CCU treatment.
• Administer drug as soon as patient's eligibility is established and his hemodynamic condition has stabilized. Reduction of mortality appears to be most significant during the first 24 hours after infarct.
• Dosage adjustments may be required in patients with renal failure.
• During administration, monitor patient's blood pressure, heart rate, and ECG readings. Stop drug if significant hypotension or bradycardia occurs.

atracurium besylate

Tracrium◇

Pregnancy Risk Category: C

INDICATIONS & DOSAGES
Facilitation of endotracheal (ET) intubation and muscle relaxation during surgery or mechanical ventilation—
Adults: initially, 0.4 to 0.5 mg/kg (represents double the dose needed for nearly complete neuromuscular blockade); maintenance dose of 0.08 to 0.10 mg/kg, p.r.n., depends on response to peripheral nerve stimulation or observation of muscle tone recovery, spontaneous breathing, and coughing, or if patient resists ET tube.

Children ages 1 month to 2 years: initially, 0.3 to 0.4 mg/kg. Frequent maintenance doses may be needed.
  Note: Dosage must be individualized.

PREPARATION & STORAGE
Atracurium is available in 5- and 10-ml ampules. Each milliliter contains 10 mg of drug. Dilute the drug with D_5W or 0.9% NaCl for intermittent or continuous infusion. Refrigerate at 36° to 46° F (2° to 8° C). Do not freeze.

Incompatibility
Incompatible with alkaline solutions because of drug's acid pH.

ADMINISTRATION
Only staff trained in giving IV anesthetics and managing adverse reactions should give drug.
Direct injection: Inject rapidly into an IV line containing a free-flowing, compatible solution.
Intermittent infusion: Infuse diluted drug into IV line containing a compatible solution, as needed, during procedure.
Continuous infusion: After direct injection, give a 0.02% to 0.05% solution at 7.5 mcg/kg/minute during procedure.

CONTRAINDICATIONS & CAUTIONS
• Contraindicated in patients hypersensitive to drug.
• Use cautiously in patients with history of severe anaphylactic reaction, asthma, or disorders exacerbated by substantial histamine release.
• Also use cautiously in patients with bronchogenic carcinoma and such neuromuscular diseases as myasthenia gravis and Eaton-Lambert syndrome because drug potentiates neuromuscular blockade.
• Use cautiously in patients with hypotension, pulmonary impairment, or electrolyte imbalance or dehydration.

SPECIAL CONSIDERATIONS
• Keep emergency resuscitation equipment available at all times.
• Maintain a patent airway.
• To treat overdose, maintain a patent airway and assist breathing, as needed. Administer fluids and vasopressors for hypotension and edrophonium, neostigmine, or pyridostigmine for neuromuscular blockade. Usually reverses in 8 to 10 minutes.
• Ensure corneas are protected because patient will be unable to blink.
• Know that patient will not have usual reflexes such as cough and gag reflexes, except for pupillary constriction to light, while under effects of drug.

atropine sulfate

Pregnancy Risk Category: C

INDICATIONS & DOSAGES
Symptomatic bradycardia—
Adults: 0.5 to 1 mg q 5 minutes until desired heart rate is reached (usually, 60 beats/minute). Maximum total dose is 3 mg; minimum dose is 0.5 mg. Lower dose could cause paradoxical bradycardia by vagal stimulation.
Ventricular asystole in advanced life support—
Adults: 1 mg q 5 minutes if asystole persists.
Adolescents and children: 0.02 mg/kg (in children, minimum 0.1 mg; maximum 1 mg) q 5 minutes, if needed. In adolescents, maximum total dose is 2 mg.
Blocked muscarinic effects of anticholinesterase agents—
Adults: 0.6 to 1.2 mg for each 0.5 to 2.5 mg of neostigmine methylsulfate or each 10 to 20 mg of pyridostigmine bromide.
Antidote for anticholinesterase toxicity—
Adults: initially, 1 to 2 mg, then 2 mg q 5 to 60 minutes until symptoms subside. In severe cases, initial

dose may be as much as 6 mg q 5 to 60 minutes, p.r.n.

PREPARATION & STORAGE
Available in single-dose ampules or vials of 0.1 mg/ml, 0.4 mg/ml, 0.5 mg/ml, 1 mg/ml, and 1.2 mg/ml; in multidose 20-ml vials of 0.4 mg/ml; and in prefilled syringes containing 0.5 and 1 mg of drug. Store at room temperature.

Incompatibility
Incompatible with alkalides, bromides, floxacillin, iodides, isoproterenol, metaraminol bitartrate, methohexital, norepinephrine, pentobarbital sodium, and sodium bicarbonate.

ADMINISTRATION
Direct injection: Inject prescribed amount of undiluted drug into vein or IV tubing over 1 to 2 minutes.

CONTRAINDICATIONS & CAUTIONS
• Contraindicated in glaucoma, except for cases of open-angle glaucoma being treated with miotics.
• Also contraindicated in myasthenia gravis, obstructive uropathy, and unstable CV status caused by acute hemorrhage.
• Patients sensitive to other belladonna alkaloids or salicylates may show atropine intolerance.
• In benign prostatic hyperplasia, other obstructive uropathy, and autonomic neuropathy, administer carefully because drug may cause urine retention.
• In obstructive GI disease, intestinal atony, paralytic ileus, and ulcerative colitis, give carefully because of impaired motility.
• Use cautiously in children with brain damage, in Down syndrome, in reflux esophagitis, in fever, in hepatic or renal impairment, in hypertension and pregnancy-induced hypertension, in hyperthyroidism, and in xerostomia. Use cautiously in tachycardia that threatens to cause cardiac decompensation.

SPECIAL CONSIDERATIONS
• Encourage fluids and provide mouth care when appropriate.
• To treat overdose, give fluids for shock, diazepam for CNS irritability, pilocarpine for mydriasis, and cooling blanket for hyperthermia. Provide respiratory support and possibly give physostigmine to treat delirium, hallucinations, coma, or supraventricular tachycardia.
• Monitor blood pressure closely to evaluate drug tolerance.
• Initial drug bolus may cause bradycardia, which usually resolves in 1 to 2 minutes.
• Monitor ECG for patients receiving drug for bradycardia or heart block. Watch for heart rate exceeding 100 beats/minute, increased PVCs, and ventricular tachycardia. Notify doctor if these occur.

aztreonam

Azactam

Pregnancy Risk Category: B

INDICATIONS & DOSAGES
Infections of the respiratory or GU tract, and bone, skin, and soft tissues caused by susceptible organisms—
Adults: 500 mg to 2 g q 8 to 12 hours. For severe systemic or life-threatening infections, 2 g q 6 to 8 hours may be given. Maximum daily dosage is 8 g.
    Dosage may need to be adjusted for renal impairment.

PREPARATION & STORAGE
Available in 15-ml vials or 100-ml piggyback infusion bottles containing 500 mg, 1 g, or 2 g of drug. For direct injection, add 6 to 10 ml of sterile water for injection to vial and shake well. For infusion, add at least 3 ml sterile water for each gram of drug. Dilute with 50 to 100 ml of 0.9% NaCl, D_5W, dextrose 5% in 0.9% NaCl injection, or lactated Ringer's solution. Solutions reconstituted with 0.9% NaCl or sterile wa-

ter retain potency for 48 hours at room temperature and for 7 days if refrigerated. Slight pink tint does not affect potency.

Before reconstitution, store at room temperature. After reconstitution, promptly use any solution over 2% concentration and discard the unused amount.

Incompatibility
Incompatible with ampicillin, amsacrine, cephradine, metronidazole, nafcillin, and vancomycin. Do not mix with other drugs.

ADMINISTRATION
Direct injection: Using a 21G to 23G needle, inject reconstituted drug over 3 to 5 minutes into vein or IV line containing a free-flowing, compatible solution.
Intermittent infusion: Over 20 to 60 minutes, infuse into IV tubing of a free-flowing, compatible solution or give using a volume-control device. If a volume-control device is being used, final dilution should not exceed 2% (20 mg/ml).

CONTRAINDICATIONS & CAUTIONS
• Contraindicated in patients hypersensitive to aztreonam. Use cautiously in patients hypersensitive to penicillins or cephalosporins.
• Use cautiously in elderly patients and in renal impairment.

SPECIAL CONSIDERATIONS
• Obtain specimens for culture and sensitivity testing before giving first dose. Therapy may start before results are available.
• In cases of overdose, aztreonam may be cleared from serum by hemodialysis, peritoneal dialysis, or both.
• Monitor for phlebitis at infusion site.
• Monitor BUN and creatinine levels during therapy.
• Observe patient for fungal and bacterial superinfection with prolonged use.

bleomycin sulfate

Blenoxane◆

Pregnancy Risk Category: D

INDICATIONS & DOSAGES
Malignant lymphoma, lymphosarcoma, reticulum cell sarcoma; squamous cell carcinomas of oropharynx, buccal mucosa, cervix and vulva, epiglottis, gingivae, head, larynx, lips, mouth, nasopharynx, neck, palate, paralarynx, penis, sinuses, skin, tongue, tonsils; testicular cancer—
Adults: 0.25 to 0.5 U/kg once or twice weekly. Because of risk of anaphylactoid reactions, give patient with lymphoma 2 U or less for the first two doses. If tolerated, follow above dosage schedule.
Hodgkin's disease—
Adults: 0.25 to 0.5 U/kg once or twice weekly. After tumor is reduced by 50%, administer 1 U daily or 5 U weekly.

PREPARATION & STORAGE
Preparation is associated with carcinogenic, mutagenic, and teratogenic risks. Follow institutional policy to reduce risks.

Vials contain 15 or 30 U of drug. For IM or SC use, reconstitute 15-unit vial with 1 ml or 30-U vial with 5 ml of sterile water for injection, bacteriostatic water for injection, or 0.9% NaCl.

For IV use, dilute the 15- or 30-U vials with at least 5 to 10 ml, respectively, of 0.9% NaCl.

Diluted solution is stable for 24 hours at room temperature. Because preparation does not contain preservatives, manufacturer recommends use within 24 hours. Discard unused portion.

Incompatibility
Incompatible with solutions containing divalent and trivalent cations, especially calcium salts and copper, because drug causes chelation. Also incompatible with amino acids, aminophylline, ascorbic acid injection,

B

cephalosporins, diazepam, drugs containing sulfhydryl groups, furosemide, hydrocortisone, methotrexate, mitomycin, penicillin, riboflavin, and terbutaline sulfate.

Do not dilute with dextrose-containing fluids, which results in loss of potency of drug.

ADMINISTRATION
Direct injection: Using a 23G or 25G butterfly needle, inject reconstituted drug over 10 minutes at a new IV site.
Intermittent infusion: Using a secondary line, infuse dose into an established line containing a free-flowing, compatible solution.

CONTRAINDICATIONS & CAUTIONS
• Contraindicated in bleomycin hypersensitivity.
• Use cautiously in patients with pulmonary impairment. Elderly patients are also at risk for pulmonary toxicity.
• Also use cautiously in hepatic or renal impairment.
• Safety and effectiveness in pediatric patients have not been established.
• After administration of bleomycin, lung damage can occur at oxygen concentrations lower than those usually considered safe.

SPECIAL CONSIDERATIONS
• Assess respiratory function carefully before each treatment, especially if patient is at high risk for pulmonary toxicity. Signs include dyspnea, bibasilar crackles, and a nonproductive cough.
• Monitor patient closely during infusion and for 1 hour after.
• Obtain BUN and creatinine clearance levels, liver and pulmonary function tests, ECG, and chest X-rays before and during treatment. Expect drug to be stopped if tests show marked deterioration.
• In patients prone to posttreatment fever, give acetaminophen before treatment and for 24 hours after.
• Monitor patient's blood pressure.

• Instruct patient that if he is ever to receive anesthesia, he must inform the anesthesiologist of prior treatment with bleomycin.

bretylium tosylate

Bretylate◇, Bretylol
Pregnancy Risk Category: C

INDICATIONS & DOSAGES
Ventricular fibrillation or hemodynamically unstable ventricular tachycardia—
Adults: 5 mg/kg given undiluted over 1 minute. If persistent, follow with 10 mg/kg q 5 to 30 minutes p.r.n. Maximum dosage is 30 to 35 mg/kg/day.
Persistent ventricular tachycardia—
Adults: 5 to 10 mg/kg infused over 8 to 10 minutes. Maintenance dosage is 5 to 10 mg/kg over 8 minutes or more, repeated q 6 to 8 hours; or continuous infusion at rate of 1 to 2 mg/minute.
Other life-threatening arrhythmias—
Adults: 5 to 10 mg/kg over at least 8 minutes repeated at 1- to 2-hour intervals if persistent. Maintenance dosage is 5 to 10 mg/kg q 6 hours or continuous infusion at a rate of 1 to 2 mg/minute.

PREPARATION & STORAGE
Supplied as single-dose, 10-ml ampule containing 500 mg drug. For infusion, dilute with at least 50 ml of D_5W or 0.9% NaCl.

Store at 59° to 86° F (15° to 30° C). Diluted drug remains stable for 48 hours at room temperature, 7 days if refrigerated.

Prediluted, commercially prepared solutions are also available.

Incompatibility
None reported.

ADMINISTRATION
Direct injection: Using a 20G to 22G needle, inject undiluted over about 8 to 10 minutes into IV line.

Intermittent infusion: Dilute to at least 50 ml with D₅W or 0.9% NaCl injection and infuse ordered dose over 8 minutes or more.
Continuous infusion: Give diluted drug at rate of 1 to 2 mg/minute.

CONTRAINDICATIONS & CAUTIONS
• Contraindicated in digitalized patients unless they have a life-threatening arrhythmia that is not caused by cardiac glycoside therapy. Avoid simultaneous initiation of bretylium and cardiac glycoside therapy.
• Use cautiously in patients with impaired cardiac output, aortic stenosis, and pulmonary hypertension.
• Reduce dosage in patients with renal impairment.

SPECIAL CONSIDERATIONS
• Subtherapeutic doses (below 5 mg/kg) may cause hypotension.
• Rapid administration may cause severe nausea and vomiting.
• Increase dosage interval in patients with impaired renal function.
• To manage overdose, administer nitroprusside or another short-acting antihypertensive to treat initial hypertensive effects. Treat hypotension with fluids and dopamine or norepinephrine. Drug is not removed by dialysis.
• Closely monitor ECG, heart rate, pulse, and blood pressure.
• Keep patient supine until he develops tolerance to hypotension, which may occur after several days of therapy. Notify doctor immediately of significant change.

bumetanide

Bumex

Pregnancy Risk Category: C

INDICATIONS & DOSAGES
Edema associated with heart failure and hepatic or renal disease—
Adults: initially, 0.5 to 1 mg daily. Repeat q 2 to 3 hours, if needed, up to maximum of 10 mg daily.

Adjunctive treatment to enhance drug or toxin elimination in intoxication—
Adults: dosage varies, depending on desired response. Maximum dosage is 10 mg daily.

PREPARATION & STORAGE
Available with premixed preservative in 2-ml (0.25 mg/ml) ampules and 2-, 4-, and 10-ml (0.25 mg/ml) vials. Drug can be further diluted for IV infusion using D₅W, 0.9% NaCl, or lactated Ringer's solution in both glass and plastic containers. Prepare solution for IV infusion within 24 hours of use. Protect drug from light to avoid discoloration. Store at room temperature.

When large doses are required, use vials to prevent glass particles from broken ampules from entering the solution. If ampules must be used, add a filter to IV tubing.

Incompatibility
Incompatible with dobutamine.

ADMINISTRATION
Direct injection: Using a 21G or 23G needle, inject desired dose of 0.25 mg/ml solution over 1 to 2 minutes.
Intermittent infusion: Give diluted drug through an intermittent infusion device or piggyback into an IV line containing a free-flowing, compatible solution. Infuse at ordered rate.

CONTRAINDICATIONS & CAUTIONS
• Contraindicated in hepatic impairment and severe electrolyte depletion; in severe renal impairment; anuria; and in bumetanide hypersensitivity.
• Give cautiously to patients with sulfonamide sensitivity.
• Also give cautiously to patients with an increased risk of hypokalemia; those receiving cardiac glycosides and diuretics for heart failure; those with hepatic cirrhosis and ascites; those in states of aldosterone excess with normal renal function;

and to patients with history of ventricular arrhythmias.

• Administer carefully in patients with gout or hyperuricemia because drug elevates serum uric levels.

• Use cautiously in patients with acute MI because excessive diuresis can precipitate shock.

• Too vigorous diuresis may result in profound water loss and dehydration, especially in elderly patients.

• Safety and effectiveness in patients under age 18 have not been established.

SPECIAL CONSIDERATIONS

• Initiate therapy with small doses, adjusting dose carefully, and using an intermittent dosage schedule if possible.

• If excessive diuresis or electrolyte imbalance occurs, expect drug to be stopped or dosage reduced until imbalance returns to normal.

• Drug may contain benzyl alcohol.

• In cases of overdose, monitor urine output and serum and urine electrolyte levels to determine symptomatic care. Provide replacement fluids and electrolytes, as needed.

• Monitor blood pressure and pulse rate during rapid diuresis. Use cautiously with other potassium-wasting drugs.

• Monitor serum electrolytes, BUN, creatinine, and carbon dioxide frequently.

• Observe for signs of hypokalemia, such as weakness, dizziness, confusion, anorexia, vomiting, and cramps.

calcitriol

Calcijex♦

Pregnancy Risk Category: C

INDICATIONS & DOSAGES

Management of hypocalcemia in patients undergoing chronic renal dialysis—
Adults: 0.5 mcg three times weekly, approximately every other day.

Dosage may be increased by 0.25 to 0.5 mcg at 2- to 4-week intervals. Maintenance dose is 0.5 to 3 mcg three times weekly.

PREPARATION & STORAGE

Available in ampules containing 1 or 2 mcg/ml. Store at room temperature. Avoid freezing. Discard unused portions immediately because calcitriol injection does not contain a preservative.

Incompatibility
None reported.

ADMINISTRATION

Direct injection: Aspirate solution from ampule and inject directly into vein or into IV tubing containing a free-flowing, compatible solution.

CONTRAINDICATIONS & CAUTIONS

• Contraindicated in hypercalcemia or vitamin D toxicity; do not use with preparations containing vitamin D.

• Give cautiously to patients taking cardiac glycosides.

SPECIAL CONSIDERATIONS

• Avoid vitamin D and its metabolites during therapy.

• Administer oral calcium supplement as needed to ensure appropriate daily intake of calcium.

• In cases of overdose, provide supportive care. Calcitonin administration may help to reverse hypercalcemia. Drug may be removed by peritoneal dialysis using a calcium-free dialysate.

• Monitor serum calcium and phosphorus at least twice weekly early in treatment and during dosage adjustment.

• Monitor serum magnesium, alkaline phosphatase, and 24-hour urine calcium and phosphorus periodically during treatment.

calcium chloride, calcium gluceptate, calcium gluconate

C

Pregnancy Risk Category: C

INDICATIONS & DOSAGES
Emergency treatment of hypocalcemia—
Adults: 7 to 14 mEq.
Children: 1 to 7 mEq.
Infants: less than 1 mEq; repeated q 1 to 3 days p.r.n.
Hypocalcemic tetany—
Adults: 4.5 to 16 mEq.
Children: 0.5 to 0.7 mEq/kg t.i.d. or q.i.d. or until tetany is controlled.
Infants: 2.4 mEq/kg daily in divided doses.
Hyperkalemia with secondary cardiac toxicity—
Adults: 2.25 to 14 mEq given while monitoring ECG; repeated in 1 to 2 minutes p.r.n.
Advanced cardiac life support—
Adults: 0.027 to 0.054 mEq/kg calcium chloride, 4.5 to 6.3 mEq calcium gluceptate, or 2.3 to 3.7 mEq calcium gluconate; repeated p.r.n.
Children: 0.27 mEq/kg calcium chloride; repeated in 10 minutes p.r.n.
Magnesium toxicity—
Adults: 7 mEq; subsequent doses based on response.
Transfusion of citrated blood—
Adults: 1.35 mEq/dl of citrated blood.
Neonates: 0.45 mEq/dl of citrated blood.

PREPARATION & STORAGE
Calcium chloride comes in a 10-ml ampule, vial, and syringe of 10% solution containing 1.36 mEq calcium/ml. Calcium gluceptate comes in a 5-ml ampule and in 50- and 100-ml bulk containers of a 22% solution containing 0.9 mEq calcium/ml. Calcium gluconate is available in 10-ml ampules and vials and 20-ml vials as a 10% solution containing 0.45 to 0.48 mEq calcium/ml. Calcium salts may be diluted with compatible solutions, including most IV and total parenteral nutrition solutions, before infusion.

Store between 59° and 86° F (15° and 30° C), unless otherwise specified by the manufacturer. Use only clear solutions. If crystals are present in calcium gluceptate, discard solution. If crystals are present in calcium gluconate, warm solution to 86° to 104° F (30° to 40° C) to dissolve them.

Warm injection to body temperature before administering in nonemergencies.

Incompatibility
All three calcium salts are precipitated by carbonates, bicarbonates, phosphates, sulfates, and tartrates. Chelation occurs when calcium salts are mixed with tetracyclines.

Calcium chloride is incompatible with amphotericin B, cephalothin sodium, chlorpheniramine maleate, dobutamine, and magnesium sulfate. Calcium gluceptate is incompatible with cefamandole nafate, cephalothin sodium, magnesium sulfate, prednisolone sodium phosphate, and prochlorperazine edisylate. Calcium gluconate is incompatible with amphotericin B, cefamandole nafate, cephalothin sodium, dobutamine, indomethacin sodium trihydrate, magnesium sulfate, methyl-prednisolone sodium succinate, and prochlorperazine edisylate.

ADMINISTRATION
Direct injection: Administer slowly through a small needle into a large vein or through an IV line containing a free-flowing, compatible solution at a rate not exceeding 1 ml/minute (1.5 mEq/minute) for calcium chloride, 1.5 to 5 ml/minute for calcium gluconate, and 2 ml/minute for calcium gluceptate. Do not use scalp veins in children.

Intermittent infusion: Infuse diluted solution through an IV line containing a compatible solution. Maximum rate of 100 mg/minute for calcium chloride or 200 mg/minute suggested for calcium gluceptate and calcium gluconate.

Continuous infusion: Infuse after addition of large volume of fluid at a maximum rate of 100 mg/minute for calcium chloride or 200 mg/minute for calcium gluceptate and calcium gluconate.

CONTRAINDICATIONS & CAUTIONS
• Contraindicated in digitalis toxicity and ventricular fibrillation; in hypercalciuria, calcium renal calculi, or hypercalcemia; and in sarcoidosis.
• Use cautiously in renal impairment, dehydration, electrolyte imbalance, and cardiac disease.
• Use calcium chloride carefully in cor pulmonale, respiratory acidosis, renal disease, or respiratory failure.

SPECIAL CONSIDERATIONS
• Infiltration into intramuscular or subcutaneous tissue may cause burning, sloughing, and necrosis of tissue. If infiltration does occur, discontinue infusion, infiltrate area with 1% procaine and hyaluronidase to reduce vasospasm and dilute calcium, and apply local heat.
• After IV injection, keep patient briefly in a recumbent position.
• If serum calcium level exceeds 12 mg/dl, give 0.9% NaCl, IV fluids, and furosemide or ethacrynic acid to promote calcium excretion. Closely monitor serum potassium and magnesium levels, blood pressure, and ECG to detect complications.
• Hypocalcemia may cause muscle twitching and spasms; hypercalcemia may cause bradycardia, depressed nervous and neuromuscular function, arrhythmias, and impaired renal function.
• Tell patient that tingling sensations, heat waves, and a calcium or chalky taste after drug administration may occur.

carboplatin

Paraplatin♦

Pregnancy Risk Category: D

INDICATIONS & DOSAGES
Ovarian carcinoma—
Adults: 360 mg/m^2 on day 1 q 4 weeks, as indicated. Reduce dose 25% if platelet count is below 50,000/mm^3 or neutrophil count is below 500/mm^3. Dose may be increased by 25% if platelet count is over 100,000/mm^3 and neutrophil count is over 2,000/mm^3. Do not repeat dose unless neutrophil count is at least 2,000/mm^3 and platelet count is at least 100,000/mm^3.

If creatinine clearance is between 41 and 59 ml/minute, adjust dose to 250 mg/m^2; if it is between 16 and 40 ml/minute, adjust dose to 200 mg/m^2.

PREPARATION & STORAGE
To avoid mutagenic, teratogenic, and carcinogenic risks, use extreme caution when preparing or administering carboplatin. Use a biological containment cabinet, wear gloves and mask, and use syringes with luer-lock fittings to prevent leakage of drug solution. Also correctly dispose of needles, vials, and unused drug and avoid contaminating work surfaces. Avoid inhalation of dust or vapors and contact with skin or mucous membranes.

Available in vials containing 50, 150, and 450 mg. Immediately before use, reconstitute with D$_5$W, 0.9% NaCl, or sterile water for injection to a concentration of 10 mg/ml.

Dilute reconstituted carboplatin with 0.9% NaCl injection or D$_5$W to a concentration as low as 0.5 mg/ml.

Store unopened vials at room temperature and protect from light. Once reconstituted and diluted, solution remains stable at room temperature for 8 hours. Because the drug does not contain antibacterial preservatives, discard unused drug after 8 hours.

Do not use needles or IV administration sets containing aluminum because carboplatin may precipitate and lose potency.

Incompatibility
Incompatible with aluminum, fluorouracil, mesna, and sodium bicarbonate.

ADMINISTRATION
Intermittent infusion: Usually infused over 15 minutes or longer into vein or with a free-flowing, compatible IV solution.

CONTRAINDICATIONS & CAUTIONS
• Contraindicated in patients with history of hypersensitivity to cisplatin, platinum-containing compounds, or mannitol.
• Also contraindicated in severe bone marrow depression or bleeding.
• Use cautiously in patients with creatinine clearance below 60 ml/minute and in those over age 65.
• Safety and effectiveness in children have not been established.
• Breast-feeding should be discontinued during therapy.
• Advise women of childbearing age to avoid becoming pregnant during therapy and to consult a doctor before becoming pregnant.

SPECIAL CONSIDERATIONS
• Drug can produce severe emesis. Administer antiemetic therapy before drug therapy.
• Have epinephrine, corticosteroids, and antihistamines available for use with hypersensitivity reactions.
• Because aluminum reacts adversely with carboplatin, do not use aluminum-containing IV sets or needles in preparation or administration.
• Observe closely for hypersensitivity reactions, which may occur within minutes of administration.
• Monitor vital signs during infusion.

• Determine serum electrolytes, creatinine, BUN, CBC, and creatinine clearance levels before the first infusion and before each course.
• Monitor CBC and platelet count frequently during therapy and, when indicated, until recovery.
• Advise patient to watch for signs of infection (fever, sore throat, fatigue) or bleeding (easy bruising, melena, bleeding gums, nosebleeds). Tell patient to take temperature daily.

carmustine (BCNU)

BiCNU◆

Pregnancy Risk Category: D

INDICATIONS & DOSAGES
Brain and hepatic tumors, Hodgkin's disease, lymphomas, malignant melanoma, multiple myeloma—
Adults and children: 150 to 200 mg/m^2 given as a single dose or divided into daily injections, such as 75 to 100 mg/m^2 on two successive days. Repeat full dose q 6 to 8 weeks if WBC count exceeds 3,000/mm^3 and platelet count exceeds 75,000/mm^3. Give 70% of dose if WBC count is between 2,000/mm^3 and 3,000/mm^3 and platelet count is between 25,000/mm^3 and 75,000/mm^3. Give 50% of previous dose for WBC counts below 2,000/mm^3 and platelet counts below 25,000/mm^3.

PREPARATION & STORAGE
Take special precautions during preparation because of the drug's mutagenic, teratogenic, and carcinogenic effects. When preparing drug, wear gloves and mask, use a biological containment cabinet, and prevent work surface con-tamination. Avoid contact with skin because drug will cause burning and a brown stain. If contact occurs, wash the area immediately and thoroughly. Correctly dispose of all equipment and unused drug.

C

Drug comes as a powder in 100-mg vials. Before preparation, check for oily film at bottom of vial (sign of decomposition) and discard if present.

Dilute 100 mg with 3 ml of sterile, dehydrated ethyl alcohol supplied by the manufacturer. After dissolving, add 27 ml of sterile water for injection to produce a clear, colorless to yellow solution with a concentration of 3.3 mg carmustine/ml of 10% alcohol. Preparation remains stable for 8 hours at room temperature and for 24 hours if refrigerated. Protect from light. Reconstituted solution may be further diluted with 250 to 500 ml of D_5W or 0.9% NaCl for infusion. If refrigerated and protected from light, this solution remains stable for 48 hours if prepared in a glass container; solution becomes unstable in plastic IV bag. Store in original container, protected from light, at 36° to 46° F (2° to 8° C).

Incompatibility
Incompatible with sodium bicarbonate.

ADMINISTRATION
Intermittent infusion: Infuse diluted solution (250 to 500 ml) over 1 to 2 hours. If patient reports pain, dilute drug further or slow infusion.

CONTRAINDICATIONS & CAUTIONS
• Contraindicated in carmustine hypersensitivity. Also contraindicated in chickenpox (or recent exposure) and herpes zoster.
• Dosage may need to be reduced in patients receiving drug in combination with other myelosuppressant drugs.
• Use cautiously in myelosuppression, existing infection, and renal, hepatic, or pulmonary impairment.
• Also use cautiously in smokers and patients with previous radiation (especially to mediastinum) or cytotoxic drug therapy.
• Safety and effectiveness in children have not been established.

• Advise women of childbearing age to avoid becoming pregnant during treatment.
• Breast-feeding should be discontinued during drug therapy.

SPECIAL CONSIDERATIONS
• Give antiemetics before carmustine.
• Administration over less than 1 to 2 hours may produce severe pain and burning at the injection site and along the vein.
• Check CBC weekly for at least 6 weeks following dose to monitor extent of myelosuppression.
• Avoid immunizing patient or exposing him to recipients of live-virus vaccine.
• Perform baseline pulmonary function tests, then monitor function during therapy. Risk of pulmonary toxicity increases with cumulative doses exceeding 1,400 mg/m².

cefamandole nafate

Mandol◆

Pregnancy Risk Category: B

INDICATIONS & DOSAGES
Severe infections caused by susceptible organisms—
Adults: 500 mg to 1 g q 4 to 8 hours.
Children age 1 month and older: 50 to 100 mg/kg/day in equally divided doses q 4 to 8 hours.
Severe, life-threatening infections; infections caused by less-susceptible organisms—
Adults: up to 2 g q 4 hours; maximum, 12 g/day.
Children age 1 month and older: 150 mg/kg daily in divided doses q 4 to 8 hours; maximum dosage is 12 g daily.
Surgical prophylaxis—
Adults: 1 to 2 g 30 to 60 minutes before surgery and 1 to 2 g q 6 hours for 24 to 48 hours after surgery.

C

Children age 3 months and older:
50 to 100 mg/kg/day 30 to 60
minutes before surgery and 50 to
100 mg/kg/day in divided doses q
6 hours for 24 to 48 hours after it.
   Note: Dosage in renal failure reflects creatinine clearance.
Adults with less severe infections:
for creatinine clearance under 2 ml/
minute, dosage is 250 to 500 mg q
12 hours; between 2 and 10 ml/
minute, 500 to 750 mg q 12 hours;
10 and 25 ml/minute, 500 mg to
1 g q 8 hours; 25 and 50 ml/
minute, 750 mg to 1.5 g q 8 hours;
50 and 80 ml/minute, 750 mg to
1.5 g q 6 hours; and if it exceeds
80 ml/minute, 1 to 2 g q 6 hours.
Adults with severe infections: for
creatinine clearance under
2 ml/minute, dosage is 500 mg q 8
hours or 750 mg q 12 hours; between 2 and 10 ml/minute, 670 mg
q 8 hours or 1 g q 12 hours; 10 and
25 ml/minute, 1 g q 6 hours or
1.25 g q 8 hours; 25 and 50 ml/
minute, 1.5 g q 6 hours or 2 g q 8
hours; 50 and 80 ml/minute, 1.5 g
q 4 hours or 2 g q 6 hours; and if it
exceeds 80 ml/minute, give usual
adult dose.

PREPARATION & STORAGE
Available in 1-, 2-, and 10-g vials.
Before reconstitution, store drug between 59° and 86° F (15° and
30° C).
   For direct injection, reconstitute
with 10 ml of sterile water for injection, D_5W, or 0.9% NaCl. Reconstitute just before use because carbon
dioxide buildup in the syringe can
cause leakage.
   For intermittent infusion, further
dilute with 100 ml of a compatible
solution. For continuous infusion,
dilute with a larger amount. Compatible solutions include amino acid
solutions; dextran; D_5W or dextrose
10% in water; 0.9% NaCl; dextrose
5% and Ionosol B; dextrose 5% and
Isolyte E; mannitol 5%, 10%, or 20%
in water; and 1/6 M sodium lactate.
Shake well until dissolved. Solution
remains stable for 24 hours at room

temperature and for 96 hours if refrigerated.

Incompatibility
Incompatible with aminoglycosides,
amiodarone hydrochloride, calcium
glucceptate, calcium gluconate, cimetidine, hetastarch, Isolyte M, and
magnesium and calcium ions (including Ringer's injection and lactated Ringer's injection).

ADMINISTRATION
Direct injection: Give over 3 to 5
minutes through a large vein or an
IV line containing a free-flowing,
compatible solution.
Intermittent infusion: Give 100 ml
over 15 to 30 minutes through an
intermittent infusion device or an IV
line containing a free-flowing, compatible solution.
Continuous infusion: Over 24 hours,
infuse solution diluted into appropriate amounts of fluid.

CONTRAINDICATIONS & CAUTIONS
• Contraindicated in cephalosporin
hypersensitivity; also give carefully to
patients with hypersensitivity to
penicillins or other drugs.
• Use cautiously in patients with GI
disease, renal impairment, or history
of bleeding disorders.
• Also use cautiously in patients with
vitamin K deficiency or predisposition to it.

SPECIAL CONSIDERATIONS
• Discontinue drug if severe diarrhea
occurs because pseudomembranous
colitis may occur.
• Administer with vitamin K in elderly or debilitated patients or those
with vitamin K deficiency.
• Monitor PT. Check for ecchymosis
and easy bruising.
• If diarrhea persists during therapy,
collect stool specimens to rule out
possible pseudomembranous colitis.
• Monitor BUN, liver enzyme levels,
and creatinine clearance in patients
with potential renal impairment.

C

• With large doses or prolonged therapy, monitor for superinfection, especially in high-risk patients.
• Use a glucose enzymatic test strip for urine glucose determinations to prevent spurious results.
• Advise patient to avoid alcohol during therapy and for 46 to 72 hours after treatment ends.

cefazolin sodium

Ancef✦, Kefzol✦

Pregnancy Risk Category: B

INDICATIONS & DOSAGES
Septicemia, endocarditis, and infections of the respiratory tract, GU tract, skin, soft tissue, biliary tract, bones, and joints caused by susceptible organisms—
Adults: in mild infection, 250 to 500 mg q 8 hours; in moderate to severe infection, 500 mg to 1 g q 6 to 8 hours; in life-threatening infection, 1 to 1.5 g q 6 hours. Maximum daily dosage is 12 g.
Children over age 1 month: 25 to 50 mg/kg daily in three or four equally divided doses; in life-threatening infection; 100 mg/kg daily may be required.
Surgical prophylaxis—
Adults: 1 g 30 to 60 minutes before surgery; during surgery, 0.5 to 1 g q 2 hours; after surgery, 0.5 to 1 g q 6 to 8 hours for 24 hours.
Note: Dosage in renal failure reflects creatinine clearance.
Adults: if creatinine clearance is 10 ml/minute or less, dosage is half usual dose q 18 to 24 hours; between 11 and 34 ml/minute, dosage is half usual dose q 12 hours; 35 and 54 ml/minute, dosage is full dose q 8 hours or less frequently; and if it exceeds 55 ml/minute, give usual adult dose.
Children: if creatinine clearance is 5 to 20 ml/minute, dosage is 10% of the usual daily dose q 24 hours; between 20 and 40 ml/minute, 25% of the usual daily dose divided equally q

12 hours; 40 and 70 ml/minute, 60% of the usual daily dose divided equally q 12 hours; and if it exceeds 70 ml/minute, give usual pediatric dose.

PREPARATION & STORAGE
Available in 500-mg and 1-g vials. To reconstitute, add 2 ml of 0.9% NaCl or sterile or bacteriostatic water to the 500-mg vial or 2.5 ml to the 1-g vial. Shake well. This dilution yields a concentration of 225 and 330 mg/ml, respectively. Further dilute reconstituted Ancef with 5 ml and Kefzol with 10 ml of compatible solution for direct injection.

For intermittent infusion, add reconstituted drug to 50 to 100 ml of compatible solution, such as D_5W; dextrose 5% in lactated Ringer's; dextrose 5% in 0.2%, 0.45%, or 0.9% NaCl; dextrose 5% and Normosol-M; or dextrose 5% and Ionosol B or Plasma-Lyte.

Reconstituted and diluted drug remains stable for 24 hours at room temperature or for 10 days if refrigerated.

Solutions reconstituted with sterile water or bacteriostatic water or 0.9% NaCl injection are stable for 12 weeks when stored at –4° F (–20° C). Do not use a cloudy or precipitated solution. Do not refreeze thawed solutions.

Incompatibility
Incompatible with aminoglycosides, amiodarone, amobarbital sodium, ascorbic acid injection, bleomycin sulfate, calcium gluceptate, calcium gluconate, cimetidine hydrochloride, colistimethate sodium, erythromycin gluceptate, hydrocortisone, idarubicin hydrochloride, lidocaine hydrochloride, norepinephrine, oxytetracycline, pentobarbital sodium, polymyxin B, ranitidine, tetracycline, theophylline, and vitamin B complex with C.

ADMINISTRATION
Direct injection: Inject the solution into a vein over 3 to 5 minutes or

into IV tubing containing a free-flowing, compatible solution. *Intermittent infusion:* Insert a 21G or 23G needle into port of primary tubing and infuse 50 to 100 ml of solution over 30 minutes.

CONTRAINDICATIONS & CAUTIONS
• Contraindicated in hypersensitivity to cephalosporins, penicillins, or penicillin-like products.
• Give cautiously in patients with renal disease to prevent toxicity.
• Also give cautiously in patients with history of ulcerative colitis, regional enteritis, or antibiotic-associated colitis.
• Safety and efficacy in premature infants and those under age 1 month have not been established.

SPECIAL CONSIDERATIONS
• If seizures occur, promptly discontinue drug; administer anticonvulsants as ordered.
• In cases of overdose, dialysis may help to remove drug.
• Check for previous penicillin or cephalosporin hypersensitivity. Expect to treat anaphylaxis with epinephrine.
• Monitor BUN and serum creatinine levels to assess renal function.
• Observe patient for fungal and bacterial superinfection with prolonged use.

cefepime hydrochloride

Maxipime
Pregnancy Risk Category: B

INDICATIONS & DOSAGES
Mild to moderate uncomplicated or complicated urinary tract infections, including pyelonephritis—
Adults and children age 12 and older: 0.5 to 1 g q 12 hours for 7 to 10 days.

Severe uncomplicated or complicated urinary tract infections, including pyelonephritis—
Adults and children age 12 and older: 2 g q 12 hours for 10 days.
Moderate to severe pneumonia—
Adults and children age 12 and older: 1 to 2 g q 12 hours for 10 days.
Moderate to severe uncomplicated skin and skin structure infections—
Adults and children age 12 and older: 2 g q 12 hours for 10 days.
   Note: Dosage in renal failure requires adjustment. Recommended initial dose should be the same as in normal renal function. Recommended maintenance doses reflect creatinine clearance. If creatinine clearance is 30 to 60 ml/minute, give usual dose q 24 hours; between 11 and 29 ml/minute, dose is half usual dose q 24 hours unless the usual recommended dose is 500 mg q 12 hours, in which case patient should receive 500 mg q 24 hours; and if it is 10 ml/minute or less, give one-fourth of usual dose q 24 hours unless recommended usual dosage is 500 mg q 12 hours, in which case patient should receive 250 mg q 24 hours.

PREPARATION & STORAGE
Available in 500-mg, 1-, and 2-g vials; 1-g ADD-Vantage vials; and 1- and 2-g piggyback bottles. For intermittent infusion, reconstitute the 1- or 2-g piggyback bottle with 50 or 100 ml of 0.9% NaCl injection, 5% and 10% dextrose injection, 1/6 M sodium lactate injection, 5% dextrose and 0.9% NaCl injection, lactated Ringer's and 5% dextrose injection, or Normosol-R and Normosol-M in 5% dextrose injection. Alternatively, reconstitute 500-mg vial with 5 ml, 1-g vial with 10 ml, or 2-g vial with 10 ml and add an appropriate quantity of the resulting solution to an IV container with one of the compatible fluids.
   Reconstitute ADD-Vantage only with 50 or 100 ml of 5% dextrose injection or 0.9% NaCl chloride in-

C

jection in ADD-Vantage flexible diluent containers.

Reconstituted solution is stable for 24 hours at controlled room temperature (68° to 77° F [20° to 25° C]) or for 7 days when refrigerated (36° to 46° F [2° to 8° C]).

Incompatibility
Incompatible with aminophylline, gentamicin, metronidazole, netilmicin sulfate, tobramycin, and vancomycin.

ADMINISTRATION
Intermittent infusion: Infuse reconstituted solution over 30 minutes.

CONTRAINDICATIONS & CAUTIONS
• Contraindicated in patients who have shown immediate hypersensitivity reactions to cefepime or cephalosporin antibiotics, penicillins, or other beta-lactam antibiotics.
• Use cautiously in patients with renal or hepatic impairment, poor nutritional state, or those receiving a protracted course of antimicrobial therapy.
• Also, use cautiously in patients with history of GI disease.

SPECIAL CONSIDERATIONS
• In cases of overdose, provide supportive treatment. Drug may be removed by hemodialysis.
• Check for previous penicillin or cephalosporin hypersensitivity.
• If diarrhea persists during therapy, collect stool specimens to rule out possible pseudomembranous colitis.
• With large doses or prolonged therapy, monitor for superinfection, especially in high-risk patients.
• Monitor PT in patients at risk for altered prothrombin activity.
• Monitor BUN and liver enzyme levels and creatinine clearance in patients with potential renal or hepatic impairment.

cefmetazole sodium
Zefazone

Pregnancy Risk Category: B

INDICATIONS & DOSAGES
Mild to moderate infections caused by susceptible organisms—
Adults: 2 g IV q 6 to 12 hours for 5 to 14 days.
Severe to life-threatening infections caused by susceptible organisms—
Adults: 2 g IV q 6 hours.
Complicated and uncomplicated urinary tract infections—
Adults: 2 g IV q 12 hours.
Prophylaxis in patients undergoing vaginal hysterectomy—
Adults: 2 g IV 30 to 90 minutes before surgery as a single dose; or 1 g IV 30 to 90 minutes before surgery, repeated in 8 and 16 hours.
Prophylaxis in patients undergoing abdominal hysterectomy—
Adults: 1 g IV 30 to 90 minutes before surgery, repeated in 8 and 16 hours.
Prophylaxis in patients undergoing cesarean section—
Adults: 2 g IV as a single dose after clamping cord; or 1 g IV after clamping cord, repeated after 8 and 16 hours.
Prophylaxis in patients undergoing colorectal surgery—
Adults: 2 g IV as a single dose 30 to 90 minutes before surgery; or 2 g IV 30 to 90 minutes before surgery, repeated in 8 and 16 hours.
Prophylaxis in patients undergoing cholecystectomy (high risk)—
Adults: 1 g IV 30 to 90 minutes before surgery, repeated in 8 and 16 hours.
Note: Adult dosage in renal failure is based on creatinine clearance. If it is below 10 ml/minute, dosage is 1 to 2 g IV q 48 hours; between 10 and 30 ml/minute, 1 to 2 g IV q 24 hours; 30 and 50 ml/minute, 1 to 2 g IV q 16 hours; and 50 and 90 ml/minute, 1 to 2 g IV q 12 hours.

C

PREPARATION & STORAGE

Available in 1- and 2-g vials. Reconstitute drug with bacteriostatic water for injection, sterile water for injection, or 0.9% NaCl for injection. Shake to dissolve drug, then let solution stand until clear. Add 3.7 ml to the 1-g vial to make a solution with an average concentration of 250 mg/ml. Add 10 ml to the 1-g vial to make a solution of about 100 mg/ml. Add 7 ml to the 2-g vial to form a solution of 250 mg/ml. Add 15 ml to the 2-g vial to make a solution of 125 mg/ml.

Store powder at controlled room temperature (59° to 86° F [15° to 30° C]). Reconstituted solutions are stable for 24 hours at room temperature (77° F [25° C]) or for 1 week if refrigerated (46° F [8° C]). Alternatively, solutions may be frozen for up to 6 weeks (–4° F [–20° C]). Thaw by gradual warming at room temperature (77° F). Do not use a microwave oven or warm water bath.

Solution should be clear after thawing. If it is cloudy or a precipitate forms at room temperature, do not use. Thawed solutions should not be refrozen; they are stable for 24 hours.

Incompatibility
Incompatible with aminoglycoside antibiotics and heparin sodium.

ADMINISTRATION

Direct injection: Temporarily discontinue medications being administered at the same site. Administer over 3 to 5 minutes.
Intermittent infusion: Reconstituted drug may be further diluted to concentrations of 1 to 20 mg/ml by adding 0.9% NaCl injection, D_5W, or lactated Ringer's injection. Infuse diluted drug over 10 to 60 minutes.

CONTRAINDICATIONS & CAUTIONS

• Contraindicated in hypersensitivity to cefmetazole or cephalosporins.

• Use cautiously in hypersensitivity to penicillin, renal impairment, or in patients with history of GI disease.

SPECIAL CONSIDERATIONS

• Prolonged use may result in overgrowth of nonsusceptible organisms.
• Check for previous cephalosporin or penicillin hypersensitivity before administering first dose. Expect to treat life-threatening hypersensitivity reactions with epinephrine, IV corticosteroids or antihistamines, pressor agents, or IV fluids.
• Monitor patient for superinfection.
• Monitor PT and administer vitamin K, as ordered.
• Monitor patient with renal impairment frequently for signs of toxicity.
• Advise patient to avoid alcohol during therapy and for 48 to 72 hours after end of treatment.

cefonicid sodium

Monocid
Pregnancy Risk Category: B

INDICATIONS & DOSAGES

Septicemia and infections of the lower respiratory and urinary tracts, skin and skin structure, and bone and joints caused by susceptible organisms—
Adults: 1 g q 24 hours. For uncomplicated infection, 0.5 g q 24 hours; in life-threatening infections, 2 g q 24 hours.
Surgical prophylaxis—
Adults: 1 g 60 minutes before surgery; may give 1 g q 24 hours for 2 days.
Prophylaxis for cesarean section—
Adults: 1 g after umbilical cord is clamped.
   Note: Adjust dosage in renal failure. In adults, adjust dosage if creatinine clearance falls below 60 ml/minute.

PREPARATION & STORAGE

Reconstitute 500-mg vial with 2 ml of sterile water for injection (yields a

C

concentration of 225 mg/ml) and 1-g vial with 2.5 ml of sterile water for injection (yields a concentration of 325 mg/ml). Shake well. Reconstitute piggyback vials with 50 to 100 ml of compatible solution.

Compatible solutions include dextrose 5% and 0.15% potassium chloride; dextrose 5% in 0.2%, 0.45%, or 0.9% NaCl; dextrose 5% in lactated Ringer's; dextrose 5% or 10% in water; Ringer's injection; lactated Ringer's; 0.9% NaCl; and 1/6 M sodium lactate.

Solution remains stable for 24 hours at room temperature and for 72 hours if refrigerated. Protect from light.

Incompatibility
Incompatible with hetastarch and sargramostim.

ADMINISTRATION
Direct injection: Using a 21G or 23G needle, inject reconstituted drug into vein over 3 to 5 minutes. Or, inject reconstituted drug into IV tubing containing a free-flowing, compatible solution.
Intermittent infusion: Infuse 50 to 100 ml of diluted drug over 20 to 30 minutes into the tubing of a free-flowing, compatible solution.

CONTRAINDICATIONS & CAUTIONS
• Contraindicated in hypersensitivity to cephalosporins.
• Use with caution in patients with allergies to penicillin or penicillin-like drugs and in those with history of allergies, especially to drug.
• Use cautiously in the elderly and in patients with renal impairment or history of GI disease.
• Also, use cautiously in breast-feeding patients.
• Give cautiously to children because safe use has not been established.

SPECIAL CONSIDERATIONS
• If patient is undergoing dialysis, maintain prescribed dosage. Only small amounts of drug are removed by dialysis.

• Check for previous penicillin or cephalosporin hypersensitivity.
• If diarrhea persists during therapy, collect stool specimens to rule out pseudomembranous colitis.
• Monitor BUN and serum creatinine levels to assess renal function. Adjust dosage accordingly.
• Observe patient for fungal and bacterial superinfection with prolonged use.

cefoperazone sodium

Cefobid ♦

Pregnancy Risk Category: B

INDICATIONS & DOSAGES
Septicemia, peritonitis, and gynecologic, skin, and urinary and respiratory tract infections caused by susceptible organisms—
Adults: 2 to 4 g daily in divided doses q 12 hours. For severe infections, 6 to 12 g/day in divided doses b.i.d., t.i.d., or q.i.d., ranging from 1.5 to 4 g/dose.

Note: Adjust dosage in renal failure. For adults, adjustment is usually not necessary; however, dosages of 4 g/day may be given cautiously to patients with hepatic impairment. Patients with both hepatic and renal impairment should not receive more than 1 to 2 g (base) daily without serum level determinations.

PREPARATION & STORAGE
Reconstitute 1 g of drug with 5 ml of compatible diluent. Shake vial vigorously until drug dissolves. Let vial stand to allow foam to dissipate before drawing up.

After reconstitution, dilute further by adding 20 to 40 ml of compatible diluent for intermittent infusion and enough diluent to make a solution of 2 to 25 mg/ml for a continuous infusion. Compatible solutions include D_5W or dextrose 10% in water, lactated Ringer's, dextrose 5% in lactated Ringer's, dextrose 5% in 0.2% or 0.9% NaCl,

Normosol-R, dextrose 5% and Normosol-M, and 0.9% NaCl. Solutions are stable for 24 hours at room temperature and for 72 hours if refrigerated.

Incompatibility
Incompatible with aminoglycosides, doxapram hydrochloride, hetastarch, labetalol hydrochloride, meperidine hydrochloride, ondansetron hydrochloride, perphenazine, promethazine hydrochloride, and sargramostim.

ADMINISTRATION
Intermittent infusion: Infuse solution over 15 to 30 minutes into IV tubing containing a compatible solution.
Continuous infusion: Infuse solution containing 2 to 25 mg/ml at ordered rate.

CONTRAINDICATIONS & CAUTIONS
• Contraindicated in cephalosporin hypersensitivity.
• Use with caution in penicillin-allergic patients because of risk of cross-reactivity and in history of allergies, especially to medication.
• Use cautiously in hypoprothrombinemia, bleeding disorders, ulcerative colitis, regional enteritis, antibiotic-associated colitis, and hepatic or biliary disease.
• Also use cautiously during prolonged parenteral or enteral nutrition and in patients with poor nutritional status, malabsorption, or alcohol dependence.
• Safe use has not been established in children.

SPECIAL CONSIDERATIONS
• Give prescribed dosage after hemodialysis treatment.
• Treat overdose symptomatically. Hemodialysis enhances drug removal.
• Check for cephalosporin or penicillin hypersensitivity before giving first dose.
• Monitor BUN and serum creatinine levels to assess renal function.

• Monitor CBC and PT to assess bleeding disturbances.
• Observe patient for fungal and bacterial superinfection with prolonged use.
• Culture stool to rule out *Clostridium difficile* infection if persistent diarrhea occurs.
• Advise patient to avoid alcohol during therapy and for 48 to 72 hours after treatment ends.

cefotaxime sodium

Claforan ◆

Pregnancy Risk Category: B

INDICATIONS & DOSAGES
Severe life-threatening infections caused by susceptible organisms—
Adults: 2 g q 4 hours; maximum dosage, 12 g daily.
Moderate to severe infections caused by susceptible organisms—
Adults and children weighing 110 lb (50 kg) or more: 1 to 2 g q 6 to 8 hours.
Children ages 1 month to 12 years (weighing under 110 lb): 50 to 180 mg/kg daily in four to six equally divided doses.
Neonates ages 1 to 4 weeks: 50 mg/kg q 8 hours.
Neonates under age 1 week: 50 mg/kg q 12 hours.
Uncomplicated infections caused by susceptible organisms—
Adults: 1 g q 12 hours.
Disseminated gonorrhea—
Adults: 1 g q 8 hours for 7 days.
Children weighing under 99 lb (45 kg): 50 mg/kg daily in divided doses for 7 days.
Neonates: 25 to 50 mg/kg b.i.d. or t.i.d. for 7 days.
Gonococcal meningitis—
Children weighing under 99 lb: 25 to 50 mg/kg q 8 to 12 hours for 10 to 14 days.
Surgical prophylaxis—
Adults: 1 g 30 to 90 minutes before surgery.

C

Prophylaxis for cesarean section—
Adults: 1 g once umbilical cord is clamped, then 1 g 6 and 12 hours later.

Note: Adjust dosage in renal failure. Adult patients with creatinine clearance below 20 ml/minute should receive half the usual dose at the usual time interval.

PREPARATION & STORAGE
Available in vials containing 500 mg, 1 g, or 2 g and in infusion bottles containing 1 or 2 g. Reconstitute vials with 10 ml of sterile water for injection. Shake well to dissolve. IV infusion bottles can be further diluted in 50 to 100 ml of D_5W or 0.9% NaCl.

Reconstituted drug can be diluted in 50 to 1,000 ml of compatible solution for continuous infusion. These solutions include D_5W or dextrose 10% in water; 0.9% NaCl; dextrose 5% in 0.2%, 0.45%, or 0.9% NaCl; invert sugar 10% in water; lactated Ringer's; and 1/6 M sodium lactate.

Reconstituted solution remains stable for 24 hours at 77° F (25° C) and for 10 days at below 41° F (5° C).

Incompatibility
Incompatible with aminoglycosides, aminophylline, doxapram hydrochloride, fluconazole, hetastarch, and sodium bicarbonate injection.

ADMINISTRATION
Direct injection: Give over 3 to 5 minutes directly into an intermittent infusion device or through an IV line containing a free-flowing, compatible solution.
Intermittent infusion: Infuse diluted solution over 20 to 30 minutes into a butterfly or scalp vein needle or through an IV line containing a compatible solution. Interrupt flow of primary IV if piggyback method is used.
Continuous infusion: Give ordered infusion over 24 hours.

CONTRAINDICATIONS & CAUTIONS
• Contraindicated in cephalosporin hypersensitivity. Use cautiously in penicillin hypersensitivity.
• In patients with history of GI disease, administer carefully.
• Give drug cautiously in renal impairment.

SPECIAL CONSIDERATIONS
• Assess IV site for inflammation or phlebitis and change site as needed.
• Treat overdose symptomatically. Hemodialysis or peritoneal dialysis removes drug.
• Check for previous penicillin or cephalosporin hypersensitivity.
• If diarrhea persists during therapy, collect stool specimens to rule out possible pseudomembranous colitis.
• Observe patient for fungal and bacterial superinfection with prolonged use.
• Monitor CBC if course of treatment exceeds 10 days.

cefotetan disodium

Cefotan ♦

Pregnancy Risk Category: B

INDICATIONS & DOSAGES
Infections (except for urinary tract) caused by susceptible organisms—
Adults: 1 to 2 g q 12 hours; in life-threatening infections, 3 g q 12 hours.
Skin and skin structure infections—
Adults: 2 g daily or 1 g q 12 hours.
Urinary tract infection—
Adults: 500 mg q 12 hours or 1 to 2 g once daily or b.i.d.
Surgical prophylaxis—
Adults: 1 to 2 g 30 to 60 minutes before surgery. For cesarean section, give dose as soon as umbilical cord is clamped. Maximum daily dosage is 6 g.

Note: Adjust dosage in renal failure. Doses or frequency of administration must be modified based on the degree of renal impairment, severity of infection, and susceptibility of organisms. Adult dosage reflects creatinine clearance. If creatinine clearance is below 10 ml/minute, dosage is usual adult dose q 48 hours or one-fourth the usual dose q 12 hours; between 10 and 30 ml/minute, usual dose q 24 hours or half usual dose q 12 hours; and if it is 30 ml/minute or more, give usual adult dose.

Hemodialysis patients should be given one-fourth the usual adult dose q 24 hours on days between treatments, and half the usual dose on the day of hemodialysis.

PREPARATION & STORAGE
Available as a white to pale yellow powder in 1- and 2-g vials and infusion vials. Reconstitute vials with 10 to 20 ml of sterile water for injection. Reconstitute infusion vials with 50 to 100 ml of D_5W or 0.9% NaCl. After reconstitution, solution remains stable for 24 hours at room temperature, for 96 hours if refrigerated, and for 1 week if frozen.

Incompatibility
Incompatible with aminoglycosides, doxapram hydrochloride, and heparin sodium.

ADMINISTRATION
Direct injection: Inject reconstituted drug directly into vein over 3 to 5 minutes.
Intermittent infusion: Over 20 to 60 minutes, infuse solution through a butterfly or scalp vein needle or into the tubing of a free-flowing, compatible solution. Interrupt flow of primary IV solution during drug administration.

CONTRAINDICATIONS & CAUTIONS
• Contraindicated in cephalosporin hypersensitivity.
• Use cautiously in penicillin hypersensitivity or history of GI disease.
• Also use cautiously in renal impairment and in bleeding disorders.
• Safe use in children has not been established.

SPECIAL CONSIDERATIONS
• Treat overdose symptomatically. Hemodialysis or peritoneal dialysis may promote drug removal.
• Check for previous penicillin or cephalosporin hypersensitivity.
• If diarrhea persists during therapy, collect stool specimens to rule out possible pseudomembranous colitis.
• Observe patient for superinfection with large doses or prolonged use.
• Monitor PT in patients with renal or hepatic impairment, malnutrition, or cancer and in the elderly.
• Instruct patient to avoid alcohol within 72 hours of drug administration.

cefoxitin sodium

Mefoxin ♦

Pregnancy Risk Category: B

INDICATIONS & DOSAGES
Severe infections caused by susceptible organisms—
Adults: 1 to 2 g q 6 to 8 hours; in life-threatening infections, up to 12 g. **Children age 3 months and older:** 80 to 160 mg/kg/day divided into three to six equal doses.
Surgical prophylaxis—
Adults: 2 g 30 to 60 minutes before surgery, then 2 g q 6 hours for 1 day after surgery.
Children age 3 months and older: 30 to 40 mg/kg 30 to 60 minutes before surgery, then 30 to 40 mg/kg q 6 hours for up to 24 hours after surgery.
Prophylaxis for cesarean section—
Adults: 2 g as a single dose after cord is clamped, or 2 g after cord is clamped and 2 g 4 and 8 hours later.
Note: Adjust dosage in renal failure. Doses or frequency of administration must be adjusted based on the degree of renal impairment, severity of infection, and susceptibility of organism. Adult dosage reflects creatinine clearance. If creatinine clearance is under 5 ml/minute, dose is 500 mg to 1 g q 24 to 48 hours;

C

between 5 and 9 ml/minute, 500 mg to 1 g q 12 to 24 hours; between 10 and 29 ml/minute, 1 to 2 g q 12 to 24 hours; between 30 and 50 ml/minute, 1 to 2 g q 8 to 12 hours; and if it exceeds 50 ml/minute, give usual adult dose.

PREPARATION & STORAGE
Available in 1- and 2-g vials, PVC bags, and infusion bottles. Store vials at 86° F (30° C).

Reconstitute 1- and 2-g vials with 10 ml of sterile water for injection. For intermittent infusion, reconstitute 1- and 2-g infusion bags or bottles with 50 to 100 ml of a compatible solution. For continuous infusion, reconstitute and add up to 1 liter of a compatible solution, such as D_5W or dextrose 10% in water; dextrose 5% in 0.2%, 0.45%, or 0.9% NaCl; Ringer's injection; lactated Ringer's; 0.9% NaCl; 1/6 M sodium lactate; invert sugar 5% or 10% in water; and dextrose 5% and Ionosol B.

Solutions remain stable for 24 hours at room temperature or 48 hours refrigerated. Both powder and solutions may turn amber, but this does not indicate significant change in potency.

Incompatibility
Incompatible with aminoglycosides and hetastarch.

ADMINISTRATION
Direct injection: Inject diluted drug over 3 to 5 minutes directly into vein, through an intermittent infusion device, or into an IV line with a free-flowing, compatible solution.
Intermittent infusion: Give 50 to 100 ml solution through a butterfly or scalp vein needle, an intermittent infusion device, or a patent IV line at the ordered flow rate. Interrupt primary solution during cefoxitin infusion. Administer over 15 to 30 minutes.
Continuous infusion: Infuse up to 1 liter of solution over the prescribed duration.

CONTRAINDICATIONS & CAUTIONS
• Contraindicated in cephalosporin hypersensitivity.
• Use with caution in history of penicillin or other allergies.
• Give cautiously in patients with renal impairment or history of GI disease.

SPECIAL CONSIDERATIONS
• Incidence of thrombophlebitis decreases when butterfly or scalp vein needle is used.
• Loading dose of 1 to 2 g should be given after hemodialysis session. Maintenance doses should reflect patient's creatinine clearance.
• Check for previous penicillin or cephalosporin hypersensitivity.
• If diarrhea persists during therapy, collect stool specimens to rule out possible pseudomembranous colitis.
• Monitor intake and output and serum creatinine and BUN levels to help detect nephrotoxicity.
• Observe patient for fungal and bacterial superinfection with large doses or prolonged use.

ceftazidime

Ceptaz♦, Fortaz◇, Tazicef, Tazidime♦

Pregnancy Risk Category: B

INDICATIONS & DOSAGES
Uncomplicated infections (except for urinary tract) caused by susceptible organisms—
Adults and children over age 12: 1 g q 8 to 12 hours; maximum daily dosage, 6 g. Dosage depends on susceptibility of organism and severity of infection.
Children ages 1 month to 12 years: 25 to 50 mg/kg q 8 hours; maximum daily dosage, 6 g.
Neonates: 30 mg/kg q 12 hours.
Urinary tract infection—
Adults and children over age 12: in uncomplicated infection, 250 mg q 12 hours; in severe infection, 500 mg q 8 to 12 hours.

Bone and joint infection—
Adults and children over age 12:
2 g q 12 hours.
Uncomplicated pneumonia, mild skin and skin-structure infections—
Adults and children over age 12:
500 mg to 1 g q 8 hours.
Peritonitis, meningitis, severe gynecologic infections, other life-threatening infections—
Adults and children over age 12:
2 g q 8 hours.
Pseudomonal lung infection in patients with cystic fibrosis who have normal renal function—
Adults and children over age 12:
30 to 50 mg/kg q 8 hours; maximum daily dosage, 6 g.

Note: Adjust dosage in renal failure. For adults, give 1-g loading dose. Maintenance dosage reflects creatinine clearance. If it is between 31 and 50 ml/minute, dosage is 1-g q 12 hours; 16 and 30 ml/minute, 1 g q 24 hours; 5 and 15 ml/minute, 500 mg q 24 hours; and if it is below 5 ml/minute, give 500 mg q 48 hours.

For hemodialysis patients, give a loading dose of 1 g, then 1 g after each session. For peritoneal dialysis patients, give a loading dose of 1 g, then 500 mg q 24 hours.

PREPARATION & STORAGE
Available as a white to off-white sterile powder in 500-mg, 1-, and 2-g vials; also available in 1- and 2-g piggyback vials for infusion. Powder and solution may darken, but potency is not generally changed. Store powder at 59° to 86° F (15° to 30° C). Protect from light.

Piggyback vials are supplied under reduced pressure because carbon dioxide is released and positive pressure develops when the drug is reconstituted. Venting may be necessary. Follow reconstitution instructions for each brand.

To reconstitute a 500-mg vial, add 5 ml of sterile water for injection, yielding a concentration of 100 mg/ml. To reconstitute a 1-g vial, add 3 ml of sterile water for in-

jection to yield a concentration of 280 mg/ml, or 10 ml to yield 95 to 100 mg/ml. To reconstitute a 2-g vial, add 10 ml of sterile water for injection to yield a concentration of 180 mg/ml.

For the 1- or 2-g piggyback vial, reconstitute with 10 ml of sterile water for injection and dilute with 90 ml of a compatible IV solution. The resultant solution will contain 10 mg/ml for the 1-g vial and 20 mg/ml for the 2-g vial.

Solutions usually remain potent for 18 to 24 hours at room temperature and for 7 to 10 days when refrigerated. If stored at –4° F (–20° C) immediately after reconstitution, they usually remain potent for 3 to 6 months. Avoid heating after thawing or refreezing. Thawed solutions usually retain potency for 8 to 24 hours at room temperature and for 4 to 7 days if refrigerated. Do not use if solution is cloudy or contains a precipitate.

For infusions at concentrations between 1 and 40 mg/ml, use these solutions: 0.9% NaCl injection; 1/6 M sodium lactate injection; dextrose 5% in 0.2%, 0.45%, or 0.9% NaCl; or D_5W or dextrose 10% in water. For concentrations between 1 and 20 mg/ml, use Ringer's injection, lactated Ringer's injection, invert sugar 10% in sterile water for injection, or dextrose 5% and Normosol-M. These solutions may be stored for 24 hours at room temperature or for 7 days if refrigerated. Solutions in dextrose 5% or 0.9% NaCl remain stable for at least 6 hours at room temperature in plastic tubing, drip chambers, or volume-control devices of infusion sets.

Incompatibility
Incompatible with aminoglycosides, fluconazole, idarubicin hydrochloride, sargramostim, sodium bicarbonate solutions, and vancomycin.

ADMINISTRATION
Direct injection: First remove any carbon dioxide bubbles. Then inject

reconstituted drug directly into vein over 3 to 5 minutes. Alternatively, give through an IV line containing a free-flowing, compatible solution.
Intermittent infusion: Using a Y-type administration set, infuse solution over 15 to 30 minutes. Discontinue primary solution during ceftazidime infusion.
Continuous infusion: Infuse prescribed volume over 24 hours. Do not use thawed solutions.

CONTRAINDICATIONS & CAUTIONS
• Contraindicated in cephalosporin hypersensitivity.
• Use cautiously in patients with penicillin hypersensitivity or history of allergies.
• Give cautiously in history of GI disease and in those with hepatic or renal impairment, poor nutritional status, or those receiving protracted course of therapy.
• Because the safety of the arginine component of Ceptaz has not been established in children, use sodium bicarbonate formulations of ceftaz-idime (Fortaz, Tazicef, Tazidime) in children under age 12.

SPECIAL CONSIDERATIONS
• Monitor PT. Administer vitamin K, as ordered, for prolonged PT.
• Assess IV site for signs of inflammation and change site as needed.
• Treat overdose symptomatically. Drug is removed by dialysis.
• Check for previous penicillin or cephalosporin hypersensitivity before giving first dose.
• If diarrhea persists during therapy, collect stool specimens to rule out possible pseudomembranous colitis.
• Closely monitor renal function if patient has renal impairment or is receiving aminoglycoside antibiotics or potent diuretics.
• Observe patient for superinfection with prolonged use.

ceftizoxime sodium

Cefizox

Pregnancy Risk Category: B

INDICATIONS & DOSAGES
Life-threatening infections caused by susceptible organisms—
Adults: 3 to 4 g q 8 hours; maximum dose, 12 g/day. In renal impairment, a loading dose of 500 mg to 1 g may be given. Maintenance dose is determined by creatinine clearance. If creatinine clearance exceeds 80 ml/minute, give usual adult dosage; if it is between 50 and 79 ml/minute, 750 mg to 1.5 g q 8 hours; between 5 and 49 ml/minute, 500 mg to 1 g q 12 hours; and if it is below 5 ml/minute, give 500 mg to 1 g q 48 hours or 500 mg q 24 hours.
Children over age 6 months: 200 mg/kg daily in divided doses. Maximum dosage is 12 g daily.
Uncomplicated infections (except those of the urinary tract) to severe infections caused by susceptible organisms—
Adults: 1 to 2 g q 8 to 12 hours; maximum dosage, 12 g/day. In renal impairment, maintenance dosage is determined by creatinine clearance. If creatinine clearance exceeds 80 ml/minute, give usual adult dosage; if it is between 50 and 79 ml/minute, 500 mg q 8 hours; between 5 and 49 ml/minute, 250 to 500 mg q 12 hours; and if it is below 5 ml/minute, give 500 mg q 48 hours or 250 mg q 24 hours.
Children over age 6 months: 50 mg/kg q 6 to 8 hours.
Uncomplicated urinary tract infection caused by susceptible organisms—
Adults: 500 mg q 12 hours. Give higher dosage in *Pseudomonas aeruginosa* infection.

PREPARATION & STORAGE
Available as a white to pale yellow crystalline powder in 500-mg, 1-, and 2-g vials; protect from light and store at 59° to 86° F (15° to 30° C). Also supplied as a frozen solution in

50-ml single-dose plastic containers, equivalent to 1 or 2 g in D_5W; store frozen but not below $-4°$ F ($-20°$ C).

When reconstituting powder, add 5 ml of sterile water for injection to the 500-mg vial, 10 ml to the 1-g vial, and 20 ml to the 2-g vial. This yields a concentration of 95 mg/ml.

Reconstitute piggyback vials with 50 to 100 ml of 0.9% NaCl injection. Alternatively, use D_5W or dextrose 10% in water; dextrose 5% in 0.2%, 0.45%, or 0.9% NaCl; Ringer's injection; lactated Ringer's; invert sugar 10% in sterile water for injection; or 5% sodium bicarbonate in sterile water for injection. Shake well. For continuous infusion, add to compatible solution an amount appropriate for the patient's condition. Solution remains stable for 24 hours at room temperature or for 96 hours if refrigerated. Although it may turn yellow to amber, this color change does not affect potency. However, do not use if solution is cloudy or contains precipitate.

Thaw frozen solution at room temperature. Discard if leaks, cloudiness, precipitation, or a broken seal is detected. After thawing, the solution remains stable for 24 hours at room temperature or for 10 days if refrigerated. Do not refreeze.

Incompatibility
Incompatible with aminoglycosides.

ADMINISTRATION
Direct injection: Inject reconstituted drug over 3 to 5 minutes directly into a vein or an IV line containing a compatible solution. Do not inject commercially available frozen solutions intended for infusion.
Intermittent infusion: Infuse 50 to 100 ml of diluted drug into established IV line over 15 to 30 minutes.
Continuous infusion: Using an infusion pump, give solution over 24 hours.

CONTRAINDICATIONS & CAUTIONS
• Contraindicated in cephalosporin hypersensitivity.

• Use cautiously in patients with penicillin hypersensitivity or history of allergies.
• Use cautiously in patients with history of GI disease and in those with renal impairment.

SPECIAL CONSIDERATIONS
• Frozen solution contains dextrose 5%.
• If patient is undergoing hemodialysis, give dose after dialysis session. Supplemental doses are not required.
• Check for previous penicillin or cephalosporin hypersensitivity before giving first dose.
• If diarrhea persists during therapy, collect stool specimens to rule out possible pseudomembranous colitis.
• If patient receives high doses, takes other antibiotics (especially aminoglycosides), or has renal impairment, monitor renal function and intake and output.
• Observe patient for superinfection with larger doses or prolonged use.

ceftriaxone sodium

Rocephin

Pregnancy Risk Category: B

INDICATIONS & DOSAGES
Severe infections caused by susceptible organisms—
Adults: 1 to 2 g once daily or in divided doses q 12 hours; maximum, 4 g daily. Dosage depends on infection type and severity.
Children under age 12: 50 to 75 mg/kg daily in divided doses q 12 hours; maximum, 2 g daily.
Meningitis—
Adults and children:
100 mg/kg/day once daily or in equally divided doses q 12 hours. May give 100-mg/kg loading dose. Maximum, 4 g daily.
Disseminated gonococcal infections—
Adults: 1 g daily.
Surgical prophylaxis—
Adults: 1 g 30 minutes to 2 hours before surgery.

C

PREPARATION & STORAGE

Available as a white to yellowish orange crystalline powder in vials containing 250 mg, 500 mg, 1 g, or 2 g. Also available in 1- and 2-g piggyback vials. When reconstituted, solution turns light yellow to amber, depending on the diluent, drug concentration, and storage duration.

Reconstitute with sterile water for injection, 0.9% NaCl injection, D_5W or dextrose 10% injection, or a combination of NaCl and dextrose injection and other compatible solutions. These include sodium lactate, invert sugar 10%, sodium bicarbonate 5%, FreAmine III, dextrose 5% and Normosol-M, dextrose 5% and Ionosol B, and mannitol 5% or 10%.

Reconstitute by adding 2.4 ml diluent to the 250-mg vial, 4.8 ml to the 500-mg vial, 9.6 ml to the 1-g vial, and 19.2 ml to the 2-g vial. Reconstitute the 1-g piggyback vial with 10 ml diluent and the 2-g vial with 20 ml diluent. All reconstituted solutions yield a concentration that averages 100 mg/ml. After reconstitution, dilute further for intermittent infusion to desired concentration. Concentrations of 10 to 40 mg/ml are recommended, but lesser ones can be used. IV dilutions are stable for 24 hours to 3 days at room temperature or 3 to 10 days if refrigerated.

Incompatibility
Incompatible with aminoglycosides. Do not mix with amsacrine, clindamycin phosphate, fluconazole, or vancomycin hydrochloride.

ADMINISTRATION
Direct injection: Inject reconstituted drug over 2 to 4 minutes directly into a vein, through an intermittent infusion device, or into an IV line containing a compatible solution. *Intermittent infusion:* Give diluted drug over 15 to 30 minutes, using an intermittent infusion device or an IV line containing a compatible solution. Administer over 10 to 30 minutes in neonates or children.

CONTRAINDICATIONS & CAUTIONS

• Contraindicated in cephalosporin hypersensitivity.
• Use cautiously in patients with penicillin hypersensitivity, history of allergies, GI disease, or renal or hepatic impairment.
• Also use cautiously in patients with preexisting disease of the gallbladder, biliary tract, liver, or pancreas.

SPECIAL CONSIDERATIONS

• Continue treatment for at least 2 days after symptoms of infection disappear. Usual duration of 4 to 14 days may be prolonged in severe infection.
• High doses and rapid infusion rates increase risk of cholelithiasis.
• Discontinue drug if symptoms of gallbladder disease occur.
• Monitor PT. Administer vitamin K, as ordered, in patients with prolonged PT at risk for vitamin K deficiency.
• Check for previous penicillin or cephalosporin allergy before giving first dose.
• If diarrhea persists during therapy, collect stool specimens to rule out possible pseudomembranous colitis.
• If patient receives high doses (over 2 g daily), receives other antibiotics (especially aminoglycosides), or has renal impairment, monitor renal function and intake and output.
• Observe patient for superinfection with large doses or prolonged use.

cefuroxime sodium

Kefurox, Zinacef
Pregnancy Risk Category: B

INDICATIONS & DOSAGES
Uncomplicated urinary tract infections, skin and skin-structure infections, disseminated gonococcal infections, and uncomplicated pneumonia caused by susceptible organisms—
Adults: 750 mg q 8 hours.

Children over age 3 months: 50 to 100 mg/kg daily in divided doses q 6 to 8 hours.
Severe or complicated infections caused by susceptible organisms—
Adults: 1.5 g q 8 hours.
Bacterial meningitis—
Adults: up to 3 g q 8 hours.
Children over age 3 months: initially, 200 to 240 mg/kg/day in divided doses q 6 to 8 hours; after clinical improvement, dosage may be reduced to 100 mg/kg/day.
Life-threatening infections or infections caused by less susceptible organisms—
Adults: 1.5 g q 6 hours.
    Note: Dosage in renal failure reflects creatinine clearance. For adults with a creatinine clearance over 20 ml/minute, give 750 mg to 1.5 g q 8 hours; between 10 and 20 ml/minute, 750 mg q 12 hours; and if it is below 10 ml/minute, give 750 mg q 24 hours.
    If patient is undergoing hemodialysis, give dose at end of session.
Preoperative prophylaxis for clean-contaminated or potentially contaminated surgery—
Adults: 1.5 g 30 to 60 minutes before surgery and, during prolonged procedures, 750 mg q 8 hours. Continue drug for at least 24 hours afterward. Open-heart surgery patients should receive 1.5 g initially and q 12 hours, to total of 6 g.

PREPARATION & STORAGE
Available as a sterile powder in 750-mg and 1.5-g vials. Store vials between 59° and 86° F (15° and 30° C) and protect from light.
    Reconstitute 750-mg vial of Zinacef with 8 ml (9 ml for Kefurox) of sterile water for injection, withdrawing the entire amount (8 ml for Kefurox) for 750-mg dose. For the 1.5-g vial of Zinacef, reconstitute with 16 ml (14 ml for Kefurox) of sterile water for injection, withdrawing the entire volume for 1.5-g dose of either Zinacef or Kefurox. After reconstitution, solutions maintain

potency for 24 hours at room temperature and for 48 hours if refrigerated. Properly frozen solutions can be stored for up to 6 months.
    For infusion, dilute 750 mg or 1.5 g in 50 to 100 ml of D_5W for injection. Solution will maintain potency for 24 hours at room temperature and for 7 days if refrigerated. Other compatible solutions include dextrose 5% in 0.2%, 0.45%, or 0.9% NaCl; dextrose 10% in water; invert sugar 10%; Ringer's injection; lactated Ringer's; 0.9% NaCl; and 1/6 M sodium lactate.
    ADD-Vantage vials should be reconstituted according to the manufacturer's directions.

Incompatibility
Incompatible with aminoglycosides, doxapram hydrochloride, fluconazole, and sodium bicarbonate injection.

ADMINISTRATION
Direct injection: Give directly into vein over 3 to 5 minutes or inject into an IV line containing a free-flowing, compatible solution.
Intermittent infusion: Infuse solution over 15 to 60 minutes. Discontinue primary infusion during cefuroxime administration.
Continuous infusion: Using an established IV line, infuse the solution at the ordered rate.

CONTRAINDICATIONS & CAUTIONS
• Contraindicated in hypersensitivity to cephalosporins.
• Use cautiously in known hypersensitivity to penicillin and in ulcerative colitis, regional enteritis, antibiotic-associated colitis, and renal dysfunction.

SPECIAL CONSIDERATIONS
• Assess IV site for signs of phlebitis and change site, as needed.
• Treat overdose symptomatically. Drug can be removed by hemodialysis and peritoneal dialysis.
• Check for previous penicillin or cephalosporin hypersensitivity.

• If diarrhea persists during therapy, collect stool specimens to rule out possible pseudomembranous colitis.
• Monitor intake and output and serum creatinine and BUN levels.
• Observe patient for superinfection with large doses or prolonged use.

cephapirin sodium

Cefadyl◆

Pregnancy Risk Category: B

INDICATIONS & DOSAGES
Severe infection caused by susceptible organisms or infection caused by less susceptible organisms—
Adults: 1 to 2 g q 4 to 6 hours; maximum, 12 g daily.
Mild to moderate infection caused by susceptible organisms—
Adults: 0.5 to 1 g q 4 to 6 hours.
Children age 3 months and older: 10 to 20 mg/kg q 6 hours.
Surgical prophylaxis—
Adults: 1 to 2 g 30 to 60 minutes before surgery, repeated intraoperatively, then q 6 hours for 24 hours after surgery. Prophylaxis may continue for up to 5 days if severe complications occur.
Note: Adjust dosage in renal failure. For adults, give lower dose of 7.5 to 15 mg/kg q 12 hours.

PREPARATION & STORAGE
Available as a white powder in 1-g vials; store at 59° to 86° F (15° to 30° C). For direct injection, reconstitute with 10 ml of sterile water for injection, 0.9% NaCl, or D_5W. For infusion, add 40 to 50 ml of dextrose 5% in Ringer's injection; dextrose 5% in lactated Ringer's; dextrose 5% in 0.2%, 0.45%, or 0.9% NaCl; dextrose 5%, 10%, or 20% in water; invert sugar 20% and 0.9% NaCl; Ringer's injection or lactated Ringer's injection; 0.9% NaCl; 1/6 M sodium lactate; dextrose 10% in Ionosol G; Ionosol D-CM; Normosol-R; or dextrose 5% in Normosol-R.

Solution concentrations remain stable for 12 to 48 hours at room temperature. A concentration of 5 mg/ml is stable for 10 days if refrigerated. All solutions may be frozen in the original vial immediately after reconstitution. Thawed slowly to room temperature, solutions remain stable for at least 12 hours. Solutions may turn yellow, but this does not affect potency.

Incompatibility
Incompatible with aminoglycosides, aminophylline, ascorbic acid injection, epinephrine hydrochloride, norepinephrine tartrate, phenytoin sodium, and thiopental sodium.

ADMINISTRATION
Direct injection: Give directly into vein over 3 to 5 minutes.
Intermittent infusion: Using a Y-type administration set, infuse into an IV line containing a free-flowing, compatible solution. If a 4-g piggyback vial is used, discontinue primary infusion while giving cephapirin.
Continuous infusion: Give solution over 24 hours.

CONTRAINDICATIONS & CAUTIONS
• Contraindicated in cephalosporin hypersensitivity.
• Use with caution in hypersensitivity to penicillins or other drugs and in renal impairment or GI disease.
• Safe use in infants under age 3 months has not been established.

SPECIAL CONSIDERATIONS
• Check IV site frequently for vein irritation and phlebitis. Use of small IV needle in the larger available veins may be preferable.
• For patient receiving hemodialysis, give 7.5 to 15 mg/kg before dialysis and every 12 hours thereafter.
• Check for previous penicillin or cephalosporin hypersensitivity before giving first dose.
• If diarrhea persists during therapy, collect stool specimens to rule out possible pseudomembranous colitis.
• Monitor renal function.

• Observe patient for superinfection with large doses or prolonged use.

chlordiazepoxide hydrochloride

Librium◆

Controlled Substance Schedule IV

Pregnancy Risk Category: D

INDICATIONS & DOSAGES
Short-term management of acute or severe anxiety—
Adults: 50 to 100 mg initially, then 25 to 50 mg t.i.d. or q.i.d., p.r.n.
Children over age 12: 25 to 50 mg t.i.d. or q.i.d.
Acute alcohol withdrawal and management of associated agitation—
Adults: 50 to 100 mg initially, then repeated q 2 to 4 hours, p.r.n., up to maximum of 300 mg daily.

PREPARATION & STORAGE
Available as a dry powder in an amber ampule containing 100 mg of drug. Do not use the IM diluent provided by the manufacturer for IV reconstitution because air bubbles will form. Instead, dilute powder with 5 ml of sterile 0.9% NaCl or sterile water for injection to yield a concentration of 20 mg/ml. Gently rotate ampule until powder dissolves. Protect from light. Administer immediately and discard any unused solution.

Incompatibility
Incompatible with benzquinamide. However, manufacturer recommends that chlordiazepoxide not be mixed with any other drug.

ADMINISTRATION
Direct injection: Inject reconstituted drug into vein over at least 1 minute. Alternatively, inject drug into IV tubing at a site directly above needle or cannula insertion site. After injection, flush tubing with 0.9% NaCl.

CONTRAINDICATIONS & CAUTIONS
• Contraindicated in chlordiazepoxide or benzodiazepine hypersensitivity, shock or unstable blood pressure, coma, and acute alcohol intoxication with depressed vital signs.
• Also contraindicated in patients with history of drug dependence or emotional instability, glaucoma, hypoalbuminemia, severe depression and myasthenia gravis, severe COPD, psychosis, and hyperkinesis.
• Give cautiously in hepatic or renal impairment and in elderly or debilitated patients.

SPECIAL CONSIDERATIONS
• Do not stop drug abruptly after long-term administration because withdrawal symptoms may occur.
• Drug may contain benzyl alcohol.
• Take vital signs before therapy and monitor them carefully during and after injection. Keep resuscitation equipment readily available.
• Maintain bed rest for at least 3 hours after injection.
• Institute safety measures to prevent falls and injuries caused by hypotension, confusion, or oversedation.
• Monitor CBC and liver function studies during prolonged therapy.

chlorpromazine hydrochloride

Largactil◇, Ormazine, Thorazine

Pregnancy Risk Category: C

INDICATIONS & DOSAGES
Severe hiccups—
Adults: 25 to 50 mg infused at rate of 1 mg/minute.
Adjunctive treatment for tetanus—
Adults: 25 to 50 mg t.i.d. or q.i.d.
Children age 6 months and older: 0.55 mg/kg q 6 to 8 hours. Maximum daily dose: 40 mg for children weighing under 50 lb (22.7 kg) and

75 mg for children weighing 50 to 100 lb (22.7 to 45.5 kg).
Vomiting during surgery—
Adults: 2 mg q 2 minutes; total dose, 25 mg.
Children: 1 mg q 2 minutes; total dose, 0.275 mg/kg. May repeat dose in 30 minutes if hypotension does not occur.

PREPARATION & STORAGE
Available in 1- and 2-ml ampules and 10-ml multiple-dose vials containing 25-mg/ml concentration. Store below 104° F (40° C), preferably between 59° and 86° F (15° and 30° C). Protect from light and freezing. Discard if darker than light amber or if precipitate forms.

For direct injection, dilute with 0.9% NaCl to a 1-mg/ml concentration. For infusion, add ordered dose to 500 to 1,000 ml of 0.9% NaCl.

Incompatibility
Incompatible with aminophylline, amphotericin B, ampicillin, atropine, chloramphenicol sodium succinate, chlorothiazide, cimetidine, dimenhydrinate, heparin sodium, melphalan hydrochloride, methicillin, methohexital sodium, paclitaxel, penicillin, pentobarbital, phenobarbital, thiopental, and solutions having a pH of 4 to 5.

ADMINISTRATION
Direct injection: Slowly inject ordered amount of diluted drug (1-mg/ml concentration) into the tubing of a patent IV line at a rate of no less than 1 mg/minute in adults or 0.5 mg/minute in children. Direct injection is generally used for adjunctive treatment of tetanus and vomiting during surgery.
Continuous infusion: Slowly infuse ordered dose diluted in 500 to 1,000 ml. Used for treatment of severe hiccups.

CONTRAINDICATIONS & CAUTIONS
• Contraindicated in hypersensitivity to phenothiazines and sulfites and in patients with severe toxic CNS depression, subcortical brain damage, bone marrow depression, and severe CV disorders.
• Avoid use in neurologic disorders such as Reye's syndrome, meningitis, encephalopathy, and encephalitis.
• Use with caution in patients with alcoholism and in debilitated or elderly patients.
• Give cautiously to patients with hypocalcemia, glaucoma or a predisposition to this disorder, hepatic or renal disease, Parkinson's disease, peptic ulcer disease, urine retention, respiratory disease, seizure disorders, and symptomatic prostatic hypertrophy.
• Use carefully in patients who show severe reactions to electroconvulsive therapy.
• Caution women against breastfeeding during therapy.

SPECIAL CONSIDERATIONS
• Because of possible hypotension, give IV only to patients on bed rest or to acute ambulatory patients who can be closely monitored.
• Administer with patient in a supine position. Keep patient supine for at least 30 minutes after injection.
• Establish baseline blood pressure and heart rate, and monitor for tachycardia and hypotension.
• After drug discontinuation, notify doctor if patient experiences dizziness, nausea, or vomiting; GI upset; pain; trembling of hands and fingers; or controlled, repetitive movements of the mouth, tongue, and jaw.
• Monitor intake and output for urine retention and constipation.

cidofovir

Vistide

Pregnancy Risk Category: C

INDICATIONS & DOSAGES
CMV retinitis in patients with AIDS—
Adults: initially, 5 mg/kg once weekly for 2 weeks; maintenance

---

dose, 5 mg/kg given once q 2 weeks. Must be administered with 2 g PO probenecid 3 hours before cidofovir, followed by 1 g at 2 and 8 hours after completion of cidofovir infusion.

Note: Adjust dosage in renal failure. If creatinine clearance is between 41 and 55 ml/minute, initial dose is 2 mg/kg once weekly for 2 weeks followed by 2 mg/kg once q 2 weeks; between 30 and 40 ml/minute, initial dose is 1.5 mg/kg once weekly for 2 weeks, followed by 1.5 mg/kg once q 2 weeks; between 20 and 29 ml/minute, initial dose is 1 mg/kg once weekly for 2 weeks, followed by 1 mg/kg once q 2 weeks; and if it is 19 ml/minute or less, initial dose is 0.5 mg/ml, followed by 0.5 mg/kg once q 2 weeks.

PREPARATION & STORAGE
Available in vials containing 75 mg/ml. Dilute with 100 ml of 0.9% NaCl solution.

Administer diluted solution within 24 hours of preparation. If it is not used immediately, refrigerate at 36° to 46° F (2° to 8° C) for up to 24 hours. Allow solution to reach room temperature before use.

Incompatibility
None reported. Do not mix with other drugs or supplements.

ADMINISTRATION
Intermittent infusion: Infuse entire volume of diluted solution over 1 hour at a constant rate with an infusion device.

CONTRAINDICATIONS & CAUTIONS
• Contraindicated in hypersensitivity to drug or history of clinically severe hypersensitivity to probenecid or other sulfur-containing medication.
• Also contraindicated as an intraocular injection or in breast-feeding women.
• Do not administer to patients with baseline serum creatinine exceeding 1.5 mg/dl or calculated creatinine

clearance of 55 ml/minute or less unless potential benefits outweigh potential risks.
• Use cautiously in renally impaired patients and in the elderly.
• Safety and efficacy in children have not been established.
• Advise women of childbearing age not to become pregnant during and within 1 month of cidofovir treatment.

SPECIAL CONSIDERATIONS
• Administer 1 L of 0.9% NaCl over 1 to 2 hours immediately before each cidofovir infusion.
• Administer probenecid, as ordered.
• Because of its mutagenic properties, drug should be prepared in a class II laminar flow biological safety cabinet. Personnel preparing drug should wear surgical gloves and a closed front surgical gown with knit cuffs.
• Discontinue zidovudine therapy or reduce dosage by 50% on the days cidofovir is administered.
• In cases of overdose, hemodialysis and hydration may reduce drug plasma levels. Probenecid may reduce the potential for nephrotoxicity.
• Monitor WBC counts and differential before each dose.
• Monitor serum creatinine and urine protein levels before each dose.

cimetidine hydrochloride

Tagamet◆

Pregnancy Risk Category: B

INDICATIONS & DOSAGES
Duodenal ulcer (short-term treatment)—
Adults: 300 mg q 6 to 8 hours (q 12 hours if creatinine clearance is under 30 ml/minute); maximum daily dosage, 2,400 mg. Adjust dosage to maintain a gastric pH above 5. To increase dosage, give

300-mg doses more frequently to maximum daily dosage.

Children: 5 to 10 mg/kg q 6 to 8 hours.

Prevention of upper GI bleeding in critically ill patients—

Adults: 50 mg/hour by continuous infusion for up to 7 days. Patients with creatinine clearance below 30 ml/minute/1.73 m² should receive 25 mg/hour.

Pathologic hypersecretory conditions or intractable ulcers—

Adults: 300 mg q 6 hours.

Note: Reduced dosage may be necessary for adult patients with hepatic or renal failure.

PREPARATION & STORAGE

Available in 2-ml single-dose disposable syringes containing 300 mg cimetidine; in 8-ml multidose vials containing 300 mg/2 ml; and in PVC bags containing 300 mg/50 ml.

For direct injection, dilute dose (including the single-dose form) with 20 ml of 0.9% NaCl for injection. For infusion, dilute with 50 to 100 ml of a compatible solution, such as amino acid solution, D_5W, Ringer's injection, lactated Ringer's, invert sugar 5% in water, 0.9% NaCl, or dextrose 5% in 0.2%, 0.45%, or 0.9% NaCl.

Use reconstituted solutions within 48 hours. Check expiration dates. Protect from light and store at room temperature. Solutions become cloudy if refrigerated. Discard solutions if discolored or if precipitate appears.

Incompatibility

Incompatible with aminophylline, amphotericin B, barbiturates, cefamandole, cefazolin, cephalothin, indomethacin sodium trihydrate, pentobarbital sodium, and a combination of pentobarbital sodium and atropine sulfate.

ADMINISTRATION

Direct injection: Inject diluted drug over at least 5 minutes directly into vein or through an IV line containing a free-flowing, compatible solution. Rapid injection may increase the risk of arrhythmias and hypotension.

Intermittent infusion: Give 50 to 100 ml of diluted drug over 15 to 20 minutes, using an intermittent infusion device or infused into an IV line containing a free-flowing, compatible solution.

Continuous infusion: Dilute 900 mg of drug in 100 to 1,000 ml of compatible solution. Using an infusion pump, infuse at a rate of 37.5 mg/ hour. Patients may require more than 900 mg/day to maintain pH control. Dosage adjustments should be individualized.

CONTRAINDICATIONS & CAUTIONS
• Contraindicated in known hypersensitivity to drug.
• Use with caution in patients under age 16 because of limited data and in the elderly.
• Also use cautiously in patients with strongyloidosis infection, organic brain syndrome, or renal or hepatic impairment.
• Dosage adjustment is needed in patients with renal or hepatic failure.
• Advise women of childbearing age to avoid becoming pregnant during drug therapy.
• Caution women against breastfeeding during therapy.

SPECIAL CONSIDERATIONS
• If patient is undergoing hemodialysis, give drug after dialysis session and every 12 hours during the interdialysis period.
• Drug may be infused over at least 30 minutes to minimize the risk of adverse cardiac effects.
• In cases of overdose, treat tachycardia with a beta blocker. Hemodialysis promotes drug clearance.
• If cimetidine and coumarin anticoagulants must be given together, closely monitor PT and adjust dosage as necessary.
• Drug-induced confusion may occur in elderly patients.

• Because cimetidine alters gastric pH, it may affect the bioavailability of many oral drugs.

ciprofloxacin

Cipro IV

Pregnancy Risk Category: C

INDICATIONS & DOSAGES
Mild to moderate urinary tract infections—
Adults: 200 mg q 12 hours.
Severe to complicated urinary tract infections; mild to moderate infections of lower respiratory tract, skin and skin structure, bone and joint—
Adults: 400 mg q 12 hours.
Severe to complicated infections of lower respiratory tract, skin and skin structure, bone and joint—
Adults: 400 mg q 8 hours.
Mild, moderate, or severe nosocomial pneumonia—
Adults: 400 mg q 8 hours.
Complicated intra-abdominal infections—
Adults: 400 mg q 12 hours (given with IV metronidazole).
Note: Dosage in renal failure reflects creatinine clearance. For adults with creatinine clearance below 29 ml/minute, dosage is 200 to 400 mg q 18 to 24 hours. Duration of treatment depends on severity of infection, but usually lasts 7 to 14 days. Bone and joint infections may require treatment for 4 to 6 weeks or more.

PREPARATION & STORAGE
Available as a clear, colorless to slightly yellow solution in 200- and 400-mg vials (injection concentrate). Dilute vials before use.
Reconstitute with 0.9% NaCl injection or 5% dextrose injection to concentrations of 1 to 2 mg/ml. IV dilutions are stable for up to 14 days at room temperature or when refrigerated.
Premixed solution is also available in flexible containers of 200 mg in 100 ml 5% dextrose or 0.9% NaCl, and 400 mg in 200 ml 5% dextrose.

Incompatibility
Incompatible with aminophylline and clindamycin phosphate.

ADMINISTRATION
Intermittent infusion: Infuse diluted solution over 60 minutes into a large vein. Discontinue flow of any concurrent IV solutions temporarily while infusing drug.

CONTRAINDICATIONS & CAUTIONS
• Contraindicated in hypersensitivity to quinolone antimicrobial agents, in pregnant or breast-feeding women, and in those under age 18.
• Use with extreme caution in concurrent IV therapy with theophylline; serious (even fatal) reactions have occurred.
• Use cautiously in renal impairment or CNS disorders and in the elderly.

SPECIAL CONSIDERATIONS
• Make sure patient has adequate hydration to avoid crystalluria. Advise patient to drink sufficient fluids to ensure hydration.
• Carefully monitor ALT, AST, LD, CK, serum bilirubin, and eosinophil and platelet counts; also monitor serum creatinine, BUN, uric acid, blood glucose, and triglyceride levels.
• Observe patient for superinfection with prolonged use.
• Caution ambulatory patient of risk of dizziness.

cisatracurium besylate

Nimbex

Pregnancy Risk Category: B

INDICATIONS & DOSAGES
Note: Dosage requirements vary widely.

Adjunct to general anesthesia, to facilitate tracheal intubation, and to provide skeletal muscle relaxation during surgery—
Adults: 0.15 to 0.2 mg/kg followed by maintenance dose of 0.03 mg/kg q 40 to 60 minutes, p.r.n. Or, after initial dose, 3 mcg/kg/minute maintenance infusion may be given to counteract the spontaneous recovery of neuromuscular function, then reduced to 1 to 2 mcg/kg/minute to maintain neuromuscular block.
Children ages 2 to 12: 0.1 mg/kg, followed by 3 mcg/kg/minute maintenance infusion, reduced to 1 to 2 mcg/kg/minute p.r.n.
Maintenance of neuromuscular blockade during mechanical ventilation in intensive care unit—
Adults: 3 mcg/kg/minute (range, 0.5 to 10.2 mcg/kg/minute).

PREPARATION & STORAGE
Available in 2- and 10-mg/ml vials. Reconstitute with 5% dextrose injection, 0.9% NaCl injection, or 5% dextrose and 0.9% NaCl injection to a concentration of 0.1 to 0.2 mg/ml.
  Solutions may be refrigerated or stored at room temperature for 24 hours.

Incompatibility
Incompatible with alkaline solutions with pH above 8.5, ketorolac, lactated Ringer's injection, and propofol.

ADMINISTRATION
Direct injection: Administer reconstituted solution directly into vein or through IV line containing a free-flowing, compatible solution over 5 to 10 seconds.
Continuous infusion: Infuse diluted solution through IV line containing a compatible solution.

CONTRAINDICATIONS & CAUTIONS
• Contraindicated in patients known to have an allergic hypersensitivity to drug or other bis-benzylisoquinolinium agents.

• Use cautiously in neuromuscular disease and in patients with burns, hemiparesis, or paraparesis.
• Do not administer drug unless personnel and facilities for resuscitation and life support and an antagonist to the drug are immediately available.

SPECIAL CONSIDERATIONS
• Drug is not recommended for rapid-sequence endotracheal intubation because of its intermediate onset.
• Do not administer before patient is unconscious.
• Burn patient may require increased dosages. Administer analgesics, if appropriate.
• In cases of overdose, maintain patent airway and control ventilation until normal neuromuscular function is achieved.
• Measure neuromuscular function with a peripheral nerve stimulator during infusion.
• Monitor acid-base balance and electrolyte levels.
• Monitor patient for malignant hyperthermia.

cisplatin (cis-platinum)

Platinol✦, Platinol-AQ✦

Pregnancy Risk Category: D

INDICATIONS & DOSAGES
Metastatic testicular cancer, in combination with other agents—
Adults: 20 mg/m^2/day for 5 days q 3 weeks for three or four cycles, or 120 mg/m^2 single dose q 3 to 4 weeks for three cycles.
Metastatic ovarian cancer—
Adults: as part of combination therapy, 75 to 100 mg/m^2 q 4 weeks; as a single agent, 100 mg/m^2 q 4 weeks. Alternative dosages, 30 to 120 mg/m^2 q 3 to 4 weeks.
Advanced bladder cancer—
Adults: 50 to 70 mg/m^2 q 3 to 4 weeks. Patients who have received

C

other antineoplastic agents or radiation therapy should receive 50 mg/m² q 4 weeks.
Head and neck cancer—
Adults: as part of combination therapy, 50 to 120 mg/m² according to hospital protocol; as a single agent, 80 to 120 mg/m² q 3 weeks or 50 mg/m² on days 1 and 8 of every 4-week cycle.
Children: 60 mg/m² daily for 2 days q 3 to 4 weeks.
Cervical carcinoma—
Adults: 50 to 100 mg/m² q 3 weeks.
Non-small-cell lung carcinoma—
Adults: as part of combination therapy, 40 to 120 mg/m² q 3 to 6 weeks as directed; as a single agent, 75 to 120 mg/m² q 3 to 6 weeks or 50 mg/m² on days 1 and 8 of every 4-week cycle.
Osteogenic sarcoma, neuroblastoma—
Children: 90 mg/m² q 3 weeks or 30 mg/m² weekly.

PREPARATION & STORAGE
Use extreme caution when preparing or giving cisplatin to avoid mutagenic, teratogenic, and carcinogenic risks. Use a biological containment cabinet and avoid contact with skin. Wear mask and gloves. If solution comes in contact with skin or mucosa, immediately wash thoroughly with soap and water. Dispose of needles, syringes, vials, and unused drug carefully.

Available as a white powder in 10- and 50-mg vials. Protect unopened vials from bright sunlight; however, exposure to fluorescent light causes no problems. Store for up to 2 years at room temperature.

Reconstitute 10-mg vial with 10 ml of sterile water and 50-mg vial with 50 ml of sterile water (drug is also available as an aqueous solution of 50 mg/50 ml and 100 mg/100 ml). For intermittent infusion, dilute reconstituted drug in 2 L of 0.33% or 0.45% NaCl along with 37.5 g of mannitol.

Precipitation may cause loss of potency. To avoid this, do not use needles, syringes, or IV kits containing aluminum parts and do not refrigerate reconstituted solutions.

Reconstituted solutions remain stable for 20 hours at room temperature. Solutions prepared with bacteriostatic water for injection with benzyl alcohol or parabens are stable for 72 hours.

Incompatibility
Incompatible with aluminum, D_5W, 0.1% NaCl, and solutions with a chloride content under 2%, sodium bicarbonate, sodium bisulfate, and sodium thiosulfate.

ADMINISTRATION
Hydrate patient using 0.9% NaCl before giving drug. Maintain urine output of 150 to 400 ml/hour at onset of administration and for at least 4 to 6 hours thereafter.
Intermittent infusion: Give diluted solution through a separate IV line, using a 21G or 23G needle. Infuse over 6 to 8 hours or follow hospital protocol.
Continuous infusion: Infuse diluted solution over 24 hours or 5 days, according to hospital protocol.

CONTRAINDICATIONS & CAUTIONS
• Contraindicated in hypersensitivity to platinum-containing compounds and in those with renal disease, myelosuppression, or hearing impairment.
• Avoid use in existing or recent chickenpox or herpes zoster infections.
• Use cautiously in patients who have received cytotoxic drug or radiation therapy.
• Give cautiously to patients with existing or recent infection and in those with gout or urate calculi.
• Advise women of childbearing age to avoid becoming pregnant during therapy.

SPECIAL CONSIDERATIONS
• For an antiemetic, administer high doses of metoclopramide, diphenhy-

C

dramine, or dexamethasone before and after each dose.

• Drug can be removed by hemodialysis for 3 hours after administration.

• Determine serum magnesium, potassium, calcium, and creatinine levels and BUN and creatinine clearance levels before first infusion and each course.

• Maintain urine output of 100 to 200 ml/hour for 18 to 24 hours after therapy.

• Regularly perform neurologic examinations. Discontinue drug if neurotoxicity occurs.

• Monitor CBC and platelet count weekly.

• Monitor liver and kidney function.

• Perform audiometric tests before each course to detect high-frequency hearing loss.

cladribine (2-chloro-deoxyadenosine)

Leustatin

Pregnancy Risk Category: D

INDICATIONS & DOSAGES
Treatment of active hairy cell leukemia (defined by clinically significant anemia, neutropenia, thrombocytopenia, or disease-related symptoms)—
Adults: 0.09 mg/kg daily by continuous IV infusion for 7 consecutive days, for a total dosage of 0.63 mg/kg.

Drug can be given daily over 7 consecutive 24-hour periods or as a continuous 7-day infusion. Deviation from this dosage regimen is not recommended. Safety and efficacy have not been established in children.

PREPARATION & STORAGE
Available as a preservative-free solution of 1 mg/ml (10-mg vial). Unopened vials should be refrigerated at 36° to 46° F (2° to 8° C) and protected from light. Freezing does not

adversely affect the solution; however, a precipitate may form at low temperatures. Allowing the solution to warm to room temperature and vigorously shaking the vial resolubilizes the precipitate. Do not heat or microwave. Once thawed, the solution is stable until the labeled expiration date if refrigerated. Do not refreeze.

Drug must be diluted before infusion. For a 24-hour infusion, add the calculated dose to a 500-ml infusion bag of 0.9% NaCl injection and infuse continuously over 24 hours. Do not use solutions that contain dextrose.

Alternatively, for the 7-day infusion use bacteriostatic NaCl injection, which contains benzyl alcohol (a preservative). Because the calculated dose dilutes the benzyl alcohol preservative, the effectiveness to the preservative may be reduced in patients weighing more than 187 lb (85 kg). To minimize the risk of microbial contamination, calculate the 7-day dose of cladribine and amount of diluent needed to bring the total volume to 100 ml. First add the calculated dose of cladribine into the infusion reservoir through a sterile 0.22 micron disposable hydrophilic syringe filter; then add the calculated amount of bacteriostatic NaCl (also through the filter) to bring the total volume to 100 ml. Clamp off the line and disconnect and discard the filter. Using aseptic technique, aspirate any air bubbles from the reservoir using the syringe with a dry sterile filter or sterile vent filter assembly. Reclamp and discard the syringe and filter. Physical and chemical stability has been demonstrated with the Pharmacia Deltec medication cassettes.

Once diluted, administer promptly or store in refrigerator for no more than 8 hours before administration. Discard any unused portion using chemotherapy precautions.

Incompatibility
Limited incompatibility data are available. Do not mix with other IV drugs or additives. Do not infuse simultaneously through a common IV line with other drugs. Dextrose solutions accelerate degradation of cladribine.

ADMINISTRATION
Intermittent infusion: Infuse daily over 7 consecutive 24-hour periods.
Continuous infusion: Infuse continuously over 7 days.

CONTRAINDICATIONS & CAUTIONS
• Contraindicated in hypersensitivity to drug or its components.
• Use cautiously in patients with pre-existing bone marrow depression or known or suspected renal or hepatic impairment.
• Advise women of childbearing age to avoid becoming pregnant during therapy.
• Caution women against breast-feeding during therapy.

SPECIAL CONSIDERATIONS
• Stop or interrupt therapy if neurotoxicity or renal toxicity occurs.
• Because drug is a potent antineoplastic agent, use disposable gloves and protective clothing. If skin or mucous membrane contact occurs, wash with copious amounts of water.
• Monitor hematologic function closely, especially during the first 4 to 8 weeks of therapy.
• Monitor renal and hepatic function. There are no specific recommendations for dosage adjustments.
• Monitor for fever during first month of treatment.

clindamycin phosphate

Cleocin Phosphate, Dalacin C Phosphate◊

Pregnancy Risk Category: B

INDICATIONS & DOSAGES
Severe infections caused by susceptible organisms—
Adults: 600 mg to 2.7 g daily equally divided q 6, 8, or 12 hours or by continuous infusion to maintain serum levels of 4 to 6 mcg/ml. May increase to 4.8 g daily for life-threatening infections.
Children over age 1 month: 15 to 40 mg/kg/day equally divided q 6 to 8 hours. Single dose should not exceed 600 mg.
Children age 1 month or less: 15 to 20 mg/kg/day equally divided q 6 to 8 hours; maximum dosage, 300 mg daily.

PREPARATION & STORAGE
Available in a concentration of 150 mg/ml in 2- and 4-ml ampules and 6-ml vials. Store below 104° F (40° C), preferably between 59° and 86° F (15° and 30° C). Protect from freezing.
For a concentration of 6 mg/ml or less, add 25 ml of compatible solution to each 150 mg of clindamycin (300 mg/50 ml). Compatible solutions include D₅W or dextrose 10% in water, Isolyte H, Isolyte M and dextrose 5%, Isolyte P and dextrose 5%, Normosol-R, lactated Ringer's, and 0.9% NaCl. Solutions should be used within 24 hours.

Incompatibility
Incompatible with aminophylline, ampicillin, barbiturates, calcium gluconate, ciprofloxacin hydrochloride, idarubicin hydrochloride, magnesium sulfate, phenytoin sodium, and theophylline. Drug is also incompatible with rubber closures, such as those on IV tubing.

ADMINISTRATION
Intermittent infusion: Infuse drug diluted to a concentration of 6 mg/ ml or less through an intermittent infusion device or into an IV line containing a free-flowing, compatible solution. Infuse 300 mg/50 ml over 10 minutes, 600 mg/100 ml over 20 minutes, or 900 mg/150 ml over 30 minutes. Infuse 1,200 mg/ 100 ml over 40 minutes. Do not infuse more than 1,200 mg over 1 hour.
Continuous infusion: Administer as a single, rapid infusion, then follow with a continuous infusion, using a diluted concentration of 6 mg/ml. For serum levels above 4 mcg/ml, rapidly infuse 10 mg/minute for 30 minutes, then give maintenance dose of 0.75 mg/minute. For serum levels above 5 mcg/ml, rapidly infuse 15 mg/minute for 30 minutes, then give maintenance dose of 1 mg/ minute. For serum levels above 6 mcg/ml, rapidly infuse 20 mg/ minute for 30 minutes, then give maintenance dose of 1.25 mg/ minute.

CONTRAINDICATIONS & CAUTIONS
• Contraindicated in clindamycin or lincomycin hypersensitivity.
• Use cautiously atopic patients and in those with GI disorders and renal or hepatic impairment.
• Also use cautiously in neonates because drug contains benzyl alcohol, which in large doses can cause "fatal gasping syndrome."

SPECIAL CONSIDERATIONS
• Drug may contain benzyl alcohol.
• Severe anaphylactic reaction requires emergency treatment with epinephrine, oxygen, and corticosteroids.
• During long-term therapy, monitor kidney and liver function tests and blood cell counts.
• Colitis may not develop for several weeks after drug has been discontinued.

• If severe, persistent diarrhea occurs, discontinue drug and obtain a stool specimen for culture.
• Observe patient for superinfection with prolonged use.

colchicine

Pregnancy Risk Category: D

INDICATIONS & DOSAGES
Acute gout, gouty arthritis—
Adults: 2 mg, followed by 0.5 mg q 6 hours p.r.n. Maximum daily dose, 4 mg.

PREPARATION & STORAGE
Available in 1-mg/2 ml ampules. Dilute with 0.9% NaCl injection or sterile water for injection. Store in tight, light-resistant containers away from moisture and high temperatures. Do not use if turbid.

Incompatibility
Incompatible with 5% dextrose injection and bacteriostatic 0.9% NaCl injection.

ADMINISTRATION
Direct injection: Administer by slow IV push over 2 to 5 minutes directly into vein or through tubing with a free-flowing, compatible IV solution.

CONTRAINDICATIONS & CAUTIONS
• Contraindicated in patients with hypersensitivity to drug, blood dyscrasias, or serious CV, renal, or GI disease.
• Use cautiously in elderly or debilitated patients and in those with early signs of CV, renal, or GI disease.
• Safety and efficacy in pediatric patients have not been established.

SPECIAL CONSIDERATIONS
• Discontinue drug if nausea, abdominal pain, vomiting, or diarrhea occurs because these are the first signs of toxicity.

• Obtain baseline laboratory studies, including CBC, before initiating therapy and periodically thereafter.
• Advise patient to report rash, sore throat, fever, unusual bleeding and bruising, tiredness, weakness, numbness, or tingling.

co-trimoxazole (sulfamethoxazole-trimethoprim)

Bactrim IV Infusion, Septra IV Infusion◆

Pregnancy Risk Category: C (D if near term)

INDICATIONS & DOSAGES

Systemic bacterial infections caused by susceptible organisms—
Adults and children age 2 months and over: 8 to 10 mg/kg of trimethoprim in two to four doses q 6, 8, or 12 hours. Maximum dose is 960 mg/day.
Pneumocystis carinii *pneumonitis—*
Adults and children age 2 months and older: 15 to 20 mg/kg trimethoprim in three or four divided doses q 6 to 8 hours.
Note: Dosage in renal failure reflects creatinine clearance.
Adults: if creatinine clearance is below 15 ml/minute, use is not recommended; between 15 and 30 ml/minute, give half usual adult dose; if it is exceeds 30 ml/minute, give usual adult dose.
Children: if creatinine clearance is below 20 ml/minute, do not use; between 20 and 30 ml/minute, give half usual pediatric dose; if it exceeds 30 ml/minute, give usual pediatric dose.

PREPARATION & STORAGE

Available in 5-ml ampules and 5-, 10-, and 30-ml vials. Before infusion, add 125 ml of D_5W to dilute a 5-ml vial. New concentration contains 0.64 mg of trimethoprim and 3.2 mg of sulfamethoxazole. Diluted 1:25 solution is stable for 6 hours at room temperature. Solutions containing 0.64 to 0.83 mg of trimethoprim and 3.2 to 4 mg of sulfamethoxazole remain stable for 4 hours; those containing 0.8 to 1.1 mg of trimethoprim and 4 to 5.3 mg of sulfamethoxazole remain stable for 2 hours.

Do not refrigerate drug or solutions. Discard cloudy solutions or those that contain precipitates.

Incompatibility
Avoid diluting with any solution but D_5W because drug components lose potency. Manufacturer recommends mixing no other drugs with co-trimoxazole.

ADMINISTRATION

Intermittent infusion: Using a 21G to 23G needle, infuse appropriate dose of diluted drug into an IV line of free-flowing D_5W over 60 to 90 minutes. Or, infuse drug into a flushed and patent intermittent infusion device. If the only available site is tubing that contains incompatible solutions, flush tubing with 10 ml of sterile water for injection before and after infusion and turn off primary IV solution during co-trimoxazole administration.

CONTRAINDICATIONS & CAUTIONS

• Contraindicated in neonates because sulfonamides can cause kernicterus and in pregnant or breast-feeding women.
• Contraindicated in hypersensitivity to sulfonamides or trimethoprim.
• Also contraindicated in megaloblastic anemias.
• Use cautiously in patients with hypersensitivity to furosemide, thiazide diuretics, sulfonylureas, or carbonic anhydrase inhibitors.
• Also use cautiously in patients with renal or hepatic impairment, bronchial asthma, G6PD deficiency, folic acid deficiency, or AIDS.
• Administer carefully to elderly, malnourished, alcoholic, or debilitated patients.

• Also give carefully to patients receiving chemotherapy, to mentally retarded children, and to patients with streptococcal pharyngitis.

SPECIAL CONSIDERATIONS

• Trimethoprim and active sulfamethoxazole are partially removed by dialysis.
• Monitor BUN, serum creatinine, CBC and platelet count, PTT, PT, and electrolyte levels. Also perform urinalysis.
• Closely monitor patients with AIDS because of increased risk of severe adverse reactions.
• Observe patient for superinfection with prolonged use.
• Advise patient to increase fluid intake to maintain hydration.

cyclophosphamide

Cytoxan✦, Neosar, Procytox◇

Pregnancy Risk Category: D

INDICATIONS & DOSAGES

Lymphomas; acute leukemia (in adults); cancers of the lung, brain, breast, and reproductive organs; autoimmune diseases; and prevention of graft-versus-host disease in organ transplants—
   Note: Dosage reflects patient's disease, condition, and response as well as use of other treatments.
Adults: initially, 40 to 50 mg/kg in divided doses over 2 to 5 days. Maintenance dosage is 10 to 15 mg/kg q 7 to 10 days or 3 to 5 mg/kg twice weekly.
Children: initially, 2 to 8 mg/kg or 60 to 250 mg/m² once weekly for 6 weeks, depending on susceptibility of neoplasm. Maintenance dosage depends on patient tolerance and a WBC count of 2,500 to 4,000/mm³. Recommended maintenance dosage is 10 to 15 mg/kg q 7 to 10 days, or 30 mg/kg q 3 to 4 weeks, or when bone marrow recovers.

PREPARATION & STORAGE

To avoid mutagenic, teratogenic, and carcinogenic risks, use a biological containment cabinet, wear gloves and mask, and use syringes with tight fittings (luer-lock) to prevent leakage. Dispose of needles, syringes, vials, and unused drug correctly.
   Available in 100-mg, 200-mg, 500-mg, 1-g, and 2-g vials. Reconstitute with sterile water for injection or bacteriostatic water for injection (parabens-preserved only) to a concentration of 20 mg/ml. If prepared with sterile water for injection, use solution within 6 hours. Powder contains enough NaCl to produce an isotonic solution. Shake vigorously. Unreconstituted drug stays stable at room temperature; reconstituted drug remains stable for 24 hours at room temperature and for 6 days if refrigerated. Discard unused drug after 24 hours.
   Other compatible solutions include dextrose 5% in lactated Ringer's, dextrose 5% in 0.9% NaCl, lactated Ringer's, 0.45% or 0.9% NaCl, and 1/6 M sodium lactate.

Incompatibility
None known.

ADMINISTRATION

Direct injection: Using a 23G to 25G winged-tip needle, inject reconstituted drug directly into vein over 2 to 3 minutes.
Intermittent infusion: Using a 23G to 25G winged-tip needle, infuse diluted drug over 15 to 20 minutes.

CONTRAINDICATIONS & CAUTIONS

• Contraindicated in patients with previous hypersensitivity to drug.
• Contraindicated in existing or recent chickenpox or herpes zoster and in severe leukopenia or thrombocytopenia.
• Use cautiously in patients with bone marrow depression, tumor infiltration of bone marrow, previous therapy with radiation or other cytotoxic agents, or impaired hepatic or renal function.

C

• Also use cautiously in patients with history of gout or urate renal stones.
• Caution women against breast-feeding during therapy.
• Advise male and female patients to consult with doctor before becoming pregnant or fathering an infant.

SPECIAL CONSIDERATIONS
• If symptoms of cystitis (hematuria, painful urination) occur, discontinue drug immediately.
• Use a new site for each injection or infusion. Heparin locks are not recommended.
• Infuse slowly to prevent facial flushing.
• High IV dosage may cause SIADH leading to hyponatremia.
• Drug can be removed by dialysis.
• Monitor CBC, kidney and liver function, and uric acid levels.
• Monitor for infection in patients with leukopenia.
• To avoid hemorrhagic cystitis, encourage patient to void every 1 to 2 hours while awake and to drink plenty of fluids before, during, and for 72 hours after treatment.
• Instruct patient to avoid OTC medications that contain aspirin.

cyclosporine

Sandimmune◆

Pregnancy Risk Category: C

INDICATIONS & DOSAGES
Prophylaxis and treatment of organ tissue rejection—
Adults and children: 5 to 6 mg/kg daily, beginning 4 to 12 hours before surgery and continuing after surgery until patient can tolerate oral form. Adjust dose to maintain plasma trough levels of 100 to 300 ng/ml.

PREPARATION & STORAGE
Available in 5-ml ampules containing a concentration of 50 mg/ml. For infusion, dilute each milliliter of drug in 20 to 100 ml of 0.9% NaCl

or D_5W. Reconstituted solutions remain stable for up to 24 hours in D_5W injection and for 6 to 12 hours in 0.9% NaCl injection (6 hours in polyvinyl chloride containers and 12 hours in glass containers). Store below 104° F (40° C), preferably at 59° to 86° F (15° to 30° C). Do not freeze or expose to light.

Incompatibility
None reported.

ADMINISTRATION
Continuous infusion: Infuse diluted drug slowly over 2 to 6 hours or up to 24 hours. Know that significant amounts of drug are lost when given through polyvinyl chloride tubing.

CONTRAINDICATIONS & CAUTIONS
• Contraindicated in hypersensitivity to cyclosporine or diluent (polyoxyl 35 castor oil) and in patients with existing or recent chickenpox or herpes zoster infection.
• Use cautiously in patients with hyperkalemia, infection, and hepatic or renal impairment.

SPECIAL CONSIDERATIONS
• Always use drug with a corticosteroid.
• If infusing drug during home care, protect solution from light.
• Monitor patient continuously for the first 30 minutes and then at frequent intervals because of risk of anaphylaxis. Keep resuscitation equipment nearby.
• Perform liver and renal function tests routinely.
• Monitor blood pressure; hypertension can develop within a few weeks of initiation of therapy.

cytarabine (arabinoside, ARA-C, cytarabine arabinoside)

Cytosar◇, Cytosar-U

Pregnancy Risk Category: D

INDICATIONS & DOSAGES
Induction of remission in acute myelogenous or lymphocytic leukemia—
Adults and children: 200 mg/m² daily for 5 days by continuous infusion, then 2 weeks off the drug; maintenance dosage, 70 to 200 mg/m² daily for 2 to 5 days at monthly intervals. Dosage varies, depending on regimen.
Refractory leukemia or malignant lymphoma—
Adults and children: 3 g/m² q 12 hours for up to 12 doses.

PREPARATION & STORAGE
To avoid mutagenic, teratogenic, and carcinogenic risks, use a biological containment cabinet, wear gloves and mask, and use syringes with tight fittings (luer-lock) to prevent drug leakage. Dispose of needles, syringes, vials, and unused drug correctly.

Drug is available in 100-mg, 500-mg, 1-g, and 2-g vials. Reconstitute 100-mg vial with 5 ml of bacteriostatic water for injection (with benzyl alcohol) for a concentration of 20 mg/ml. Reconstitute 500-mg vial with 10 ml of bacteriostatic water for injection (with benzyl alcohol) for a concentration of 50 mg/ml. Reconstitute 1-g vial with 10 ml of bacteriostatic water for injection (with benzyl alcohol) for a concentration of 100 mg/ml. Reconstitute 2-g vial with 20 ml of bacteriostatic water for injection (with benzyl alcohol) for a concentration of 100 mg/ml. However, avoid using benzyl alcohol as a diluent when preparing high-dose cytarabine. Reconstituted solution remains stable for 48 hours at room temperature. Discard if cloudy.

For infusion, dilute with D₅W or with 0.9% NaCl; solution stays stable for 8 days at room temperature. Other compatible solutions include dextrose 5% in 0.9% NaCl and dextrose 5% in lactated Ringer's.

Incompatibility
Incompatible with cephalothin, fluorouracil, heparin sodium, methylprednisolone sodium succinate, nafcillin, oxacillin, and penicillin.

ADMINISTRATION
Direct injection: Give directly into vein or through a winged-tip needle, an intermittent infusion device, or an IV line containing a free-flowing, compatible solution.
Intermittent infusion: Infuse diluted solution over 1 hour or as ordered.
Continuous infusion: Infuse diluted solution over ordered duration, usually 5 days.

CONTRAINDICATIONS & CAUTIONS
• Contraindicated in hypersensitivity to drug and in patients with existing or recent chickenpox or herpes zoster infection.
• Use cautiously in preexisting myelosuppression, hepatic or renal impairment, and history of gout or urate renal calculi.
• Advise women of childbearing age to avoid becoming pregnant during treatment.
• Caution women against breastfeeding during therapy.

SPECIAL CONSIDERATIONS
• If toxicity occurs, withhold next dose of cytarabine and notify doctor.
• Many doctors order prophylactic ophthalmic steroid solutions and pyridoxine (100 mg daily) for patients receiving high-dose therapy.
• Treat skin reactions resulting from high-dose cytarabine with agents used in burn therapy.
• If diarrhea develops, give meticulous skin care to avoid or treat perirectal abscess. Be alert for elec-

trolyte imbalance, malabsorption, and pressure ulcers.

• Prevent or minimize uric acid nephropathy by providing good hydration, alkalinizing urine, or administering allopurinol.

• When giving high-dose cytarabine, perform a thorough neurologic assessment before every dose.

• Monitor kidney and liver function and WBC and platelet counts.

cytomegalovirus immune globulin intravenous, human (CMV-IGIV)

CytoGam

Pregnancy Risk Category: C

INDICATIONS & DOSAGES

To attenuate primary CMV disease in seronegative kidney transplant recipients who receive a kidney from a CMV seropositive donor—

Adults: administer according to the following schedule: within 72 hours of transplant, 150 mg/kg; 2 weeks after transplant, 100 mg/kg; 4 weeks after transplant, 100 mg/kg; 6 weeks after transplant, 100 mg/kg; 8 weeks after transplant, 100 mg/kg; 12 weeks after transplant, 50 mg/kg; and 16 weeks after transplant, 50 mg/kg.

Administer initial dose at 15 mg/kg/hour. Increase to 30 mg/kg/hour after 30 minutes if no untoward reactions occur; then increase to 60 mg/kg/hour after another 30 minutes if no untoward reactions occur. Volume should not exceed 75 ml/hour. Subsequent doses may be administered at 15 mg/kg/hour for 15 minutes, increasing at 15-minute intervals in a stepwise fashion to 60 mg/kg/hour.

PREPARATION & STORAGE

CMV immune globulin is available in a single-dose vial containing about 2,500 mg of lyophilized immunoglobulin. Store in refrigerator at 36° to 46° F (2° to 8° C). Do not store reconstituted drug.

To prepare, remove tab and swab rubber stopper with 70% alcohol or equivalent. Reconstitute with 50 ml sterile water for injection. Final concentration is about 50 mg/ml. *Do not shake; avoid foaming.* Use a double-ended transfer needle or large syringe to add diluent. If using a double-ended transfer needle, first insert one end into the vial of water because the lyophilized powder is in an evacuated vial and the water will transfer by suction. After the water is transferred, release any residual vacuum to hasten dissolving process.

Gently rotate the container to wet any undissolved powder. Allow 30 minutes for dissolution to occur. Reconstituted solution should appear colorless and translucent. Further dilution is not recommended.

Incompatibility
Do not mix with other drugs.

ADMINISTRATION

Intermittent infusion: 15 mg/kg/hour by continuous infusion device; may increase to 30 mg/kg/hour after 30 minutes if no adverse effects; may increase to 60 mg/kg/hour after 30 minutes if no adverse effects. Volume not to exceed 75 ml/hour.

Administer through a separate IV line using a continuous infusion pump. When this is not possible, piggyback into preexisting line of 0.9% NaCl injection, dextrose 2.5% in water, D_5W, $D_{10}W$, or $D_{20}W$. Dextrose solutions may or may not have NaCl added. Do not dilute more than 1:2 with any of the above solutions. Filters are not necessary.

CONTRAINDICATIONS & CAUTIONS
• Contraindicated in patients with history of prior severe reaction associated with this or other human immunoglobulin preparations.
• Anaphylactic reactions may result if administered to patients with selective immunoglobulin A (IgA) deficiency who may have developed antibodies to IgA.

SPECIAL CONSIDERATIONS
• Begin infusions within 6 hours of reconstitution and end within 12 hours.
• If anaphylaxis or hypotension occurs, stop infusion and administer supportive therapy, including diphenhydramine and epinephrine.
• Adverse reactions are usually related to rate of administration. Slow or stop infusion if minor adverse reactions occur.
• Monitor vital signs before infusion, midway through infusion, after infusion, and before any rate increase.
• Instruct patient to defer live-virus vaccinations for at least 3 months after administration.

dacarbazine

DTIC◇, DTIC-Dome
Pregnancy Risk Category: C

INDICATIONS & DOSAGES
Metastatic malignant melanoma—
Adults: 2 to 4.5 mg/kg/day for 10 days, repeated q 4 weeks; or 250 mg/m²/day for 5 days, repeated q 3 weeks.
Hodgkin's disease as second-line therapy—
Adults: 150 mg/m²/day for 5 days (in combination with other drugs), repeated q 4 weeks; or 375 mg/m² on day 1 (in combination with other drugs), repeated q 15 days.

PREPARATION & STORAGE
Use caution when preparing drug to avoid mutagenic, teratogenic, and carcinogenic risks. Use a biological containment cabinet and wear gloves and mask. Use syringes with tight fittings (luer-locks) to prevent drug leakage, and dispose of needles, syringes, vials, and unused drug correctly. Avoid contaminating work surfaces.

Drug comes as a powder in 100- and 200-mg vials that require refrigeration at 36° to 46° F (2° to 8° C) and protection from light. Reconstitute by adding 9.9 ml of sterile water to 100-mg vial or 19.7 ml of sterile water to 200-mg vial. Dilute further for infusion by mixing reconstituted solution with 250 ml of either D_5W or 0.9% NaCl for infusion. Reconstituted drug remains stable for 8 hours at room temperature and for up to 72 hours if refrigerated. Diluted solutions remain stable for 8 hours at room temperature and for up to 24 hours if refrigerated. Protect drug from light during infusion. If color of solution changes to pink, this indicates decomposition.

Incompatibility
Incompatible with cefepime, hydrocortisone sodium succinate, piperacillin, and tazobactam sodium.

ADMINISTRATION
Direct injection: Using a 21G or 23G needle, inject drug directly into vein or through an intermittent infusion device over 1 minute. Apply hot packs to injection site to alleviate pain or burning.
Intermittent infusion: Using a 21G or 23G needle, infuse diluted drug over 15 to 30 minutes.

CONTRAINDICATIONS & CAUTIONS
• Contraindicated in hypersensitivity to dacarbazine.
• Also contraindicated in recent or existing chickenpox or herpes zoster infection.

• Use cautiously in patients with hepatic or renal impairment and myelosuppression.

SPECIAL CONSIDERATIONS
• Avoid extravasation. If it occurs, stop drug and give at another site. Apply ice to area for 24 to 48 hours.
• Administering antiemetics before giving dacarbazine may help decrease nausea.
• Some doctors recommend that patient be well hydrated 1 hour before receiving drug.
• When possible, give by infusion; injection can be painful.
• Restrict patient's food and fluids 4 to 6 hours before giving drug to help reduce nausea and vomiting.
• In cases of overdose, provide supportive care and monitor blood counts.
• Monitor hematologic status carefully.
• Monitor kidney and liver function carefully; dysfunction can delay drug excretion. Avoid IM injections when platelet counts are below 100,000/mm³.

dactinomycin (actinomycin D)

Cosmegen◆

Pregnancy Risk Category: C

INDICATIONS & DOSAGES
Note: Dosage varies, depending on patient tolerance, size and location of tumor, and use of other treatments; in obese or elderly patients, dosage should be based on body surface area.
Choriocarcinoma, Ewing's sarcoma, rhabdomyosarcoma, testicular cancer, uterine cancer, Wilms' tumor—
Adults: 500 mcg/day for maximum of 5 days.
Children over age 6 months: 15 mcg/kg/day for 5 days or total dose of 2.5 mg/m² over 1 week.

Both adults and children may have a second course after 3 weeks if toxic effects have subsided.

PREPARATION & STORAGE
Because of mutagenic, teratogenic, and carcinogenic risks, use a biological containment cabinet during drug preparation. Wear gloves and mask, use syringes with tight fittings (luer-locks) to prevent drug leakage, and avoid contamination of work surface. Properly dispose of needles, syringes, vials, and unused drug.
To prepare drug, reconstitute each 500-mcg vial with 1.1 ml of sterile water *without preservative* to yield 0.5 mg/ml; use 2.2 ml to yield 0.25 mg/ml. For infusion, dilute the clear, gold-colored reconstituted drug with D₅W or 0.9% NaCl. Product does not contain any preservative; discard unused portion of reconstituted solution. Store intact vials below 85° F (30° C).

Incompatibility
Incompatible with diluents containing preservatives (causes precipitation) and with filgrastim.

ADMINISTRATION
Direct injection: Inject 500 mcg over a few minutes, preferably through a side port in an IV line containing freely flowing D₅W or 0.9% NaCl. Assess vein patency frequently. After injection, run the IV solution for 2 to 5 minutes or inject 5 to 10 ml of IV solution through tubing to remove residual drug. Use of some in-line cellulose ester filters may partially remove active drug from the IV solution.
Intermittent infusion: Infuse diluted dose over 10 to 15 minutes into tubing of a free-flowing IV solution.

CONTRAINDICATIONS & CAUTIONS
• Contraindicated in recent or active chickenpox or herpes zoster infection, and in children age 6 months and less.

D

• Use cautiously in patients with gout or history of urate renal calculi and in myelosuppressed patients.

SPECIAL CONSIDERATIONS
• If extravasation occurs, discontinue infusion and aspirate as much drug as possible. Infiltrate area with 4 ml of isotonic sodium thiosulfate (1 g/10 ml) diluted with 6 ml of sterile water for injection, 50 to 100 mg of hydrocortisone sodium succinate, or ascorbic acid injection. Cover with sterile gauze and apply cold compresses.
• Alkalinizing urine or administering allopurinol may prevent or minimize uric acid nephropathy.
• Monitor CBC and platelet count.
• Monitor renal and hepatic function.
• Encourage patient to maintain adequate hydration.

daunorubicin hydrochloride (daunomycin hydrochloride)

Cerubidine◆

Pregnancy Risk Category: D

INDICATIONS & DOSAGES
Remission induction in acute non-lymphocytic leukemia in adults and acute lymphocytic leukemia in both adults and children, in combination with other chemotherapeutic agents—
Adults: 30 or 45 mg/m²/day on days 1, 2, and 3 of first course and, for acute nonlymphocytic leukemia only, give also on days 1 and 2 of subsequent courses.
Children: 25 mg/m² weekly in combination with other chemotherapeutic drugs.
Induction of remission in acute myelogenous leukemia—
Adults: 60 mg/m²/day for 3 days, repeated q 3 to 4 weeks. Maximum total lifetime dosage, 550 mg/m².

Previous chest radiation therapy requires a limit of 450 mg/m².
   In patients with hepatic or renal impairment, the manufacturer recommends that 75% of usual daily dose be given if serum bilirubin concentrations are 1.2 to 3 mg/dl and 50% of usual daily dose be given if serum bilirubin or creatinine concentrations are above 3 mg/dl.

PREPARATION & STORAGE
Because of mutagenic, teratogenic, and carcinogenic risks, use a biological containment cabinet and wear gloves and mask. Use syringes with tight fittings (luer-locks) to prevent drug leakage, and dispose of needles, syringes, vials, and unused drug correctly. Avoid contaminating work surfaces.
   Available in 20-mg glass vials. Reconstitute with 4 ml of sterile water for injection; then withdraw desired dose into syringe containing 10 to 15 ml of 0.9% NaCl. Reconstituted solution remains stable for 48 hours if refrigerated and for 24 hours at room temperature if protected from direct sunlight.

Incompatibility
Incompatible with heparin and dexamethasone. Drug should not be mixed with other medications.

ADMINISTRATION
Direct injection: Give drug through the side port of a newly started IV line, preferably using a 23G or 25G winged-tip needle. Inject a 10- to 15-ml solution over 2 to 3 minutes. After administration, flush vein with primary IV solution.
   Closely monitor for signs of infiltration and instruct the patient to promptly report changes in sensation, such as burning at the IV site. Extravasation can cause slow, progressive necrosis of skin and painful ulcers. If it occurs, stop injection and aspirate as much of drug as possible. Then immediately infiltrate the area with 50 to 100 ml of hydrocortisone sodium succinate or

sodium bicarbonate and apply cold compresses.
Intermittent infusion: Infuse a 100-ml solution over 30 to 45 minutes. Flush and monitor site as above.

CONTRAINDICATIONS & CAUTIONS
• Contraindicated in existing or recent chickenpox or herpes zoster infection.
• Give cautiously to patients with preexisting myelosuppression or cardiac disease or to those who have had previous therapy with doxorubicin, cyclophosphamide, dacarbazine, dactinomycin, or mitomycin.
• Use carefully in renal or hepatic impairment and history of gout or urate renal calculi.
• Advise women of childbearing age to avoid becoming pregnant during therapy.

SPECIAL CONSIDERATIONS
• Give antiemetic before treatment, as ordered, to prevent nausea and vomiting.
• Drug can reactivate radiation-induced skin lesions.
• Keep patient well hydrated; alkalinizing urine and possibly administering allopurinol can prevent or minimize uric acid nephropathy.
• Monitor ECG (before treatment and monthly during therapy), CBC, and hepatic function.
• Tell patient that urine may appear red for 1 to 2 days and does not indicate presence of blood.

desmopressin acetate

DDAVP Injection◆, Octostim◇, Stimate
Pregnancy Risk Category: B

INDICATIONS & DOSAGES
Nonnephrogenic diabetes insipidus—
Adults and children age 12 and over: usual maintenance dosage is 2 to 4 mcg daily given in two divided doses. Dosage adjustment depends on changes in urine volume and osmolality.
Hemophilia A and von Willebrand disease—
Adults and children age 3 months and older: 0.3 mcg/kg by slow IV infusion.

PREPARATION & STORAGE
Available in 10-ml multidose vials, 1-ml ampules (concentration of 4 mcg/ml), and 1- and 2-ml ampules (concentration of 15 mcg/ml).
For infusion, dilute the appropriate dose in 50 ml of 0.9% NaCl (for adults and children weighing over 22 lb [10 kg] or in 10 ml of 0.9% NaCl (for children weighing 22 lb or less). Store at 39° F (4° C) unless manufacturer specifies otherwise; protect from freezing.

Incompatibility
None reported.

ADMINISTRATION
Intermittent infusion: Infuse diluted drug over 15 to 30 minutes. Rapid administration may produce hypotension.

CONTRAINDICATIONS & CAUTIONS
• Contraindicated in hypersensitivity to desmopressin.
• Do not use in type IIB form of von Willebrand disease or pseudo von Willebrand disease because of risk of thrombocytopenia and platelet aggregation.
• Do not use IV form in infants under age 3 months. Safety of IV form as an antidiuretic has not been established for children under age 12.
• Use cautiously in patients with coronary artery insufficiency or hypertensive CV disease.

SPECIAL CONSIDERATIONS
• Decrease fluid intake to avoid water intoxication and hyponatremia.
• In cases of overdose, reduce desmopressin dosage. If fluid overload is severe, give furosemide.
• During infusion, monitor patient's blood pressure and pulse. After infu-

sion, monitor intake and output and serum sodium level.
• If patient has a hemorrhagic disorder, monitor factor VIII, factor VIII:R co-factor, factor VIII antigen levels, and APTT.
• If patient has diabetes insipidus, monitor urine volume and osmolality. Also periodically monitor serum osmolality.

dexamethasone sodium phosphate

Dalalone, Decadron Phosphate✦, Decaject, Dexameth, Dexasone, Dexone, Hexadrol Phosphate, Solurex

Pregnancy Risk Category: C

INDICATIONS & DOSAGES
Adjunctive treatment of shock—
Adults: 1 to 6 mg/kg in a single dose, 40 mg q 2 to 6 hours p.r.n., or 20 mg in a single dose followed by 3 mg/kg over 24 hours in a continuous infusion.
Adjunctive treatment of cerebral edema—
Adults: 10 mg IV initially, then 4 mg IM q 6 hours. For inoperable or recurrent brain tumors, 2 mg IV maintenance dose may be given b.i.d. or t.i.d.
Allergic reactions—
Adults: 4 to 8 mg IM on day 1, followed by oral medication starting on day 2.

PREPARATION & STORAGE
Available in concentrations of 4, 10, and 24 mg/ml in vials and syringes in a range of sizes. The solution is clear but may appear yellow at higher concentrations.
    Dilute drug in D_5W or 0.9% NaCl for intermittent or continuous infusion. Protect from light and freezing.

Incompatibility
Incompatible with daunorubicin, doxorubicin, and vancomycin.

ADMINISTRATION
Direct injection: Give undiluted drug over at least 1 minute.
Intermittent infusion: Give diluted drug as ordered.
Continuous infusion: Infuse diluted drug over 24 hours.

CONTRAINDICATIONS & CAUTIONS
• Contraindicated in sensitivity to any component of drug, including sulfites.
• Also contraindicated in peptic ulcers (except if life-threatening).
• Use cautiously in diverticulitis and nonspecific ulcerative colitis if risk of perforation, abscess, or other pyogenic infection exists; in recent intestinal anastomoses; and in seizure disorders, diabetes mellitus, osteoporosis, and bacterial, viral, or fungal infections.
• Also use cautiously in hypothyroidism, cirrhosis, cardiac disease, heart failure, renal insufficiency, hypertension, and thromboembolic disease.
• Administer carefully in ocular herpes simplex; in patients with history of tuberculosis or with positive skin tests; in glaucoma; in hepatic impairment or hypoalbuminemia; and in hyperlipidemia.
• Use cautiously in hyperthyroidism and hypothyroidism.

SPECIAL CONSIDERATIONS
• IV administration is usually followed by use of IM or PO route.
• Long-term therapy may retard bone growth in infants and children and should be closely monitored.
• Keep emergency resuscitation equipment nearby before starting therapy.

---

dexrazoxane

Zinecard
Pregnancy Risk Category: C

INDICATIONS & DOSAGES
Reduction in the incidence and severity of doxorubicin-induced cardiomyopathy in women with metastatic breast cancer who have received a cumulative dose of 300 mg/m² but would benefit from continued doxorubicin therapy—
Adults: dosage ratio of dexrazoxane to doxorubicin is 10:1 (for example, 500 mg/m² of dexrazoxane to 50 mg/m² of doxorubicin). After reconstitution, administer dexrazoxane by slow IV push or rapid IV infusion. After completion of dexrazoxane administration and before 30 minutes have elapsed from its start, give IV injection of doxorubicin.

PREPARATION & STORAGE
Drug must be diluted with diluent supplied with drug (0.167 M sodium lactate injection) to give concentration of 10 mg dexrazoxane per 1 ml sodium lactate. Reconstituted drug may be further diluted with either 0.9% NaCl solution or D₅W to a concentration range of 1.3 to 5 mg/ml in IV infusion bags. Resultant solutions are stable for 6 hours at 59° to 86° F (15° to 30° C). Discard unused solutions.

When handling and preparing reconstituted solution, wear gloves and use same precautions as those for handling antineoplastic drugs. If drug powder or solution contacts skin or mucosa, immediately wash affected area thoroughly with soap and water.

Incompatibility
Do not mix drug with other medications.

ADMINISTRATION
Direct injection: Administer by slow IV push or rapid IV infusion.

Intermittent infusion: Administer by rapid IV infusion.

CONTRAINDICATIONS & CAUTIONS
• Contraindicated in patients not receiving anthracycline as part of the chemotherapy regimen and in pregnant or breast-feeding women.
• Drug is not recommended for use until after patient has an accumulated doxorubicin dose of 300 mg/m² and continuation of doxorubicin therapy is desired. With combination therapy, dexrazoxane should be administered before doxorubicin.
• Use cautiously in all patients because additive effects of immunosuppression may occur from concomitant administration of cytotoxic drugs.

SPECIAL CONSIDERATIONS
• In cases of overdose, there is no known antidote. Treatment consists of supportive care until resolution of myelosuppression and related conditions is complete.
• Monitor CBC closely. Institute infection control and bleeding precautions as indicated by CBC results.
• Instruct patient to report signs of infection and bleeding.
• Take temperature daily.

dextran

Low-molecular-weight dextran 40: 10% Dextran 40 in 5% Dextrose Injection, 10% Dextran 40 in 0.9% NaCl Injection, 10% Gentran 40 in 5% Dextrose Injection, 10% Gentran 40 in 0.9% NaCl Injection, 10% LMD in 5% Dextrose Injection, 10% LMD in 0.9% NaCl Injection, 10% Rheomacrodex in 5% Dextrose Injection, 10% Rheomacrodex in 0.9% NaCl Injection
High-molecular-weight dextran 70 and 75: 6% Dextran 70 in 5% Dextrose Injection, 6%

Dextran 70 in 0.9% NaCl Injection, 6% Dextran 75 in 5% Dextrose Injection, 6% Dextran 75 in 0.9% NaCl Injection, 6% Gentran 70 in 0.9% NaCl Injection, Macrodex in 0.9% NaCl Injection

Pregnancy Risk Category: C

INDICATIONS & DOSAGES

Adjunctive treatment of shock from hemorrhage, burns, surgery, or other trauma—
Adults and children: dosage reflects fluid loss and resultant hemoconcentration. Total dosage of 10% low-molecular-weight solution should not exceed 2 g/kg (20 ml/kg) for first 24 hours, then 1 g/kg (10 ml/kg) daily for 4 days. Total dosage of 6% high-molecular-weight solution should not exceed 1.2 g/kg (20 ml/kg) for first 24 hours, then 0.6 g/kg (10 ml/kg) daily, p.r.n.
Prophylaxis of venous thrombosis and pulmonary embolism—
Adults: 50 to 100 g (500 to 1,000 ml) of 10% low-molecular-weight solution during surgery, then 50 g daily for 2 to 3 days, followed by 50 g q 2 or 3 days for up to 2 weeks.

PREPARATION & STORAGE

Low-molecular-weight dextran is available in 500-ml bottles as a 10% solution diluted in 0.9% NaCl or D_5W. High-molecular-weight dextran comes in 500-ml bottles as a 6% solution diluted in 0.9% NaCl or D_5W. Store solutions at a constant temperature, preferably 77° F (25° C). Crystals may form at low temperatures. If this occurs, submerge bottle in warm water to dissolve crystals before infusing. Do not administer cloudy solutions. Preparation has no preservatives; discard partially used containers.

Incompatibility
Incompatible with ascorbic acid, phytonadione, promethazine, and protein hydrolysate. Do not add any drug to a bottle of dextran.

ADMINISTRATION

Intermittent infusion: Rapidly infuse first 500 ml of low-molecular-weight dextran over 15 to 30 minutes. Slowly infuse remainder based on patient response. In an emergency, infuse high-molecular-weight dextran at 1.2 to 2.4 g (20 to 40 ml)/minute. In normovolemic patient, do not exceed 0.24 g (4 ml)/minute.
Continuous infusion: Infuse over 24 hours based on patient condition and response.

CONTRAINDICATIONS & CAUTIONS

• Contraindicated in hypersensitivity to dextran.
• Also contraindicated in pulmonary edema; marked thrombocytopenia, coagulation defects, and bleeding disorders; and renal disease with severe oliguria or anuria.
• In extreme dehydration, avoid using low-molecular-weight dextran.
• Give cautiously (especially NaCl solutions) in heart failure, cardiac decompensation, and hemorrhage.

SPECIAL CONSIDERATIONS

• Discontinue infusion at first sign of an allergic reaction, but maintain IV access. Keep resuscitation equipment available.
• Maintain hydration with additional IV fluids.
• Slow or discontinue the infusion if CVP increases rapidly (normal CVP, 7 to 14 cm H_2O) or if patient is anuric or oliguric after receiving 500 ml of dextran. Give mannitol to help increase urine flow.
• Change IV tubing or flush well with 0.9% NaCl before transfusing blood. Dextran may cause blood to coagulate in the tubing.
• Monitor pulse, blood pressure, CVP, and urine output every 5 to 15 minutes for first hour and then hourly.

dextrose in NaCl solutions

Pregnancy Risk Category: C

COMPOSITION
These solutions contain combinations of hypotonic or isotonic concentrations of dextrose and NaCl. Solutions of dextrose 2.5% or 5% and 0.45% NaCl are hypotonic. Others are isotonic.

INDICATIONS & CONCENTRATIONS
Temporary treatment of circulatory insufficiency and shock when plasma volume expander is not available; fluid replacement in burned, dehydrated, and other patients—
Adults and children: concentration and infusion rate reflect patient's age, weight, condition, and fluid, electrolyte, and acid-base balance.

PREPARATION & STORAGE
Available in 250-, 500-, and 1,000-ml bottles and polyvinyl chloride bags. Dextrose 5% in 0.2% NaCl also comes in 150-ml containers. Concentrations include dextrose 2.5% in 0.45% NaCl; dextrose 5% in 0.11%, 0.2%, 0.225%, 0.3%, 0.45%, or 0.9% NaCl; and dextrose 10% in 0.2% or 0.9% NaCl. Store solutions in a cool, dry place, and protect from freezing or extreme heat. Do not administer cloudy solutions.

Incompatibility
Incompatible with amphotericin B, ampicillin sodium, amsacrine, diazepam, erythromycin lactobionate, mannitol, and phenytoin.

ADMINISTRATION
Continuous infusion: Infuse through a peripheral or central vein at ordered rate.

CONTRAINDICATIONS & CAUTIONS
• Contraindicated in diabetic coma or allergy to corn or corn products.
• Avoid use or give with extreme caution during concurrent corticosteroid therapy and in heart failure, severe renal insufficiency, and edema with sodium retention.
• Use cautiously in renal impairment; in urinary obstruction; and in diabetes mellitus or carbohydrate intolerance.

SPECIAL CONSIDERATIONS
• Give electrolyte supplements as needed.
• Monitor changes in fluid balance, electrolyte levels, and acid-base balance during prolonged parenteral therapy.
• Watch closely for fluid overload (exacerbated hypertension, signs of heart failure or pulmonary edema), especially in elderly patients or in patients with renal or cardiac disease.

dextrose in water solutions (glucose solutions)

Pregnancy Risk Category: C

COMPOSITION
Containing glucose and water, these solutions vary in tonicity and concentration. Solutions of 2.5% are hypotonic, solutions of 5% are isotonic, and solutions over 10% are hypertonic.

INDICATIONS & CONCENTRATIONS
Provision of calories and water to meet metabolic and hydration needs—
Adults and children: 2.5%, 5%, or 10% solution.
Hyperkalemia and conditions that require adequate calories but little water—
Adults and children: 20% solution.
Promotion of diuresis—
Adults and children: 20% to 50% solution.
Base solution for IV hyperalimentation—
Adults and children: 10% to 70% solution.
Adjunctive treatment of shock—

Adults and children: 40% to 70% solution.
Cerebral edema, pregnancy-induced hypertension, renal disease, acute hypoglycemia, and as a sclerosing agent—
Adults and children: 50% solution.
Acute symptomatic hypoglycemia—
Infants and neonates: 10% to 25% solution.

PREPARATION & STORAGE
Available in 50-, 100-, 150-, 250-, 500-, and 1,000-ml bottles or polyvinyl chloride bags in the following concentrations: 2.5%, 5%, 7.7%, 10%, 11.5%, 20%, 25%, 30%, 38%, 38.5%, 40%, 50%, 60%, and 70%. Because dextrose is an excellent medium for bacterial growth, store solutions in a cool, dry place. Protect from freezing and extreme heat. Do not administer cloudy solutions.

Incompatibility
Incompatible with ampicillin sodium, cisplatin, diazepam, erythromycin lactobionate, fat emulsions (10% and 25% solutions), phenytoin, procainamide, thiopental (solutions of 10% and above), and whole blood.

ADMINISTRATION
Direct injection: Give 50 ml of 50% solution at 3 ml/minute.
Continuous infusion: Give isotonic solutions through a peripheral vein, hypertonic solutions through a central venous line. Rate depends on solution's concentration and patient's age and condition. An hourly rate above 0.5 g/kg may cause glycosuria in healthy people. Maximum rate should not exceed 0.8 g/kg/hour.

CONTRAINDICATIONS & CAUTIONS
• Hypertonic solutions are contraindicated in neurosurgical procedures, delirium tremens with dehydration, intracranial or intraspinal hemorrhage, and anuria.
• All dextrose solutions are contraindicated in diabetic coma and in allergies to corn or corn products.

• Use dextrose solutions cautiously in patient with renal disease, cardiac disease, and hypertension; in overt or subclinical diabetes mellitus; in urinary obstruction; and in carbohydrate intolerance.

SPECIAL CONSIDERATIONS
• Avoid extravasation because tissue sloughing and necrosis can occur. Never infuse hypertonic solutions rapidly because this can cause hyperglycemia and fluid shift.
• Give electrolyte supplements, as needed.
• To avoid rebound hypoglycemia, substitute dextrose 5% or 10% after discontinuing hypertonic solutions.
• Monitor intake and output and weight, and watch for signs of fluid overload.
• Monitor serum glucose levels.
• Monitor serum electrolyte and acid-base balance during prolonged administration.

diazepam

Valium ✦

Controlled Substance Schedule IV

Pregnancy Risk Category: D

INDICATIONS & DOSAGES
Short-term, symptomatic relief of acute anxiety or as skeletal muscle relaxant in patients who cannot take oral medication—
Adults and children over age 12: 2 to 10 mg (0.4 to 2 ml) q 3 to 4 hours. May repeat in 1 hour, with maximum of 30 mg in 8 hours. Give 2 to 5 mg to elderly patients or when another sedative has been given.
Cardioversion—
Adults: 5 to 15 mg (1 to 3 ml) just before procedure as amnesic agent.
Endoscopy—
Adults: up to 20 mg before procedure, then titrated to achieve desired effect. May produce anterograde amnesia.

Tetanus—
Adults and children age 5 and older: 5 to 10 mg. May repeat dose in 3 to 4 hours.
Infants over age 1 month: 1 to 2 mg q 3 to 4 hours.
Status epilepticus and recurrent seizures—
Adults: 5 to 10 mg by slow IV push at 2 to 5 mg/minute. May repeat dose q 10 to 15 minutes up to maximum of 30 mg. Give 2 to 5 mg to elderly or debilitated patients; in recurrent seizures, dose may be repeated in 20 to 30 minutes.
Children age 5 and older: 0.5 to 1 mg q 2 to 5 minutes up to total dose of 10 mg. May be repeated in 2 to 4 hours.
Infants over age 1 month: 0.2 to 0.5 mg q 2 to 5 minutes up to a total dose of 5 mg. May be repeated in 2 to 4 hours.

PREPARATION & STORAGE
Available in 10-ml vials (5 mg/ml), prefilled syringes, and 2-ml ampules. Protect vials from light.

Because of incompatibility, the manufacturer warns against diluting drug before administration. However, several studies indicate that diazepam infusions may be prepared using 0.9% NaCl injection. The concentration should not exceed 10 mg/100 ml, and only glass bottles should be used. Avoid polyvinyl chloride infusion sets, and use an in-line filter. Do not store in plastic syringes. Check with a pharmacist for more information.

Incompatibility
Incompatible with *all* other drugs and most IV solutions.

ADMINISTRATION
Direct injection: Slowly inject undiluted drug into large vein or catheter at a rate of less than 5 mg/minute for adults and 0.25 mg/kg of body weight over 3 minutes for children. Avoid extravasation. If drug is injected into tubing, choose a site directly above the needle or catheter inser-

tion site. Afterward, flush with 0.9% NaCl.

CONTRAINDICATIONS & CAUTIONS
• Contraindicated in hypersensitivity to drug, in acute narrow-angle glaucoma or untreated chronic open-angle glaucoma, in shock or coma, and in acute alcohol intoxication.
• Also contraindicated in pregnant women and infants under age 30 days.
• Give with extreme caution to patients with limited pulmonary reserve. Also give with extreme caution for endoscopy.
• Give diazepam cautiously to psychotic or depressed patients, and to patients with myasthenia gravis or porphyria.
• Also administer cautiously to patients with renal or hepatic impairment; to patients with hypoalbuminemia; to elderly or debilitated patients; and to addiction-prone patients.

SPECIAL CONSIDERATIONS
• Always keep emergency resuscitation equipment nearby when giving IV diazepam.
• If patient is receiving a narcotic, reduce its dosage by at least one-third.
• Discontinue drug if paradoxical reaction occurs, typified by anxiety, acute excitation, hallucinations, increased muscle spasticity, insomnia, or rage.
• Abrupt withdrawal after high doses or extended use can cause seizures and delirium.
• In cases of overdose, provide supportive care. Maintain airway patency and give IV fluids. Administer dopamine, norepinephrine, and metaraminol for hypotension.
• Obtain baseline blood pressure and respiratory rate before administration.
• Instruct patient to maintain bed rest for 3 hours after parenteral administration.

D

digoxin

Lanoxin✦

Pregnancy Risk Category: C

INDICATIONS & DOSAGES

Heart failure, atrial flutter and fibrillation, atrial tachycardias (including paroxysmal atrial tachycardia)—
Adults and children over age 10: loading dose, 0.5 to 1 mg (alternatively, 0.008 to 0.012 mg/kg); maintenance dose, 0.125 to 0.5 mg daily (usual dose, 0.25 mg).
Children ages 5 to 10: loading dose, 0.015 to 0.03 mg/kg; maintenance dose, 25% to 35% of loading dose.
Children ages 2 to 5: loading dose, 0.025 to 0.035 mg/kg; maintenance dose, 25% to 35% of loading dose.
Children ages 1 month to 2 years: loading dose, 0.03 to 0.05 mg/kg; maintenance dose, 25% to 35% of loading dose.
Full-term neonates under age 1 month: loading dose, 0.02 to 0.03 mg/kg; maintenance dose, 25% to 35% of loading dose.
Premature infants: loading dose, 0.015 to 0.025 mg/kg; maintenance dose, 20% to 30% of loading dose.

PREPARATION & STORAGE

Available in 1- and 2-ml ampules (0.25 mg/ml) for adults and in 1-ml ampules (0.1 mg/ml) for children. Store drug at room temperature.

Dilute with 10 ml of D_5W, 0.9% NaCl, or sterile water, or give undiluted. Drug can precipitate if less than a fourfold dilution is used. Give diluted drug immediately.

Incompatibility

Incompatible with dobutamine, doxapram, fluconazole, and foscarnet. The manufacturer recommends not mixing digoxin (or administering in the same IV line) with other drugs.

ADMINISTRATION

Direct injection: Inject undiluted drug over at least 5 minutes as close to IV insertion site as possible.

CONTRAINDICATIONS & CAUTIONS

• Contraindicated in patients with digitalis-induced toxicity and in patients with ventricular fibrillation.
• Use with extreme caution in renal insufficiency and in heart failure.
• Use cautiously in the elderly and in patients with acute MI, incomplete AV block, severe heart failure, hypothyroidism, or chronic constrictive pericarditis.
• Use cautiously in patients who have received a cardiac glycoside preparation within the past 3 weeks and in those with acute myocarditis, renal insufficiency, severe pulmonary disease, hypoxia, sick sinus syndrome, myxedema, or Wolff-Parkinson-White syndrome with atrial fibrillation.
• Also administer cautiously in idiopathic hypertrophic subaortic stenosis, hypokalemia, hypomagnesemia, hypercalcemia, heightened carotid sinus sensitivity, and renal impairment.

SPECIAL CONSIDERATIONS

• Divide the loading dose over 24 hours, as ordered.
• Discontinue drug at first sign of toxicity (anorexia, diarrhea, nausea, and vomiting in adults; in children, the most common sign is cardiac arrhythmias). Monitor ECG continuously and maintain patient's serum potassium level between 3.5 and 5 mEq/L.
• Check patient's apical pulse for 1 minute before each dose. Report significant changes (irregular beats or pulse rate below 60 beats/minute or above 100 beats/minute). Also report blood pressure changes and anticipate an order for a 12-lead ECG.
• Use a continuous ECG to monitor patients on IV digoxin for development or improvement of arrhythmias.
• Therapeutic serum levels are 0.5 to 2 ng/ml. Measure peak serum levels

at least 4 hours after a dose; trough levels just before the next dose.

digoxin immune FAB

Digibind

Pregnancy Risk Category: C

INDICATIONS & DOSAGES
Potentially life-threatening cardiac glycoside toxicity—
Adults and children: dosage based on ingested amount or serum level of digoxin or digitoxin.

For digoxin tablets, solution, or IM injection, find the antidote dose (in mg) by multiplying the ingested amount by 0.8; divide answer by 0.5 and multiply by 38. For digitoxin tablets, digoxin capsules, or IV digoxin or digitoxin, find the antidote dose (in mg) by dividing the ingested dose (in mg) by 0.5 and multiplying by 38.

If the serum digoxin or digitoxin level is known, determine the dosage as follows: multiply the serum digoxin level (in ng/ml) by patient's weight (in kg), divide by 100, and multiply by 38. Or, multiply the serum digitoxin level (in ng/ml) by the patient's weight (in kg), divide by 1,000, and multiply by 38.
Acute toxicity, or if estimated ingested amount or serum digoxin level is unknown—
Adults and children: consider administering 20 vials (760 mg) of digoxin immune FAB and observing patient's response. Dosage should be effective in most life-threatening ingestions in adults and children, but may cause volume overload in young children.

PREPARATION & STORAGE
Available in 38-mg vials. Reconstitute with 4 ml of sterile water for injection. For infusion, further dilute solution with 0.9% NaCl. For children or other patients who need small doses, reconstitute 38-mg vial with 38 ml of 0.9% NaCl for 1 mg/

ml concentration. Use reconstituted solution promptly. If not used immediately, refrigerate for up to 4 hours.

Incompatibility
None reported.

ADMINISTRATION
Direct injection: If cardiac arrest is imminent, rapidly inject directly into vein or IV line containing a free-flowing, compatible solution, using a 0.22-micron filter needle.
Continuous infusion: Infuse diluted solution over 15 to 30 minutes through a 0.22-micron filter needle.

CONTRAINDICATIONS & CAUTIONS
• Experience with drug is limited. It is recommended only for life-threatening situations.
• Use cautiously in heart failure; cardiac glycoside levels may fall below effective inotropic concentrations.

SPECIAL CONSIDERATIONS
• If patient is allergic to sheep proteins (or has previously reacted to digoxin immune FAB) and his condition is not life-threatening, consider skin testing. Dilute 0.1 ml of reconstituted drug in 10 ml of sterile NaCl solution. Inject 0.1 ml of this solution intradermally, and examine site after 20 minutes. Urticarial wheal surrounded by erythema indicates positive result.
• Do not attempt redigitalization until the elimination of Digibind (which can take up to 1 week) is complete.
• Overly high doses can cause allergic reaction, febrile reaction, or delayed serum sickness.
• Obtain serum digoxin or digitoxin levels before giving digoxin immune FAB because serum studies will be difficult to interpret afterward.

D

dihydroergotamine mesylate

D.H.E. 45
Pregnancy Risk Category: X

INDICATIONS & DOSAGES
Rapid control of vascular headaches (including migraine and cluster headaches)—
Adults: 1 mg IM at start of attack, then 1 mg IM in 1 hour, p.r.n. until relief of headache; not to exceed 3 mg/day. When more rapid response is needed, drug may be given IV to maximum of 2 mg. Do not exceed IM or IV dose of 6 mg weekly.

PREPARATION & STORAGE
Available as a colorless solution in 1 mg/ml vials. Drug does not need dilution for IV use. Protect from light, freezing, and heat. Store at 59° to 86° F (15° to 30° C). Do not administer discolored solutions.

Incompatibility
None reported.

ADMINISTRATION
Direct injection: IM or IV at the first warning sign of a headache.

CONTRAINDICATIONS & CAUTIONS
• Contraindicated in patients with history of hypersensitivity to ergot alkaloids and in those with peripheral vascular disease, coronary artery disease, severe hypertension, hepatic or renal impairment, infection, or sepsis.
• Contraindicated in pregnant and breast-feeding women.
• Also contraindicated in children because safety and efficacy have not been proven.
• Use cautiously in elderly patients.

SPECIAL CONSIDERATIONS
• Give drug when prodromal signs occur or as soon as possible after headache begins. Dosage and speed of relief may be directly related to prompt administration.
• In cases of overdose, provide symptomatic care. Treat seizures with IV diazepam or barbiturates, as ordered. Support respirations as needed. For severe vasospasm, apply warmth to ischemic extremities to prevent tissue damage. Carefully administer vasodilators (such as nitroprusside, prazosin, or tolazoline) because they can cause hypotension.
• Instruct patient to immediately report numbness or tingling in extremities, weakness, chest pain, changes in heart rate, edema, or itching.

diltiazem hydrochloride

Cardizem Injectable
Pregnancy Risk Category: C

INDICATIONS & DOSAGES
Temporary control of rapid ventricular rate in atrial fibrillation or atrial flutter; rapid conversion of paroxysmal supraventricular tachycardia—
Adults: initially, 0.25 mg/kg as a bolus given over 2 minutes; if inadequate, a second bolus dose of 0.35 mg/kg may be given after 15 minutes. Subsequent IV bolus doses should be individualized. Low–body weight patient should be dosed on a body-weight basis: some may respond to 0.15 mg/kg; however, duration of action is shorter. For continued reduction of heart rate, a continuous infusion of 10 mg/hour may be started immediately following the bolus doses. The initial infusion rate may be increased by 5 mg/hour up to a maximum rate of 15 mg/hour, p.r.n. Infusions continued beyond 24 hours or at a rate exceeding 15 mg/hour are not recommended.

PREPARATION & STORAGE
Available as a 5-mg/ml solution in 5- and 10-ml single-dose vials. Re-

---

frigerate at 36° to 46° F (2° to 8° C). Drug may be stored at room temperature for up to 1 month; after 1 month it must be destroyed.

To prepare bolus injection, withdraw calculated dose from vial. To prepare continuous infusion, aseptically transfer calculated dose to desired volume of 0.9% NaCl, D₅W, or dextrose 5% in 0.45% NaCl. Mix thoroughly and use within 24 hours. Refrigerate until ready to use.

Incompatibility
Incompatible when mixed directly with diazepam, furosemide, heparin, phenytoin, and rifampin.

ADMINISTRATION
Direct injection: Give ordered dose via patent IV line. Do not inject with incompatible drugs or solutions.
Continuous infusion: Administer via an infusion control device. Infuse over 24 hours at rate not exceeding 15 mg/hour.

CONTRAINDICATIONS & CAUTIONS
• Contraindicated in patients with sick sinus syndrome and second- or third-degree AV block (except with a functioning ventricular pacemaker), severe hypotension, cardiogenic shock, hypersensitivity to drug, atrial fibrillation, or atrial flutter associated with Wolff-Parkinson-White syndrome.
• Use cautiously in patients with impaired hepatic or renal function, impaired ventricular function, or those taking other drugs that decrease peripheral resistance, intravascular volume, myocardial contractility, or conduction.
• Safety and efficacy for use in children have not been established.

SPECIAL CONSIDERATIONS
• Duration of infusion should not exceed 24 hours. Patient should be transitioned to other antiarrhythmic agents.
• Do not administer IV diltiazem and IV beta blockers together or within a few hours of each other.

• Discontinue drug if dermatologic events progressing to erythema multiforme or exfoliative dermatitis occur or persist.
• When using continuous infusion, continuously monitor ECG. Frequently monitor blood pressure. Have a defibrillator and emergency equipment readily available.

diphenhydramine hydrochloride

Benadryl◆, Hyrexin-50, Nordryl
Pregnancy Risk Category: B

INDICATIONS & DOSAGES
Parkinsonism and drug-induced extrapyramidal reaction in elderly patients unable to tolerate more potent agents; mild cases of parkinsonism (including drug-induced) with centrally acting anticholinergic agents; treatment of allergic reactions, nausea, and vertigo—
Adults: 10 to 50 mg, up to 100 mg if required. Maximum daily dose is 400 mg.
Children: 5 mg/kg/day or 150 mg/m² divided into four doses. Maximum daily dose is 300 mg.

PREPARATION & STORAGE
Available in 10- and 50-mg/ml vials. Store in light-resistant containers at 59° to 86° F (15° to 30° C), and avoid freezing. Further dilution is not required for direct injection.

Incompatibility
Drug is compatible with most IV solutions. Compatibility depends on several factors (including concentration of drugs, specific diluents, pH, temperature). Consult specialized references for specific compatibility information.

D

ADMINISTRATION
Direct injection: Inject drug over 3 to 5 minutes directly into vein or into an IV line containing a free-flowing, compatible solution.
Intermittent infusion: After diluting appropriate dosage, infuse slowly.

CONTRAINDICATIONS & CAUTIONS
• Contraindicated in antihistamine hypersensitivity.
• Also contraindicated in neonates and premature infants.
• Use cautiously in patients with lower respiratory tract symptoms (including asthma), narrow-angle glaucoma, stenosing peptic ulcer, pyloroduodenal obstruction, symptomatic prostatic hypertrophy, bladder neck obstruction, CV disease, or hypertension.

SPECIAL CONSIDERATIONS
• Keep patient in supine position during drug administration.
• Withdraw drug 4 days before skin tests.
• Monitor vital signs and level of consciousness during infusion.

dobutamine hydrochloride

Dobutrex ◆

Pregnancy Risk Category: B

INDICATIONS & DOSAGES
Short-term treatment of cardiac decompensation resulting from depressed contractility in heart disease or cardiac surgery—
Adults: 2.5 to 15 mcg/kg/minute.

PREPARATION & STORAGE
Supplied in 20-ml vials containing 250 mg drug. Before reconstitution, store at room temperature. Reconstitute with 10 ml of sterile water or D_5W (25 mg/ml). Reconstituted solution remains potent for 6 hours at room temperature and for 48 hours if refrigerated.

Before administration, further dilute with at least 50 ml of solution, using one of the following as diluent: D_5W, dextrose 5% in 0.45% NaCl, 0.9% NaCl, 10% dextrose injection, Isolyte M with 5% dextrose injection, Ringer's injection, Normosol-M in D_5W, 20% Osmitrol in water for injection, or sodium lactate injection. For a concentration of 250 mcg/ml, mix 250 mg of drug in 1,000 ml of solution; for 500 mcg/ml, mix 250 mg in 500 ml of solution; for 1 mg/ml, mix 250 mg in 250 ml of solution. Maximum concentration for infusion is 5 mg/ml.

Use diluted solution within 24 hours. Solution may turn pink from slight drug oxidation, but this does not significantly affect its potency. Avoid freezing; solution may crystallize.

Incompatibility
Incompatible with acyclovir, alkaline solutions, alteplase, aminophylline, bretylium, bumetanide, calcium chloride, calcium gluconate, cefamandole, cefazolin, cephalothin (neutral), diazepam, doxapram, foscarnet, hydrocortisone, indomethacin sodium trihydrate, insulin (regular), magnesium sulfate, penicillin, phenytoin, phytonadione, sodium bicarbonate, sodium ethacrynate, and verapamil.

ADMINISTRATION
Continuous infusion: Administer via a central IV line, using an infusion pump for most accurate titration. Titrate appropriately diluted infusion, using the guidelines given below:

Drug delivery rate (mcg/kg/min)	Infusion rate (ml/kg/min)
250 mcg/ml†	
2.5	0.01
5	0.02
7.5	0.03
10	0.04
12.5	0.05
15	0.06

(continued)

Drug delivery rate (mcg/kg/min)	Infusion rate (ml/kg/min)
500 mcg/ml†	
2.5	0.005
5	0.01
7.5	0.015
10	0.02
12.5	0.025
15	0.03
1,000 mcg/ml†	
2.5	0.0025
5	0.005
7.5	0.0075
10	0.01
12.5	0.0125
15	0.015

†concentration

CONTRAINDICATIONS & CAUTIONS
• Contraindicated in dobutamine or sulfite hypersensitivity and in idiopathic hypertrophic subaortic stenosis.
• Give cautiously in atrial fibrillation, hypertension, hypovolemia, PVCs, and after MI.
• Safety and efficacy in children have not been established.

SPECIAL CONSIDERATIONS
• Before treatment, correct hypovolemia with a volume expander and, as ordered, digitalize patient who has a rapid ventricular response to atrial fibrillation.
• Signs of overdose include tachycardia or excessive alteration in blood pressure. Reduce rate or discontinue therapy until patient is stable.
• Monitor blood pressure and heart rate and rhythm continuously. Also monitor cardiac output and pulmonary artery wedge pressure.

docetaxel

Taxotere

Pregnancy Risk Category: D

INDICATIONS & DOSAGES
Treatment of patients with locally advanced or metastatic breast cancer who have progressed during anthracycline-based therapy or have relapsed during anthracycline-based adjuvant therapy—
Adults: 60 to 100 mg/m² IV over 1 hour q 3 weeks.

PREPARATION & STORAGE
Available as a 20-mg vial with diluent vial of 1.83 ml and 80-mg vial with diluent vial of 7.33 ml.

Wear gloves during preparation and administration. If solution contacts skin, wash immediately and thoroughly with soap and water. If drug contacts mucous membranes, flush thoroughly with water.

Reconstitute drug vials with entire contents of their respective diluent vials, yielding a concentration of 10 mg/ml. Allow drug and diluent to stand at room temperature 5 minutes before mixing. After mixing, allow foam to dissipate before proceeding to next step.

Solution is further diluted for infusion in 250 ml of either 0.9% NaCl solution or 5% dextrose to produce a final concentration of 0.3 to 0.9 mg/ml.

If dose greater than 240 mg is desired, use a larger volume of infusion solution. Do not exceed a concentration exceeding 0.9 mg/ml of solution. Mix infusion thoroughly by manual rotation.

Store unopened vials at 36° to 46° F (2° to 8° C). Protect from light.

Incompatibility
None reported.

ADMINISTRATION
Intermittent infusion: Administer as 1-hour infusion at room temperature and under ambient light.

CONTRAINDICATIONS & CAUTIONS
• Contraindicated in patients with history of severe hypersensitivity to drug or other formulations containing polysorbate 80 and in those with neutrophil counts below 1,500 cells/mm³.

• Advise patient of childbearing age to avoid pregnancy or breast-feeding during therapy.

SPECIAL CONSIDERATIONS
• Do not administer drug in patients with bilirubin values above upper limits of normal. Patients with ALT or AST levels exceeding 1.5 times upper limits of normal and alkaline phosphatase levels above 2.5 times upper limits of normal generally should not receive drug.
• Premedicate all patients with oral corticosteroids, such as dexamethasone 8 mg twice daily for 5 days, starting 1 day before docetaxel administration, to reduce incidence and severity of fluid retention and hypersensitivity reactions.
• Bone marrow toxicity is the most frequent and dose-limiting toxicity. Frequent blood count monitoring is necessary during therapy.

dopamine hydrochloride

Intropin◆, Revimine◇

Pregnancy Risk Category: C

INDICATIONS & DOSAGES
Note: Dopamine infusion must be carefully adjusted to patient response.
Adjunctive treatment of shock that persists after adequate fluid volume replacement or in which oliguria is refractory to other vasopressors; to increase cardiac output, blood pressure, and urine flow—
Adults: initially, 1 to 5 mcg/kg/minute, increased by 1 to 4 mcg/kg/minute or less at 10- to 30-minute intervals until desired response is achieved. Maintenance dosage, usually under 20 mcg/kg/minute.
Chronic refractory heart failure—
Adults: 0.5 to 2 mcg/kg/minute until desired response is achieved.
Occlusive vascular disease—

Adults: therapy initiated with an infusion rate of 1 mcg/kg/minute or less.
Severe illness—
Adults: initially, 5 mcg/kg/minute, increased by 5 to 10 mcg/kg/minute at 10- to 30-minute intervals up to 50 mcg/kg/minute until desired response is achieved.

PREPARATION & STORAGE
Available in 5-ml vials, single-dose vials, and prefilled syringes of 200 mg (40 mg/ml), 400 mg (80 mg/ml), and 800 mg (160 mg/ml). Because injectable solution is light-sensitive, it is available in protective vials. Dopamine also comes premixed with D_5W for infusion in concentrations of 0.8, 1.6, and 3.2 mg/ml in 250- and 500-ml glass or polyvinyl chloride containers. Do not use discolored solutions or those darker than light yellow.
  Dilute dopamine concentrate to 200 mg/250 ml or 200 mg/500 ml using 0.9% NaCl, D_5W, dextrose 5% in 0.9% NaCl, lactated Ringer's solution, dextrose 5% in lactated Ringer's solution, or 1/6 M sodium lactate. Dilution with 250 ml yields an 800-mcg/ml solution. Protect the diluted concentration from light. It is stable for 24 hours.

Incompatibility
Incompatible with acyclovir sodium, alteplase, amphotericin B, ampicillin sodium, cephalothin, gentamicin sulfate, indomethacin sodium trihydrate, iron salts, oxidizing agents, penicillin G potassium, and sodium bicarbonate or other alkaline solutions. Do not mix additives with a dopamine and dextrose solution because of the risk of incompatibility.

ADMINISTRATION
Continuous infusion: Use an infusion control device to avoid inadvertent bolus administration of dopamine. Using an appropriately diluted concentration, administer dopamine through a long IV catheter in a large

vein, such as the antecubital fossa, rather than in a hand or ankle vein because of risk of extravasation. Continuously observe the infusion site for extravasation, which can lead to gangrene. If extravasation occurs, use a small-gauge needle to promptly infiltrate the area with 10 to 15 ml of 0.9% NaCl containing 5 to 10 mg of phentolamine.

CONTRAINDICATIONS & CAUTIONS
• Contraindicated in dopamine and sulfite hypersensitivity and in pheochromocytoma.
• Use cautiously in tachyarrhythmias or ventricular arrhythmias and in occlusive disease (Raynaud's disease, arterial embolism).
• Safety and efficacy in children have not been established.

SPECIAL CONSIDERATIONS
• Correct hypovolemia before dopamine therapy.
• When discontinuing drug, reduce infusion rate gradually to prevent severe hypotension.
• Before and during therapy, monitor heart rate, blood pressure, urine output, peripheral perfusion, central venous pressure or pulmonary artery wedge pressure, and cardiac output.

doxorubicin hydrochloride (hydroxydaunomycin hydrochloride)

Adriamycin RDF, Doxil◆, Rubex

Pregnancy Risk Category: D

INDICATIONS & DOSAGES
Solid tumors, including carcinomas, soft-tissue and osteogenic sarcomas, breast carcinoma, ovarian, transitional cell bladder carcinoma, small-cell lung carcinoma, gastric carcinoma, neuroblastoma, Wilms' tumor, lymphomas, acute lymphocytic leukemia, acute myelocytic leukemia—
Adults: 60 to 75 mg/m² as a single dose at 21-day intervals; 20 mg/m² weekly; or 25 to 30 mg/m²/day for 2 or 3 consecutive days q 3 to 4 weeks. Total lifetime dose should not exceed 550 mg/m² because of risk of cumulative cardiotoxicity.
Children: 30 mg/m² for 3 consecutive days q 4 weeks.
    Note: Reduce dosage in hepatic impairment. If serum bilirubin level is 1.2 to 3 mg/dl, reduce dosage by 50%; if above 3 mg/dl, reduce dosage by 75%.

PREPARATION & STORAGE
To avoid mutagenic, teratogenic, and carcinogenic risks when preparing doxorubicin, use a biological containment cabinet during preparation, wear a mask to avoid inhaling drug particles or solution, and put on gloves to avoid skin contact. If drug comes in contact with skin or mucosa, immediately wash the area with soap and water.
    Dispose of needles, vials, and unused drug correctly. Use syringes with luer-lock fittings to prevent drug leakage. Avoid contamination of work surfaces. Clean spills with 5% sodium hypochlorite (household bleach) to inactivate drug.
    Doxorubicin is supplied as a powder in 10-, 20-, 50-, 100-, and 150-mg vials. Store in a dry place, away from sunlight. Reconstitute with 0.9% NaCl, D$_5$W, or sterile water for injection. Avoid using diluents containing preservatives or having a pH less than 3 or greater than 7.
    To reconstitute drug, add 5 ml of diluent to 10-mg vial, 10 ml to 20-mg vial, 25 ml to 50-mg vial, 50 ml to the 100-mg vial, or 75 ml to the 150-mg vial. When using sterile water for injection, add 2 to 3 volumes of 0.9% NaCl to drug to make solution isotonic. Shake vial to help dissolve drug. Reconstituted drug remains stable for 24 hours at room temperature and for 48 hours

D

at 39° to 50° F (4° to 10° C). For best results, use within 8 hours of reconstitution. Discard unused drug.

Incompatibility
Incompatible with aluminum, aminophylline, bacteriostatic diluents, cephalothin sodium, dexamethasone sodium phosphate, diazepam, fluorouracil, furosemide, heparin sodium, and hydrocortisone sodium succinate.

ADMINISTRATION
Direct injection: Using a 21G or 23G winged-tip needle, inject drug into a large vein over 3 to 5 minutes. Or, inject drug into tubing of free-flowing IV line containing 0.9% NaCl or D_5W. Avoid injecting into veins over joints or extremities with compromised venous return or impaired lymphatic drainage. Flush administration set with 0.9% NaCl after use.

CONTRAINDICATIONS & CAUTIONS
• Contraindicated in myelosuppression and in patients who have received a total lifetime dose of 550 mg/m². Avoid giving a lifetime dose exceeding 400 mg/m² to patients who have received chest radiation therapy, a related tetracyclic chemotherapeutic drug (such as daunorubicin), or cyclophosphamide.
• Also contraindicated in chickenpox or herpes zoster infection.
• Use cautiously in gout, heart disease, bone marrow depression, and history of urate stones.

SPECIAL CONSIDERATIONS
• Prevent or minimize uric acid nephropathy through hydrating, alkalinizing urine, or giving allopurinol.
• Reduce administration rate if patient develops facial flushing or local erythema.
• Some degree of toxicity occurs with a therapeutic response.

• Cardiotoxicity may be more common in children under age 2, in elderly patients, in patients who have received chest radiation therapy, and in those whose cumulative dose exceeds 550 mg/m².
• In cases of overdose watch for increased toxic effects (mucositis, leukopenia, and thrombocytopenia).
• Regularly monitor ECG in patients who have received 300 mg/m² or more of drug. Also monitor CBC and liver function tests for signs of toxicity.
• Watch for early signs of heart failure; drug-induced condition often fails to respond to therapy.

droperidol

Inapsine✦

Pregnancy Risk Category: C

INDICATIONS & DOSAGES
Preoperative sedation and prevention or alleviation of nausea and vomiting—
Adults and children over age 12: 2.5 to 10 mg given 30 to 60 minutes before surgery.
Children ages 2 to 12: 0.088 to 0.165 mg/kg given 30 to 60 minutes before surgery.
Adjunct to induction in general anesthesia—
Adults and children over age 12: 0.22 to 0.275 mg/kg.
Maintenance in general anesthesia—
Adults and children over age 12: 1.25 to 2.5 mg.
Children ages 2 to 12: 0.088 to 0.165 mg/kg.
Conscious sedation for diagnostic procedures—
Adults and children over age 12: 1.25 to 2.5 mg IV titrated to patient response, after IM premedication.
Adjunct in regional anesthesia—
Adults: 2.5 to 5 mg.

PREPARATION & STORAGE
Available in concentrations of 2.5 mg/ml in 1-, 2-, and 5-ml am-

pules and in 10-ml multidose vials. Protect from light and store at room temperature. Drug is compatible with all IV solutions.

Incompatibility
Incompatible with barbiturates, fluorouracil, foscarnet sodium, furosemide, heparin, leucovorin calcium, methotrexate sodium, and nafcillin sodium.

ADMINISTRATION
Direct injection: Inject directly into vein in small incremental boluses or into an established IV line containing a free-flowing solution.

CONTRAINDICATIONS & CAUTIONS
• Contraindicated in hypersensitivity to drug.
• Use cautiously in elderly, debilitated, and other high-risk patients.
• Use cautiously in hepatic or renal impairment, and in hypotensive or hypovolemic patients.

SPECIAL CONSIDERATIONS
• Keep resuscitation equipment available during administration.
• When giving an opioid analgesic with droperidol, reduce narcotic dosage by one-fourth to one-third for up to 12 hours or until patient becomes fully alert.
• Watch for signs of an extrapyramidal reaction, such as akathisia or dystonia. Call doctor immediately if such signs occur.
• Frequently monitor patient's vital signs.

enalaprilat

Vasotec IV
Pregnancy Risk Category: C

INDICATIONS & DOSAGES
Mild to severe hypertension—
Adults: 1.25 mg over a 5-minute period q 6 hours. Dose for patients being converted from PO to IV dose is the same.

Concurrent diuretic therapy—
Adults: 0.625 mg over a 5-minute period q 6 hours. If after 1 hour there is an inadequate clinical response, dose may be repeated.
Note: Adjust dosage in renal impairment. For adults with a creatinine clearance below 30 ml/minute, initial dose is 0.625 mg. Gradually titrate dose based on response. Patients undergoing hemodialysis should receive a supplemental dose on dialysis days.

PREPARATION & STORAGE
Available as a clear, colorless solution in 1- and 2-ml vials containing 1.25 mg/ml. May be diluted with up to 50 ml of the following compatible solutions: 5% dextrose injection, 0.9% NaCl injection, 0.9% NaCl injection in 5% dextrose, 5% dextrose in lactated Ringer's injection, or Isolyte E. Diluted solutions maintain full activity for 24 hours at room temperature. Store below 86° F (30° C).

Incompatibility
Incompatible with amphotericin B and phenytoin sodium.

ADMINISTRATION
Direct injection: Administer as provided or dilute with up to 50 ml of a compatible diluent. Infuse slowly over at least 5 minutes.

CONTRAINDICATIONS & CAUTIONS
• Contraindicated in hypersensitivity to drug and history of angioedema related to previous treatment with ACE inhibitors.
• Use with caution in patients with collagen vascular disease or immune system disorders and in those taking drugs that may depress immune function or cause a decrease in WBC count.
• Use cautiously in patients taking potassium-sparing diuretics, potassium supplements, and salt substitutes.
• Use with caution in patients with vascular insufficiency, recent MI,

E

cerebrovascular disease, and renal impairment
• Use cautiously when administering drug to breast-feeding women.
• Advise pregnant patient in second and third trimesters to have ultrasound examinations.

SPECIAL CONSIDERATIONS
• If hypotension occurs, place patient in a supine position and infuse 0.9% NaCl, as ordered.
• Observe patient for facial swelling and difficulty breathing, which may indicate angioedema. If angioedema of the face, extremities, lips, tongue, glottis, or larynx occurs, discontinue treatment immediately. Institute appropriate therapy: epinephrine solution 1:1,000 (0.3 to 0.5 ml) SC and measures to ensure a patent airway. Monitor patient carefully until signs and symptoms disappear.
• Monitor WBC count and liver and kidney functions.

epinephrine hydrochloride

Adrenalin Chloride◆, EpiPen Auto-Injector, EpiPen Jr., Sus-Phrine

Pregnancy Risk Category: C

INDICATIONS & DOSAGES
Bronchospasm and hypersensitivity reactions—
Adults: 0.1 to 0.25 mg (1 to 2.5 ml of 1:10,000 dilution) slowly over 5 to 10 minutes. May be followed by an infusion of 1 to 4 mcg/minute.
Children: 0.1 mg (10 ml of 1:100,000 dilution) slowly over 5 to 10 minutes. May be followed by an infusion of 0.1 mcg/kg/minute, increased p.r.n. to a maximum of 1.5 mcg/kg/minute.
Cardiac arrest—
Adults: 0.1 to 1 mg (1 to 10 ml of 1:10,000 dilution) repeated q 5 minutes p.r.n. May be followed by

an infusion of 1 mcg/minute, increased p.r.n. to 4 mcg/minute.
Children: 0.01 mg/kg (0.1 ml/kg of a 1:10,000 dilution) repeated q 5 minutes p.r.n. May be followed by an infusion of 0.1 mcg/kg/minute, increased p.r.n. by 0.1 mcg/kg/minute to a maximum of 1 mcg/kg/minute.
Neonates: 0.01 to 0.03 mg/kg (0.1 to 0.3 ml/kg of 1:10,000 dilution) repeated q 5 minutes p.r.n.

PREPARATION & STORAGE
Available in 1- and 30-ml vials in concentrations of 0.1 mg/ml (1:10,000), 0.5 mg/ml (1:2,000), and 1 mg/ml (1:1,000). Also available in prefilled syringes containing 1 to 2 ml of 1 mg/ml concentration, 10 ml of 0.1 mg/ml, and 5 ml of 0.01 mg/ml. To obtain a solution of 4 mcg/ml, add 1 mg of drug to 250 ml of D_5W or 0.9% NaCl, dextrose 10% in water, dextrose 5% in lactated Ringer's injection, or dextrose 5% in Ringer's injection. Compatible with most other IV solutions.
Protect epinephrine from light. (Keep ampules in carton until ready to use.) Discard brown solutions or solutions that contain a precipitate.

Incompatibility
Rapidly destroyed by alkalies or oxidizing agents, including halogens, nitrates, nitrites, permanganates, sodium bicarbonate, and salts of easily reducible metals (such as iron, copper, and zinc). Incompatible with aminophylline, ampicillin sodium, cephapirin, furosemide, hyaluronidase, and mephentermine sulfate.

ADMINISTRATION
Direct injection: Slowly inject drug (0.1 mg over 5 to 10 minutes) directly into a vein or into an IV line containing a free-flowing, compatible solution.
Intermittent infusion: Using an appropriately diluted solution, piggyback drug into a compatible solution and infuse over 5 to 10 minutes.

Continuous infusion: Using an appropriately diluted solution, infuse drug at a rate of 0.1 to 1.5 mg/kg/minute with an infusion pump.

CONTRAINDICATIONS & CAUTIONS
• Contraindicated in shock (except anaphylactic shock); in organic brain damage, cerebral arteriosclerosis, organic heart disease, cardiac dilation, coronary insufficiency, and most arrhythmias; and in narrow-angle glaucoma.
• Give cautiously in hyperthyroidism, especially in elderly patients; diabetes mellitus; and CV disorders, such as angina pectoris, tachycardia, heart failure, coronary artery disease, and hypertension.
• Also use cautiously in sensitivity to sulfites or sympathomimetic amines; in psychoneurosis; and in Parkinson's disease.

SPECIAL CONSIDERATIONS
• Overdose may cause renal shutdown and circulatory collapse. Overdose or prolonged use can produce severe metabolic acidosis because of elevated lactic acid levels.
• Monitor vital signs. Drug can widen pulse pressure.

epoetin alfa (erythropoietin)

Epogen, Eprex◇, Procrit
Pregnancy Risk Category: C

INDICATIONS & DOSAGES
Treatment of anemia associated with chronic renal failure—
Adults: initially, 50 to 100 U/kg three times weekly. Patients receiving dialysis should be given drug IV; those with chronic renal failure not on dialysis may receive drug SC.
  Reduce dosage when target hematocrit is reached or if hematocrit increases more than 4 points within 2-week period. Increase dosage if hematocrit does not increase by 5 to 6

points after 8 weeks of therapy and target range of 30% to 33% has not been reached. Individualize dosage for maintenance range.
Treatment of anemia associated with zidovudine (AZT) therapy in patients infected with HIV and low endogenous erythropoietin levels—
Adults: initiate therapy with 100 U/kg three times weekly for 8 weeks. If response is not adequate, increase dosage to 150 or 200 U/kg three times weekly. Reevaluate response q 1 to 2 months and increase dosage by 50 to 100 U/kg three times weekly, p.r.n. Response is unlikely to dosages above 300 U/kg three times weekly. Adjust doses cautiously based on concurrent infections or changes in AZT therapy.

PREPARATION & STORAGE
Available in vials of 2,000, 3,000, 4,000, and 10,000 U/ml. Vials also contain 2.5 mg of human albumin. Refrigerate at 36° to 46° F (2° to 8° C). Do not shake because this may denature glycoprotein. Do not dilute solution. Single-dose vials do not contain preservative. Use only one dose per vial. Also available as 2-ml multidose vial containing 10,000 U/ml, which contains preservative.

Incompatibility
Avoid mixing with other drugs.

ADMINISTRATION
Direct injection: Administer through the IV access site (after dialysis session).

CONTRAINDICATIONS & CAUTIONS
• Contraindicated in patients hypersensitive to mammalian cell-derived products or to human albumin, and in those with uncontrolled hypertension.

SPECIAL CONSIDERATIONS
• Determine endogenous erythropoietin levels in patient receiving drug for AZT-induced anemia before therapy. He is unlikely to respond to drug therapy if endogenous levels exceed 500 milliunits/ml.

E

• A rapid increase in hematocrit can cause loss of control of blood pressure. Reduce dosage so hematocrit does not increase by more than 4 points within a 2-week period. Drug may have to be withheld until blood pressure is controlled.

• Discontinue drug if hematocrit increases beyond target range of 30% to 33%.

• Hemodialysis patients being treated with epoetin alfa may require increased heparin dosage to reduce risk of clogging dialysis machine.

• Drug therapy may result in increased hematocrit and decreased plasma volume, which may reduce effectiveness of dialysis treatments.

• In case of overdose drug therapy can result in polycythemia if hematocrit is not carefully monitored and dose appropriately adjusted.

epoprostenol sodium

Flolan

Pregnancy Risk Category: B

INDICATIONS & DOSAGES

Long-term IV treatment of primary pulmonary hypertension in New York Heart Association class III and class IV patients—
Adults: initially, 2 ng/kg/minute infusion, increased by 2 ng/kg/minute q 15 minutes or longer until dose-limiting pharmacologic effects occur. Begin maintenance dosing with 4 ng/kg/minute less than the maximum tolerated rate determined during initial dosing. If the maximum rate is less than 5 ng/kg/minute, the maintenance infusion is started at one-half the maximum rate. Subsequent adjustments are made based on persistence, recurrence, or worsening of the symptoms. Such increases should be made gradually in increments of 1 to 2 ng/kg/minute q 15 minutes or longer. Occurrence of adverse events from excessive dosage may require a gradual decrease in dosage in decre-

ments of 2 ng/kg/minute q 15 minutes or longer.

PREPARATION & STORAGE
Reconstitute drug only as directed, using sterile diluent for Flolan. Do not reconstitute or mix with other parenteral medications or solutions before or during administration.

Follow manufacturer's guidelines for reconstituting drug. The prescribed concentration should be compatible with the infusion pump's minimum and maximum flow rates and reservoir capacity, and with other criteria recommended by the manufacturer. When used for maintenance infusion, drug should be prepared in a drug delivery reservoir appropriate for the infusion pump, with a total reservoir volume of at least 100 ml. Drug should be prepared using two vials of sterile diluent for use during 24 hours.

Protect reconstituted solutions from light and refrigerate at 36° to 46° F (2° to 8° C); do not freeze. Discard frozen solution or solution that has been refrigerated longer than 48 hours.

Incompatibility
Do not infuse drug with other medications or IV solutions.

ADMINISTRATION
Continuous infusion: Administer by ambulatory infusion pump via a central catheter. Peripheral infusion may be done on a temporary basis until central access is established.

CONTRAINDICATIONS & CAUTIONS
• Contraindicated in hypersensitivity to drug or structurally related compounds.
• Chronic use is contraindicated in patients with heart failure due to severe left ventricular systolic dysfunction, and in those who develop pulmonary edema during initial dosing.
• Use cautiously in the elderly and pregnant or breast-feeding patients.
• Safety and efficacy in children have not been established.

SPECIAL CONSIDERATIONS
• Avoid abrupt withdrawal of drug or sudden large reductions in infusion rate.
• To facilitate extended use at ambient temperatures above 77° F (25° C), a cold pouch with frozen gel packs can be used. The pouch must be able to maintain a temperature of 36° to 46° F (2° to 8° C) for 12 hours. When such a pouch is used, the reconstituted solution should be used for more than 24 hours.
• Administer anticoagulant therapy during maintenance infusion, unless contraindicated.
• Monitor standing and supine blood pressure and heart rate for several hours to ensure tolerance.

ergonovine maleate

Ergotrate Maleate♦

Pregnancy Risk Category: NR

INDICATIONS & DOSAGES
Emergency treatment of postpartum or postabortion hemorrhage caused by uterine atony or subinvolution—
Adults: 0.2 mg in a single dose, repeated q 2 to 4 hours, if necessary, up to five doses.

PREPARATION & STORAGE
Supplied in 1-ml ampules containing 0.2 mg/ml. Dilute with 5 ml of 0.9% NaCl before infusion. Store below 46° F (8° C) in light-resistant containers. Discard discolored ergonovine injections (normally clear and colorless) or those that contain a precipitate. Avoid freezing.

Incompatibility
None reported, but drug should not be mixed with any IV infusions.

ADMINISTRATION
Direct injection: Inject diluted drug directly into vein over at least 60 seconds. Avoid rapid injection because of severe CV effects.

CONTRAINDICATIONS & CAUTIONS
• Contraindicated before placental expulsion.
• Contraindicated for induction of labor; in threatened spontaneous abortion; and in hypersensitive or idiosyncratic reaction to ergonovine or methylergonovine.
• Also contraindicated in hypertension, heart disease, AV shunts, mitral valve stenosis, and obliterative vascular disease.
• Use cautiously in sepsis, hepatic or renal impairment, and hypocalcemia.

SPECIAL CONSIDERATIONS
• Review patient's history. In a hypocalcemic patient, for instance, the uterus may not respond until IV calcium is administered.
• Closely monitor blood pressure and pulse.
• Closely monitor contractions and uterine tone after administration. If appropriate, give analgesics.
• Instruct patient to report sensation of tingling in fingers or toes or other sensory alterations; these may represent vasoconstriction.

esmolol hydrochloride

Brevibloc

Pregnancy Risk Category: C

INDICATIONS & DOSAGES
Supraventricular tachycardia; to lower heart rate and blood pressure in patients with acute myocardial ischemia; to produce controlled hypotension during anesthesia—
Adults: loading dose is 500 mcg/kg/minute by IV infusion over 1 minute, followed by a 4-minute maintenance infusion of 50 mcg/kg/minute. If adequate response does not occur within 5 minutes, repeat the loading dose followed by a maintenance infusion of 100 mcg/kg/minute for 4 minutes. Repeat loading dose and increase mainte-

E

nance infusion in a stepwise fashion as needed. Maximum maintenance infusion for tachycardia is 200 mcg/kg/minute.
Management of perioperative hypertension—
Adults: for immediate intraoperative control, inject 80 mg over 30 seconds. If necessary, follow with an infusion of 150 mcg/kg/minute. For gradual control of hypertension, follow dosing schedule for supraventricular tachycardia.

PREPARATION & STORAGE
Available in 10-ml ampules containing 250 mg/ml. Before infusion, reconstitute 2 ampules with 20 ml of diluent to yield a concentration of 10 mg/ml. Concentrations of 20 mg/ml or higher are associated with venous irritation and thrombophlebitis. A ready-to-use formulation containing 10 mg/ml in a 10-ml single-dose vial is also available.

Compatible solutions include D_5W, dextrose 5% in lactated Ringer's, lactated Ringer's, dextrose 5% in 0.45% NaCl, potassium chloride 40 mEq in 5% dextrose injection, and 0.45% or 0.9% NaCl. Diluted solution is stable for 24 hours at room temperature. Freezing does not alter drug effect, but do not expose to high temperatures.

Incompatibility
Incompatible with diazepam, furosemide, procainamide hydrochloride, sodium bicarbonate, and thiopental sodium.

ADMINISTRATION
Direct injection: inject intraoperative dose over 30 seconds (do not use 250-mg/ml ampule).
Continuous infusion: Using an IV catheter and an infusion pump, give loading dose over 1 minute and maintenance dose over 4 minutes. If reaction occurs at infusion site, stop infusion and resume at another site. Avoid using winged-infusion needle.

CONTRAINDICATIONS & CAUTIONS
• Contraindicated in sinus bradycardia or second- or third-degree heart block, and in cardiogenic shock or overt heart failure.
• Use cautiously in bronchospastic disease, diabetes mellitus, hypoglycemia, or renal impairment and in the elderly.
• Safe use in children has not been established.

SPECIAL CONSIDERATIONS
• Hypotension can usually be reversed within 30 minutes by decreasing the dose or, if necessary, by stopping infusion.
• Once heart rate stabilizes, substitute a longer acting antiarrhythmic, as ordered. After starting new drug, gradually reduce esmolol infusion over 1 hour.
• Closely monitor blood pressure and heart rate and rhythm, and frequently assess for signs of neurologic deficit.
• Monitor ECG and blood pressure continuously during infusion.
• Instruct patient to report respiratory or cardiac symptoms promptly.

etoposide (VP-16, VP-16-213)

VePesid♦

etoposide phosphate

Etopophos

Pregnancy Risk Category: D

INDICATIONS & DOSAGES
Induction of remission in refractory testicular cancer—
Adults: 50 to 100 mg/m²/day IV on days 1 to 5, or 100 mg/m²/day IV on days 1, 3, and 5. Repeat q 3 to 4 weeks.
Small-cell lung cancer—

Adults: 35 mg/m²/day for 4 days or 50 mg/m²/day for 5 days, repeated q 3 to 4 weeks.

Note: Dosages are for etoposide; when etoposide phosphate is given, equivalent doses should be used.

PREPARATION & STORAGE

Exercise extreme caution when preparing or giving drug to avoid mutagenic, teratogenic, and carcinogenic risks. Use a biological containment cabinet and avoid contact with skin. Wear mask and gloves. If solution comes in contact with skin or mucosa, immediately wash thoroughly with soap and water. Use syringes with luer-lock fittings to handle concentrate for injection. Dispose of needles, syringes, ampules, and unused drug correctly. Avoid contaminating work surfaces.

Etoposide is supplied in 5-ml ampules containing 20 mg/ml. Unopened ampules remain stable at room temperature for 2 years; diluted solutions are stable up to 48 hours. Dilute with D₅W or 0.9% NaCl to a concentration of 0.2 or 0.4 mg/ml. Discard solution that is discolored or contains precipitates.

Etoposide phosphate is supplied as 113.6-mg vials equivalent to 100 mg etoposide. Reconstitute each vial with 5 or 10 ml of sterile water for injection, 5% dextrose injection, 0.9% NaCl injection, bacteriostatic water for injection with benzyl alcohol, or bacteriostatic NaCl for injection with benzyl alcohol. Reconstitution with 5 ml diluent yields a concentration equivalent to 20 mg/ml; using 10 ml diluent yields a concentration of 10 mg/ml. After reconstitution, drug may be administered without further dilution or can be further diluted to concentrations as low as 0.1 mg/ml using 5% dextrose injection or 0.9% NaCl injection. Discard solution that is discolored or contains precipitates. After reconstitution, etoposide phosphate can be stored at controlled room temperature from 68° to 77° F (20° to 25° C) or under refrigeration at 36° to 46° F (2° to 8° C) for 24 hours.

Incompatibility
Incompatible with idarubicin hydrochloride.

ADMINISTRATION

Direct injection: not used because of delayed and possibly fatal toxicity.
Intermittent infusion: Give diluted etoposide over at least 30 to 60 minutes. Administer through a 21G or 23G needle directly into vein; avoid extravasation. Etoposide phosphate may be given over 5 to 210 minutes.

CONTRAINDICATIONS & CAUTIONS

• Contraindicated in hypersensitivity to drug and in known or recent chickenpox or herpes zoster infection.
• Also contraindicated in patients with platelet counts below 50,000/mm³ or with neutrophil counts below 500/mm³.
• Use with caution in patients with hepatic or renal impairment.
• Advise women of childbearing age to avoid pregnancy and breast-feeding during therapy.
• Safety and efficacy in children have not been established.

SPECIAL CONSIDERATIONS

• Have diphenhydramine, hydrocortisone, epinephrine, and emergency equipment available to establish an airway if anaphylaxis occurs.
• Do not administer through a membrane-type in-line filter because diluent may dissolve it.
• Give antiemetics to control nausea and vomiting.
• Therapeutic response to drug is usually associated with toxic effects.
• Patients with low serum albumin may be at increased risk for toxicities.
• Obtain baseline blood pressure before starting therapy.
• Monitor blood pressure every 15 minutes during infusion.

E

famotidine

Pepcid IV

Pregnancy Risk Category: B

INDICATIONS & DOSAGES

Active duodenal ulcer in patients who cannot take oral medication—
Adults: 20 mg q 12 hours.
Hypersecretory conditions, including Zollinger-Ellison syndrome and multiple endocrine adenomas—
Adults: 20 mg q 6 hours. May require up to 160 mg q 6 hours.

PREPARATION & STORAGE

Available in 2-ml single-dose vials and 4- and 20-ml multidose vials with a concentration of 10 mg/ml. Also available premixed as 20 mg/ 50 ml in 0.9% NaCl. Refrigerate vials, but avoid freezing.

For injection, reconstitute with 5 or 10 ml of diluent; for infusion, use 100 ml of diluent. Drug is compatible with sterile water for injection, 0.9% NaCl, D_5W, dextrose 10% in water, lactated Ringer's, or 5% sodium bicarbonate. Diluted solution remains stable for 48 hours at room temperature.

Incompatibility

Incompatible with cefepime, piperacillin, and tazobactam.

ADMINISTRATION

Direct injection: Inject 5 or 10 ml of reconstituted drug over at least 2 minutes, no faster than 10 mg/ minute.
Intermittent infusion: Infuse drug diluted in 100 ml over 15 to 30 minutes.

CONTRAINDICATIONS & CAUTIONS

• Contraindicated in famotidine hypersensitivity and during breast-feeding.
• Use cautiously in severe renal or hepatic impairment.

SPECIAL CONSIDERATIONS

• Discontinue drug for 24 hours before diagnostic skin tests.
• Gastric cancer must be ruled out before initiating famotidine therapy.
• Check IV site for irritation.
• Closely monitor patient with gastric ulcers.

fentanyl citrate

Sublimaze♦

Controlled Substance Schedule II

Pregnancy Risk Category: C

INDICATIONS & DOSAGES

Dosage depends on concurrently given drugs (especially anesthetics), type and anticipated length of surgery, and patient's age, weight, body size, physical status, underlying disorder, and response to drug.
Short-term perioperative analgesia—
Adults: up to 2 mcg/kg in divided doses.
General anesthesia (as sole agent with 100% oxygen)—
Adults: 50 to 100 mcg/kg; up to 150 mcg/kg may be required.
Induction and maintenance of general anesthesia—
Children ages 2 to 12: 1.7 to 3.3 mcg/kg.
Adjunct in general anesthesia—
Adults: low dose, 2 mcg/kg in divided doses; moderate dose before major surgery, 2 to 20 mcg/kg initially, then 25 to 100 mcg p.r.n.; high dose before complicated surgery, 20 to 50 mcg/kg initially, then 25 mcg to half initial dose p.r.n.
Adjunct in regional anesthesia—
Adults: 50 to 100 mcg.

PREPARATION & STORAGE

Available in 2-, 5-, 10-, 20-, 30-, and 50-ml containers in concentrations of 50 mcg/kg. Store at room temperature, avoid excessive heat or freezing, and protect from light.

Drug is compatible with most common IV solutions.

Incompatibility
Incompatible with methohexital, pentobarbital sodium, and thiopental.

ADMINISTRATION
Direct injection: Inject drug over at least 1 minute to avoid muscle rigidity. If rapid injection is necessary, administer a neuromuscular blocker first to prevent rigidity.
Continuous infusion: sometimes used for induction of general anesthesia. Use high-dose concentrations to rapidly and smoothly achieve initial induction dose.

CONTRAINDICATIONS & CAUTIONS
• Contraindicated in hypersensitivity to fentanyl derivatives and in children under age 12 or those weighing less than 33 lb (15 kg).
• Use cautiously in patients with head injury and increased intracranial pressure.
• Use cautiously in patients with hepatic, renal, or respiratory dysfunction; poor pulmonary reserve; hypothyroidism; and bradyarrhythmias.
• Administer carefully to elderly, young, or debilitated patients.

SPECIAL CONSIDERATIONS
• When used in high doses, respiratory depression may persist for several hours after the patient awakens, making ventilatory support necessary.
• Drug may cause muscle rigidity in the chest wall, leading to problems with ventilation. Note that these problems may occur during emergence from anesthesia. A neuromuscular blocking agent may be required.
• Following recovery from anesthesia, patient may experience delayed respiratory depression, respiratory arrest, bradycardia, asystole, arrhythmias, and hypotension.

filgrastim

Neupogen
Pregnancy Risk Category: C

INDICATIONS & DOSAGES
To decrease incidence of infection caused by myelosuppressive effects of cancer chemotherapy used for non-myeloid tumors—
Adults and children:
5 mcg/kg/day administered as a single daily injection. If necessary, increase dose by 5 mcg/kg/day for each cycle. Begin at least 24 hours after the last dose of chemotherapy and continue beyond nadir until neutrophil count reaches 10,000/mm^3. Discontinue at least 24 hours before next dose of chemotherapy.
To reduce duration of neutropenia and neutropenia-related clinical sequelae in patients with nonmyeloid malignancies undergoing myeloablative chemotherapy followed by bone marrow transplantation—
Adults: following bone marrow transplantation, 10 mcg/kg/day administered as an IV infusion over 4 to 24 hours or as a continuous, 24-hour SC infusion. Give first dose at least 24 hours after chemotherapy and at least 24 hours after bone marrow infusion.
To reduce the incidence and duration of sequelae of neutropenia in symptomatic patients with congenital, cyclic, or idiopathic neutropenia—
Adults: 2 to 60 mcg/kg/day infused over 30 minutes for congenital neutropenia; idiopathic or cyclic neutropenia, 0.5 to 11.5 mcg/kg daily infused over 30 minutes. Chronic administration is required to maintain clinical benefit.

PREPARATION & STORAGE
Available in 1- and 1.6-ml single-dose vials (300 mcg/ml). For infusion, drug may be diluted in 5% dextrose solution to concentrations between 5 and 15 mcg/ml. Add albumin at a final concentration of

F

F

2 mg/ml to prevent adsorption to plastic. Store in refrigerator; do not freeze. Drug is stable at room temperature for 24 hours. Do not shake.

Incompatibility
Incompatible with NaCl solutions.

ADMINISTRATION
Intermittent infusion: Infuse over 15 to 30 minutes using an established IV line containing dextrose solution. *Continuous infusion:* Infuse over 24 hours or at 10 mcg/kg/day.

CONTRAINDICATIONS & CAUTIONS
• Contraindicated in patients with hypersensitivity to products derived from *Escherichia coli.*

SPECIAL CONSIDERATIONS
• Before injection, allow vial to reach room temperature for a maximum of 24 hours. Discard after 24 hours. Use only one dose per vial; do not reenter vial.
• Obtain CBC and platelet count before therapy and twice weekly during therapy. Regularly monitor hematocrit level.
• Adult respiratory distress syndrome may occur in septic patients because of the influx of neutrophils at inflammation site. MI and arrhythmias have occurred; closely monitor patients with preexisting cardiac conditions.
• Instruct patient to promptly report signs of infection, such as fever, chills, and sore throat.

fluconazole

Diflucan

Pregnancy Risk Category: C

INDICATIONS & DOSAGES
Oropharyngeal candidiasis—
Adults: 200 mg on day 1, followed by 100 mg once daily. Therapy should continue for 2 weeks.
Children: 6 mg/kg on day 1, followed by 3 mg/kg once daily.

Esophageal candidiasis—
Adults: 200 mg on day 1, followed by 100 mg once daily. Higher doses (up to 400 mg/day) have been used, depending on patient's condition and tolerance of treatment. Patient should receive drug for at least 3 weeks or 2 weeks after symptoms resolve.
Children: 6 mg/kg on day 1, followed by 3 mg/kg once daily. Doses up to 12 mg/kg/day may be used.
Systemic candidiasis—
Adults: 400 mg on day 1, followed by 200 mg once daily. Treatment should continue for at least 4 weeks or 2 weeks after symptoms resolve.
Children: 6 to 12 mg/kg/day.
Cryptococcal meningitis—
Adults: 400 mg/day. Treatment should continue for 10 to 12 weeks after CSF cultures are negative.
Children: 12 mg/kg/day on day 1, followed by 6 mg/kg once daily.
Suppression of relapse of cryptococcal meningitis in patients with HIV infection—
Adults: 200 mg/day.
Children: 6 mg/kg/day.
Note: Adjust dosage in renal failure. For adults and children, give an initial loading dose of 50 to 400 mg. If creatinine clearance is 21 to 50 ml/minute, reduce dosage by 50%; if it is between 11 and 20 ml/minute, reduce dosage by 75%.

PREPARATION & STORAGE
Available in glass bottles or plastic IV bags with 200 mg/100 ml or 400 mg/200 ml. Store glass bottles at 41° to 86° F (5° to 30° C) and plastic bags at 41° to 77° F (5° to 25° C). Protect from freezing. Brief exposure of plastic containers to temperatures up to 104° F (40° C) will not adversely affect the drug.

IV bags of fluconazole are shipped with a protective overwrap that should not be removed until just before use. This helps ensure product sterility. The plastic container may show some opacity from moisture absorbed during sterilization. This is normal, does not affect the drug, and diminishes over time.

Incompatibility
Incompatible with amphotericin B, ampicillin sodium, calcium gluconate, cefotaxime sodium, ceftazidime, ceftriaxone sodium, cefuroxime sodium, chloramphenicol sodium succinate, clindamycin phosphate, co-trimoxazole, diazepam, digoxin, erythromycin lactobionate, furosemide, haloperidol lactate, hydroxyzine hydrochloride, imipenem-cilastatin sodium, pentamidine isethionate, piperacillin sodium, and ticarcillin disodium. Manufacturer recommends that drug not be mixed with other drugs.

ADMINISTRATION
Intermittent infusion: Administer ordered dose at a rate of approximately 200 mg/hour.

CONTRAINDICATIONS & CAUTIONS
• Contraindicated in patients hypersensitive to drug.
• Use cautiously in patients hypersensitive to other antifungal azole compounds.
• Also use cautiously in patients with abnormal liver function tests.
• Adjust dosage in patients with impaired renal function.
• Advise women receiving drug to use a form of birth control other than oral contraceptives.

SPECIAL CONSIDERATIONS
• Patients receiving regular hemodialysis treatment should receive the usual dose after each dialysis session.
• To prevent air embolism, do not connect in series with other infusions. Do not add other drugs to the solution.
• Incidence of adverse reactions appears to be greater in patients with severe underlying disease, including cancers, and in those with HIV infection, especially if they are taking other medications known to be hepatotoxic or associated with exfoliative skin disorders.

• Closely monitor patient who develops a rash in response to drug. Discontinue drug if rash worsens.

fludarabine

Fludara

Pregnancy Risk Category: D

INDICATIONS & DOSAGES
Treatment of B-cell chronic lymphocytic leukemia in patients who have either not responded or have responded inadequately to at least one standard alkylating agent regimen—
Adults: 25 mg/m² IV over 30 minutes for 5 consecutive days. Repeat cycle q 28 days. Treatment should continue for three additional cycles after maximal response is achieved; then, discontinue drug.

PREPARATION & STORAGE
Available as a 50-mg single-dose vial of lyophilized solid cake. Store in refrigerator at 36° to 45° F (2° to 8° C). To prepare, add 2 ml of sterile water for injection to the solid cake of fludarabine. Dissolution should occur within 15 seconds. Each milliliter will contain 25 mg of drug. Use within 8 hours of reconstitution. Can be diluted in 100 or 125 ml of D₅W or 0.9% NaCl.

Incompatibility
Physically incompatible with acyclovir sodium, amphotericin B, chlorpromazine hydrochloride, daunorubicin hydrochloride, ganciclovir, hydroxyzine hydrochloride, miconazole, and prochlorperazine edisylate. Compatibility may depend on concentration of drugs, specific diluents, resulting pH of solution, and temperature. Consult specialized references.

ADMINISTRATION
Intermittent infusion: Infuse 25 mg/m² over 30 minutes.

CONTRAINDICATIONS & CAUTIONS
• Contraindicated in hypersensitivity to drug or its components.
• Use cautiously and with dosage adjustments in renal insufficiency, advanced age, and bone marrow impairment.
• Advise women of childbearing age to avoid becoming pregnant during therapy and to consult a doctor before becoming pregnant.
• Caution women against breastfeeding during therapy.
• Safety and efficacy in children have not been established.

SPECIAL CONSIDERATIONS
• Severe neurologic effects are seen when high doses are used to treat acute leukemia. Irreversible CNS toxicity characterized by delayed blindness, coma, and death is associated with high doses. No specific antidote exists. Discontinue drug and provide supportive treatment.
• Monitor hematologic function frequently and closely during and after therapy.
• Instruct patient to promptly report symptoms of infection (chills, fever, cough, sore throat) or bleeding (hematuria, bleeding gums, easy bruising, melena).

flumazenil

Romazicon

Pregnancy Risk Category: C

INDICATIONS & DOSAGES
Complete or partial reversal of the sedative effects of benzodiazepines after anesthesia or short diagnostic procedures (conscious sedation)—
Adults: initially, 0.2 mg over 15 seconds. If patient does not reach the desired level of consciousness after 45 seconds, repeat dose. If needed, repeat at 1-minute intervals until a cumulative dose of 1 mg has been given (initial dose plus four additional doses). Most patients respond after 0.6 to 1 mg of drug. In case of

resedation, dosage may be repeated after 20 minutes; however, no more than 1 mg should be given at any one time, and no more than 3 mg/hour.
Management of suspected benzodiazepine overdose—
Adults: initially, 0.2 mg over 30 seconds. If patient does not reach desired level of consciousness after 30 seconds, administer 0.3 mg over 30 seconds. If patient still does not respond adequately, give 0.5 mg over 30 seconds; repeat 0.5-mg doses at 1-minute intervals until a cumulative dose of 3 mg has been given. Most patients suffering from benzodiazepine overdose respond to cumulative doses between 1 and 3 mg; rarely, patients who respond partially after 3 mg may require additional doses. Do not give more than 5 mg over 5 minutes initially. Sedation that persists after this dosage is unlikely to be caused by benzodiazepines. In case of resedation, dosage may be repeated after 20 minutes; however, no more than 1 mg should be given at any one time, and no more than 3 mg/hour.

PREPARATION & STORAGE
Available as a 0.1 mg/ml solution in 5- and 10-ml vials. To minimize pain at injection site, administer through a free-flowing IV solution into a large vein. Flumazenil is compatible with D_5W, lactated Ringer's, and 0.9% NaCl. If drawn into a syringe or mixed with any of these solutions, discard after 24 hours.

Incompatibility
None reported.

ADMINISTRATION
Direct injection: Inject over 15 to 30 seconds into an IV line in a large vein with free-flowing IV solution.

CONTRAINDICATIONS & CAUTIONS
• Contraindicated in patients hypersensitive to flumazenil or benzodiazepines, in those who have been given a benzodiazepine for a poten-

fluorouracil (5-FU)

tially life-threatening condition, and in those who show signs of serious cyclic antidepressant overdose.
• Drug should not be used during labor and delivery.
• Do not use drug as treatment for benzodiazepine dependence or management of protracted benzodiazepine abstinence syndromes.
• Use cautiously in patients with hepatic impairment or with alcohol and other drug dependencies.
• Use cautiously in patients at high risk for development of seizures, patients who have recently received multiple doses of a parenteral benzodiazepine, patients displaying some signs of seizure activity, those who may be at risk for unrecognized benzodiazepine dependence, patients with head injury, those who have received neuromuscular blockers, and psychiatric patients.
• Safety and efficacy for use in children have not been established.

SPECIAL CONSIDERATIONS

• To control the reversal of sedation to the desired end point and to minimize risk of adverse effects, administer flumazenil as a series of small injections, not as a single bolus dose.
• Patients should have a secure airway and IV access before administration; they should be awakened gradually.
• Reversal with excessively high doses of flumazenil may produce anxiety, agitation, and possibly convulsions. Treat with barbiturates, benzodiazepines, and phenytoin.
• Monitor patient closely for resedation after reversal of benzodiazepine effects. Duration of monitoring depends on the specific drug being reversed. Resedation is unlikely in patients who fail to show signs of resedation 2 hours after 1-mg dose of flumazenil.

fluorouracil (5-FU)

Adrucil◆, Fluorouracil Injection

Pregnancy Risk Category: D

INDICATIONS & DOSAGES
Dosage depends on protocol and patient weight.
Palliative treatment of colorectal, stomach, pancreas, and advanced breast cancer—
Adults: initially, 12 mg/kg/day for 4 days. Maximum dosage, 800 mg/day. If no toxicity occurs, 6 mg/kg can be given on days 6, 8, 10, and 12. No therapy is given on days 5, 7, 9, or 11. Therapy is discontinued on day 12. Maintenance dosage: initial dose repeated in 30 days, then 10 to 15 mg/kg weekly. Do not exceed 1g per week.
High-risk adults: initially, 6 mg/kg/day for 3 days. Maximum dosage, 400 mg/day. If no toxicity occurs, 3 mg/kg can be given on days 5, 7, and 9. No therapy is given on days 4, 6, or 8. Maintenance dosage is reduced.

PREPARATION & STORAGE
Exercise extreme caution when preparing fluorouracil to avoid mutagenic, teratogenic, and carcinogenic risks. Use a biological containment cabinet and wear gloves and mask. Use syringes with luer-lock tips to avoid drug leakage. Correctly dispose of needles, ampules, and unused drug, and avoid contaminating work surfaces. Manufacturer recommends cleaning spills with sodium hypochlorite 5% (household bleach) to inactivate drug.
Available in 10-ml glass ampules containing 500 mg of drug in a clear yellow aqueous solution, as well as in 10-, 20-, and 100-ml vials containing 50 mg/ml solution. Store at room temperature and protect from direct sunlight. Do not use dark yellow solutions; potency may be affected.

F

For injection, drug requires no further dilution. For infusion, dilute with D₅W or 0.9% NaCl in an appropriate volume based on the patient's condition. Use a filtered needle to prevent injection of glass particles that may enter the solution when opening the ampule.

Incompatibility
Incompatible with carboplatin, cisplatin, cytarabine, diazepam, doxorubicin, droperidol, epirubicin, filgrastim, methotrexate, and ondansetron hydrochloride.

ADMINISTRATION
Direct injection: Administer by a 23G or 25G winged infusion set at any convenient rate. Consider using distal rather than major veins to allow for repeated venipunctures, if needed. Use a new site for each injection.
Continuous infusion: Infuse appropriately diluted drug via central line over 2 to 24 hours.

CONTRAINDICATIONS & CAUTIONS
• Contraindicated in patients with serious infection, especially recent or existing chickenpox or herpes zoster.
• Also contraindicated in patients who have had surgery within the past month.
• Use cautiously in patients with hepatic or renal impairment, previous metastasis to the bone marrow, and after high-dose radiation therapy or use of alkylating agents.
• Advise women not to become pregnant during drug therapy.
• Advise both men and women to use reliable contraception during drug therapy.
• Caution women against breastfeeding during therapy.

SPECIAL CONSIDERATIONS
• Expect toxic effects with therapeutic doses of fluorouracil.
• Any form of concomitant therapy that increases stress to the patient, interferes with nutrition, or depress-

es bone marrow function increases the toxicity of fluorouracil.
• Treat anorexia and nausea with antiemetics. Stop drug if patient experiences intractable vomiting or diarrhea or if GI bleeding occurs.
• Monitor patient's hematologic function for at least 4 weeks.
• Advise patient to report bleeding or bruising.

folic acid

Folvite◆

Pregnancy Risk Category: A (C if greater than RDA)

INDICATIONS & DOSAGES
Megaloblastic and macrocytic anemias as seen in tropical sprue, anemia of nutritional origin, pregnancy, infancy, or childhood—
Adults and children: 250 mcg to 1 mg daily.

PREPARATION & STORAGE
Available in 10-ml vials containing concentrations of 5 mg/ml or 10 mg/ml. Store between 59° and 86° F (15° and 30° C). Protect from light and freezing.

For direct injection, dilute 1 ml of 5 mg/ml concentration with 49 ml of sterile water for injection to get a concentration of 0.1 mg/ml.

Incompatibility
Incompatible with calcium gluconate, 40% dextrose in water, 50% dextrose in water, doxapram hydrochloride, oxidizing and reducing agents, and heavy metal ions.

ADMINISTRATION
Direct injection: Slowly inject dose directly into vein or into the tubing of a free-flowing, compatible IV solution.

CONTRAINDICATIONS & CAUTIONS
• Contraindicated in neonates and immature infants.

• Administer with caution to patients who may also suffer from vitamin B_{12} deficiency. Folic acid can mask the diagnosis of pernicious anemia by improving hematologic measurements. Neurologic damage, however, will continue to progress. Therefore, do not use as sole treatment of pernicious anemia.

SPECIAL CONSIDERATIONS
• Use IV administration only when oral administration is not acceptable, such as with GI surgery or malabsorption syndromes.
• Monitor CBC to measure effectiveness of drug treatment.
• Tell patient to report adverse reactions promptly.

foscarnet sodium

Foscavir

Pregnancy Risk Category: C

INDICATIONS & DOSAGES
Treatment of CMV retinitis in patients with AIDS and acyclovir-resistant mucocutaneous herpes simplex virus (HSV) infection in immuno-compromised patients—
Adults: initially, 60 mg/kg IV as an induction treatment in patients with normal renal function. Administer as an IV infusion over at least 1 hour q 8 hours for 2 to 3 weeks based on clinical response. Maintenance infusion is 90 mg/kg/day administered over 2 hours, which may be increased to 120 mg/kg/day if disease shows signs of progression.
Treatment of HSV infections—
Adults: 40 mg/kg (minimum 1-hour infusion) either q 8 or 12 hours for 2 to 3 weeks or until infection resolves.

Dosage adjustment in patients with renal failure: First calculate the patient's creatinine clearance (Cr clear) using the following formulas: for male patients, use Cr clear = (140 − age)/(serum Cr X 72); for female patients, multiply the above

value by 0.85. See package insert for complete dosing information. See examples of dosing for CMV below.

Induction dose CMV (mg/kg)

Cr clear (ml/min/kg)	Equivalent to 180 mg/kg/day (60 mg/kg q 8 hr)
> 1.4	60 q 8 hr
> 1 to 1.4	45 q 8 hr
> 0.8 to 1	50 q 12 hr
> 0.6 to 0.8	40 q 12 hr
> 0.5 to 0.6	60 q 24 hr
≥ 0.4 to 0.5	50 q 24 hr
< 0.4	not recommended

Maintenance dose CMV (mg/kg)

Cr clear (ml/min/kg)	Equivalent to 90 mg/kg/day	Equivalent to 120 mg/kg/day
> 1.4	90 q 24 hr	120 q 24 hr
> 1 to 1.4	70 q 24 hr	90 q 24 hr
> 0.8 to 1	50 q 24 hr	65 q 24 hr
> 0.6 to 0.8	80 q 48 hr	105 q 48 hr
> 0.5 to 0.6	60 q 48 hr	80 q 48 hr
≥ 0.4 to 0.5	50 q 48 hr	65 q 48 hr
< 0.4	not recommended	not recommended

PREPARATION & STORAGE
Available as a 24 mg/ml solution for infusion in 250- and 500-ml glass bottles. Store at 59° to 86° F (15° to 30° C). Undiluted drug is stable for 24 months at 77° F (25° C). At a concentration of 12 mg/ml in 0.9% NaCl solution, foscarnet is stable for 30 days at 41° F (5° C). Do not freeze; precipitation is likely. Discard any frozen product.

Undiluted drug can only be administered through a central line because of possible venous irritation. For peripheral administration, dilute with an equal amount (1:1) of 5% dextrose injection or 0.9% NaCl injection for a final concentration of 12 mg/ml. To avoid accidental overdosage, calculate dose, and then remove and discard any excess before starting infusion.

Incompatibility

Incompatible with 30% dextrose, lactated Ringer's, or solution containing calcium (such as total parenteral nutrition). Use only 5% dextrose or 0.9% NaCl for dilution. Immediate precipitation occurs with acyclovir, amphotericin B, co-trimoxazole, ganciclovir, pentamidine, trimetrexate, and vancomycin. Delayed precipitation occurs with dobutamine, droperidol, haloperidol, and phenytoin. Gas production occurs with diazepam, digoxin, lorazepam, midazolam, and promethazine. Cloudiness or color change was seen when mixed with diphenhydramine, leucovorin, and prochlorperazine.

ADMINISTRATION

Intermittent infusion: 60 mg/kg or less infused over at least 1 hour; higher doses, over at least 2 hours. Administer undiluted solutions through a central line and diluted solutions through a peripheral line. Foscarnet must be administered at a constant rate by an infusion pump.

CONTRAINDICATIONS & CAUTIONS

• Contraindicated in hypersensitivity to foscarnet.
• Use cautiously in abnormal renal function and anemia.
• Safety and efficacy in children have not been established.

SPECIAL CONSIDERATIONS

• Drug is highly toxic. Because toxicity is probably dose-related, the lowest effective maintenance dose should be used.
• Hydrate patient well before and during foscarnet therapy.
• Anemia is common in up to 33% of patients receiving treatment. Transfusion may be required.
• Drug has been associated with changes in serum electrolytes, including hypocalcemia, hypophosphatemia, hyperphosphatemia, hypomagnesemia, and hypokalemia.
• Regular ophthalmologic examinations are necessary.

• Decreases in calcium may not always be reflected in patient's laboratory values. Advise patient to report perioral tingling, numbness in the extremities, and paresthesia.

fosphenytoin

Cerebyx

Pregnancy Risk Category: D

INDICATIONS & DOSAGES

Fosphenytoin should always be prescribed and dispensed in phenytoin sodium equivalent units (PE).
Status epilepticus—
Adults: 15 to 20 mg PE/kg IV at 100 to 150 mg PE/minute as loading dose, then 4 to 6 mg PE/kg/day IV as maintenance dose. Phenytoin may be used instead of fosphenytoin as maintenance, using the appropriate dose.
Prevention and treatment of seizures during neurosurgery (nonemergent loading or maintenance dosing)—
Adults: loading dose of 10 to 20 mg PE/kg IM or IV at infusion rate not exceeding 150 mg PE/minute. Maintenance dose is 4 to 6 mg PE/kg/day IV or IM
Short-term substitution for oral phenytoin therapy—
Adults: same total daily dosage equivalent as oral phenytoin sodium therapy given as a single daily dose IM or IV, at an infusion rate not exceeding 150 mg PE/minute. Some patients may require more frequent dosing.

PREPARATION & STORAGE

Available as 2-ml vial with fosphenytoin sodium 150 mg equivalent to 100 mg of phenytoin sodium and 10-ml vial containing 750 mg equivalent to 500 mg phenytoin sodium.
 Before IV infusion, dilute drug in 5% dextrose or 0.9% NaCl solution for injection to a concentration ranging from 1.5 to 25 mg PE/ml.
 Store unopened vials refrigerated at 36° to 46° F (2° to 8° C). Do not

---

store at room temperature for more than 48 hours. Discard vial containing particulate matter.

Incompatibility
Do not infuse with other drugs.

ADMINISTRATION
Direct injection: not recommended; can be administered IM. Do not use IM administration for status epilepticus because therapeutic concentrations may not be reached as quickly as with IV administration.
Intermittent infusion: Infuse drug diluted to concentration of 1.5 to 25 mg PE/ml at rate not exceeding 150 mg PE/minute. Typical infusion for a 50-kg patient takes 5 to 7 minutes.

CONTRAINDICATIONS & CAUTIONS
• Contraindicated in hypersensitivity to phenytoin, fosphenytoin, or other hydantoins.
• Contraindicated in sinus bradycardia, SA block, second- or third-degree AV block, and Adams-Stokes syndrome.
• Use cautiously in patients with porphyria and hypersensitivity to similarly structured drugs.
• Caution women against breast-feeding during therapy.
• Safety in children has not been established.

SPECIAL CONSIDERATIONS
• Phosphate load supplied by fosphenytoin (0.0037 mmol phosphate/mg PE fosphenytoin) will affect patients requiring severe phosphate restriction, such as those with renal failure.
• Abrupt withdrawal of drug may precipitate status epilepticus.
• In cases of overdose, closely monitor respiratory and CV function and provide supportive care.
• Monitor vital signs and ECG continuously during period when maximal serum phenytoin levels occur (about 10 to 20 minutes after fosphenytoin infusion ends).
• Monitor serum phosphate levels.

• If rash occurs, discontinue infusion and notify doctor.
• Monitor liver function tests. Drug should be discontinued in acute hepatotoxicity.
• Do not check serum phenytoin levels until conversion of fosphenytoin to phenytoin is complete: about 2 hours after IV administration or 4 hours after IM administration.

furosemide

F

Lasix◆, Lasix Special◇
Pregnancy Risk Category: C

INDICATIONS & DOSAGES
Edema—
Adults: initially, 20 to 40 mg, increased in 20-mg increments q 2 hours until desired response is achieved. Effective dose given once or twice daily p.r.n.
Pulmonary edema—
Adults: initially, 40 mg, increased to 80 mg in 1 hour, if needed.
Infants and children: initially, 1 mg/kg, increased by 1 mg/kg q 2 hours, if needed. Maximum daily dosage, 6 mg/kg.
Hypertensive crisis with pulmonary edema or renal failure—
Adults: 100 to 200 mg.
Heart failure and chronic renal failure—
Adults: for IV bolus injection, maximum should not exceed 1 g/day given over 30 minutes.

PREPARATION & STORAGE
Available in 2-, 4-, and 10-ml ampules and single-use vials and in syringes with a 10 mg/ml concentration. For infusion, dilute in D_5W, lactated Ringer's, dextrose 5% in lactated Ringer's, dextrose 5% in Ringer's injection, or 0.9% NaCl. Filter solution to remove any glass particles from ampules.

Store at room temperature and protect from light. Discard discolored (yellow) solution or solution that contains a precipitate.

Incompatibility
Incompatible with acidic solutions
(pH <5.5), aminoglycosides, amiodarone, amsacrine, bleomycin,
buprenorphine, chlorpromazine, diazepam, dobutamine, doxapram,
doxorubicin, droperidol, erythromycin, esmolol, fluconazole, fructose 10% in water, gentamicin, hydralazine, idarubicin, invert sugar
10% in electrolyte #2, isoproterenol,
meperidine, metoclopramide, milrinone, morphine, netilmicin, ondansetron, prochlorperazine, promethazine, quinidine, vinblastine,
and vincristine.

ADMINISTRATION
Direct injection: Inject directly into
vein or through tubing of a free-
flowing, compatible solution over 1
to 2 minutes.
Intermittent infusion: Infuse diluted
drug at appropriate rate, but not exceeding 4 mg/minute.

CONTRAINDICATIONS & CAUTIONS
• Contraindicated in anuria, in hypersensitivity to furosemide or sulfonamides, and in worsening azotemia or oliguria.
• Use cautiously in diabetes mellitus,
hyperuricemia, hepatic impairment,
acute MI, and history of gout, pancreatitis, or lupus erythematosus.

SPECIAL CONSIDERATIONS
• Drug may cause hypochloremic
metabolic alkalemia and a compensatory respiratory acidemia (increased partial pressure of carbon
dioxide).
• Give slowly; overly rapid injection
or infusion can cause ototoxicity.
• In cases of overdose, manifesta-
tions include excessive diuresis with
dehydration and electrolyte depletion. Correct fluid and electrolyte
imbalance and treat symptomatically.
• Monitor BUN, serum uric acid,
glucose, and electrolyte levels, and
liver and kidney function tests; also
monitor patient's weight, intake and
output, and vital signs.

• Instruct patient to immediately report changes in hearing, abdominal
pain, sore throat, and fever, which
may indicate furosemide toxicity.

ganciclovir

Cytovene

Pregnancy Risk Category: C

INDICATIONS & DOSAGES
Treatment of CMV retinitis—
Adults: initial dose of 5 mg/kg q 12
hours for 14 to 21 days, followed by
maintenance dose of 5 mg/kg/day
for 7 days/week or 6 mg/kg/day
for 5 days/week.
*Prevention of CMV disease in trans-
plant recipients—*
Adults: initial dose of 5 mg/kg q 12
hours for 7 to 14 days, followed by
5 mg/kg/day for 7 days/week or
6 mg/kg/day for 5 days/week. Duration of therapy depends on degree
and duration of immunosuppression.
Note: Adjust dosage in renal impairment. For adults with creatinine
clearance over 70 ml/minute, initial
dose is 5 mg/kg b.i.d. and maintenance dose is 5 mg/kg/day; if creatinine clearance is between 50 and
69 ml/minute, initial dose is
2.5 mg/kg b.i.d. and maintenance
dose is 2.5 mg/kg/day; if creatinine
clearance is between 25 and 49 ml/
minute, initial dose is 2.5 mg/kg/
day and maintenance dose is
1.25 mg/kg/day; if creatinine clearance is between 10 and 24 ml/
minute, initial dose is 1.25 mg/
kg/day and maintenance dose is
0.625 mg/kg/day; and if creatinine
clearance is below 10 ml/minute,
initial dose is 1.25 mg/kg three
times weekly after hemodialysis and
maintenance dose is 0.625 mg/kg
three times weekly following hemodialysis.

PREPARATION & STORAGE
Because ganciclovir should be considered a potential carcinogen, consider handling it according to insti-

tutional guidelines developed for cytotoxic drugs. Available in vials of 500 mg. Store between 59° and 86° F (15° and 30° C). Add 10 ml of sterile water without preservative to one 500-mg vial to produce a solution of 50 mg/ml. Shake vial until solution is clear to ensure complete dissolution of particles. After reconstitution, solutions with a concentration of 50 mg/ml retain potency for 12 hours at room temperature. Do not refrigerate.

Dilute further to a final concentration of 10 mg/ml with 100 ml of 0.9% NaCl, D$_5$W, Ringer's injection, or lactated Ringer's injection. Use diluted solutions within 24 hours. Keep diluted solutions refrigerated until use. Do not freeze.

Incompatibility
Incompatible with parabens, a bacteriostatic agent. Also incompatible with amsacrine, cytarabine, doxorubicin, fludarabine phosphate, foscarnet sodium, ondansetron hydrochloride, piperacillin sodium, sargramostim, tazobactam sodium, and vinorelbine. Do not mix with other drugs.

ADMINISTRATION
Intermittent infusion: Administer drug over 1 hour.

CONTRAINDICATIONS & CAUTIONS
• Contraindicated in hypersensitivity to ganciclovir or acyclovir.
• Because ganciclovir solutions are alkaline (pH about 11), use caution in handling and preparing drug. Latex gloves and safety glasses are recommended. If solution contacts skin or mucous membranes, wash area thoroughly with soap and water; irrigate eyes with plain water.
• Caution women against breastfeeding during therapy and for at least 72 hours after therapy.
• Advise patient to use effective birth control during therapy.
• Safety and efficacy in children have not been established.

SPECIAL CONSIDERATIONS
• Patients on dialysis should receive their dose of ganciclovir after the dialysis session.
• In cases of overdose, dialysis may be useful in reducing serum concentrations of drug. Adequate hydration should be maintained. Consider use of hematopoietic growth factors.
• Monitor CBC to detect neutropenia. This complication usually appears after about 10 days of therapy. Neutropenia is reversible but may require discontinuation of therapy. Patient may restart the drug when CBC returns to normal.
• Advise patient to immediately report signs or symptoms of infection (fever, chills, sore throat) or bleeding (easy bruising, bleeding gums, hematuria, melena).

gemcitabine hydrochloride

Gemzar
Pregnancy Risk Category: D

INDICATIONS & DOSAGES
Locally advanced or metastatic adenocarcinoma of the pancreas and in patients previously given fluorouracil—
Adults: 1,000 mg/m^2 IV over 30 minutes once weekly for up to 7 weeks, unless toxicity occurs. Therapy should be adjusted for bone marrow suppression. Treatment course of 7 weeks is followed by 1 week rest. Subsequent treatment cycles consist of one infusion weekly for 3 of 4 consecutive weeks. Dosage adjustments for subsequent cycles are based on absolute granulocyte and platelet count nadirs and degree of nonhematologic toxicities.

PREPARATION & STORAGE
Use caution in preparing and handling gemcitabine solutions. The use of gloves is recommended. If solution contacts skin or mucosa, immediately wash skin with soap and water, and

flush mucosa with copious amounts of water. Dispose of empty vials, infusion bags and sets, and syringes according to institutional policy for disposing chemotherapeutic waste.

Available as 200-mg powder in 10-ml single-use vial, and as 1-g powder in 50-ml single-use vial. Recommended diluent is 0.9% NaCl injection without preservative. The maximum concentration upon reconstitution is 40 mg/ml. Reconstitutions at greater concentrations may result in incomplete dissolution and should be avoided.

Add 5 ml 0.9 % NaCl for injection to the 200-mg vial or 25 ml to the 1-g vial to yield a gemcitabine concentration of 40 mg/ml. Shake vials to assist in dissolution. Reconstituted drug may be further diluted with 0.9% NaCl injection to concentrations as low as 0.1 mg/ml.

Inspect solution before administration and discard if discolored or if it contains particulates. When reconstituted, solutions are stable at room temperature of 68° to 77° F (20° to 25° C) for 24 hours. Do not refrigerate because crystallization may occur. Discard unused solutions.

Incompatibility
Compatibility with other drugs has not been studied. No known incompatibility with infusion bottles, polyvinyl chloride bags, or administration sets.

ADMINISTRATION
Intermittent infusion: Infuse over 30 minutes; do not prolong infusion time beyond 60 minutes.

CONTRAINDICATIONS & CAUTIONS
• Contraindicated in hypersensitivity to drug.
• Drug is not recommended for pregnant or breast-feeding patients.
• Use cautiously in patients with renal or hepatic impairment. Age, gender, and renal impairment may predispose patient to toxicity.
• Safety and effectiveness in children have not been established.

SPECIAL CONSIDERATIONS
• Prolonged infusion time (over 60 minutes) or frequency of administration of more than once weekly has been associated with increased toxicity.
• In cases of overdose, monitor patient closely and obtain blood counts; provide supportive therapy.
• Obtain patient's CBC, including differential and platelet counts, before each infusion.
• Instruct patient to report signs of infection (fever, chills, sore throat) and bleeding (easy bruising, bleeding gums, hematuria, melena) promptly.

gentamicin sulfate

Garamycin✦, Jenamicin
Pregnancy Risk Category: B

INDICATIONS & DOSAGES
Life-threatening infections caused by susceptible organisms—
Adults: 5 mg/kg/day IV in divided doses q 6 to 8 hours. Adjust dosage based on serum levels; decrease dosage to 3 mg/kg/day in divided doses as soon as possible.
Severe infections caused by susceptible organisms—
Adults: 3 mg/kg/day IV in divided doses q 8 hours.
Children age 1 and older: 2 to 2.5 mg/kg IV q 8 hours.
Infants: 2.5 mg/kg IV q 8 hours.
Neonates age 1 week and less: 2.5 mg/kg IV q 12 hours.
Endocarditis prophylaxis in GI or GU procedures (usually given in conjunction with ampicillin)—
Adults: gentamicin 1.5 mg/kg with 2 g ampicillin, given separately 30 to 60 minutes before surgery. Administer oral ampicillin after procedure.
Children: 2 mg gentamicin and 50 mg/kg ampicillin 30 to 60 minutes before procedure. Administer oral ampicillin, as ordered, after procedure.

Note: Adjust dosage in renal failure. Dosage adjustments are calculated by monitoring peak and trough levels. If patient is undergoing hemodialysis, measure serum levels after each session; dialysis may remove half of the drug. If serum levels are not measured, give 1 to 1.7 mg/kg for adults and 2 to 2.5 mg/kg for children, depending on severity of infection.

PREPARATION & STORAGE
Available as a clear, colorless to slightly yellow aqueous solution in 2-ml vials with a 10 or 40 mg/ml concentration, in 20-ml vials with a 40 mg/ml concentration, in 1.5-ml disposable syringes with a 40 mg/ml concentration, and in 2-ml disposable syringes with a 10 mg/ml concentration. Also available in 60-, 80-, and 100-ml containers (concentration, 1 mg/ml) diluted with D_5W for intermittent infusion and in 50- and 100-ml bags (with a concentration of 0.4 to 2.4 mg/ml) diluted with 0.9% NaCl for intermittent infusion. Intrathecal preparation available as 2 mg/ml preservative-free solution. Containers and bags have no preservatives and must be used promptly once the seal is broken. Discard unused portions.

Do not use discolored or precipitated solution. Store solution between 36° and 86° F (15° and 30° C). Solution is stable for 24 hours at room temperature.

Incompatibility
Incompatible with ampicillin, cefamandole, cefazolin, cefuroxime, cephalothin, cephapirin, cytarabine, dopamine, fat emulsions, furosemide, heparin, hetastarch, idarubicin, nafcillin, certain parenteral nutrition formulations, and ticarcillin. Manufacturer recommends that gentamicin not be mixed with other drugs.

ADMINISTRATION
Direct injection: not recommended, but used for adults if necessary. Inject drug directly into vein or an established IV line over 30 minutes. Do not use infusion units.
Intermittent infusion: Infuse solution (with a concentration not exceeding 1 mg/ml) over 30 minutes to 2 hours.

CONTRAINDICATIONS & CAUTIONS
• Contraindicated in aminoglycoside hypersensitivity or previous severe toxic reaction.
• Use cautiously in the elderly, infants and neonates.
• Administer cautiously in patients with renal impairment, previous aminoglycoside therapy, hearing impairment, or history of noise exposure or ear infections.
• Give cautiously to infants with botulism and to patients with neuromuscular disorders (especially myasthenia gravis).
• Use cautiously in hypomagnesemia, hypocalcemia, and hypokalemia.
• Drug may contain sulfites, which can cause allergic reaction in some patients.

SPECIAL CONSIDERATIONS
• Beta-lactam antibiotics (such as penicillins, cephalosporins) may inactivate aminoglycosides when admixed. Ticarcillin and carbenicillin have the most significant beta-lactam effect. Separate these infusions by several hours.
• Risk of neuromuscular blockade is greatest after rapid, direct injection or if given soon after anesthesia or muscle relaxants.
• In cases of overdose, support respiratory and renal function. Hemodialysis or peritoneal dialysis may help remove drug.
• Weigh patient and test renal function before therapy.
• During therapy, monitor renal function and intake and output. Keep patient well hydrated to minimize risk of toxicity and chemical irritation of renal tubules.

G

glucagon

Pregnancy Risk Category: B

INDICATIONS & DOSAGES
Severe hypoglycemia—
Adults: 0.5 to 1 mg. Larger doses may be necessary.
Children weighing under 44 lb (20 kg): 0.5 mg or dose equivalent to 20 to 30 mcg/kg.
　If patient does not respond, may repeat dose twice.
Diagnostic aid for GI, urologic, and radiologic examinations—
Adults: 0.25 to 2 mg, depending on desired onset time and duration of effect.

PREPARATION & STORAGE
Potency of glucagon is expressed in USP units. One USP unit equals 1 IU and about 1 mg.
　Available as a powder in 1- and 10-unit vials; store at room temperature. Reconstitute with provided diluent, which is clear, sterile, and contains 0.2% phenol as a preservative and 1.6% glycerin. Preparation contains lactose.
　Although reconstituted solution should be used immediately, it is stable for up to 3 months when stored at 36° to 46° F (2° to 8° C).

Incompatibility
Incompatible with NaCl solution and other solutions having a pH of 3 to 9.5 because drug may cause precipitation.

ADMINISTRATION
Direct injection: Give directly into vein or into IV tubing of a free-flowing, compatible solution over 2 to 5 minutes. Interrupt primary infusion during glucagon injection if using the same IV line.

CONTRAINDICATIONS & CAUTIONS
• Contraindicated in hypersensitivity to glucagon.
• Use cautiously in patients allergic to proteins, in those with history of insulinoma, and in pheochromocytoma.

SPECIAL CONSIDERATIONS
• If hypoglycemic patient does not respond to glucagon, give IV dextrose.
• Glucagon causes a smooth, gradual termination of insulin coma. When used to terminate insulin shock therapy in a psychiatric patient, give dose 1 hour after coma induction.
• Once hypoglycemia resolves, give carbohydrate- and protein-containing foods to prevent recurrence.
• Monitor patient's blood pressure and serum glucose levels.

glycopyrrolate

Robinul◆

Pregnancy Risk Category: B

INDICATIONS & DOSAGES
Adjunctive treatment of peptic ulcers—
Adults and children age 12 and over: 0.1 to 0.2 mg q 6 to 8 hours (maximum, 4 doses daily).
Intraoperative medication as an antiarrhythmic—
Adults: 0.1 mg, repeated q 2 to 3 minutes, p.r.n.
Children: 0.0044 mg/kg (maximum, 0.1 mg), repeated q 2 to 3 minutes, p.r.n.
Blockage of adverse muscarinic effects of neostigmine or pyridostigmine—
Adults and children: 0.2 mg for each 1 mg of neostigmine or 5 mg of pyridostigmine. Give in same syringe.

PREPARATION & STORAGE
Available as a clear, colorless sterile solution in 1-, 2-, 5-, and 20-ml vials with a concentration of 0.2 mg/ml. Drug can be given diluted or undiluted. Having a pH of 2 to 3, drug is most stable in acidic solutions and unstable in solutions with pH exceeding 6. Store at room temperature.

For infusion, solutions containing concentrations of 0.8 mg/L remain stable at room temperature for 48 hours when mixed with D_5W, dextrose 5% in 0.45% NaCl, 0.9% NaCl, or Ringer's injection. When using lactated Ringer's injection, prepare admixture immediately before use.

Incompatibility
Incompatible with drugs having an alkaline pH and with chloramphenicol sodium succinate, dexamethasone sodium phosphate, diazepam, dimenhydrinate, methohexital sodium, methylprednisolone sodium succinate, pentazocine lactate, pentobarbital sodium, secobarbital sodium, sodium bicarbonate, and thiopental sodium.

ADMINISTRATION
Direct injection: Inject drug at ordered rate into vein or into an IV line containing a free-flowing, compatible solution.
Intermittent infusion: Infuse at ordered rate or according to hospital guidelines.

CONTRAINDICATIONS & CAUTIONS
• Contraindicated in hypersensitivity to glycopyrrolate.
• Also contraindicated in severe ulcerative colitis, toxic megacolon, obstructive GI disease, cardiospasm, paralytic ileus, and intestinal atony; acute angle-closure glaucoma; and obstructive uropathy or prostatic hypertrophy.
• Use with caution in coronary artery disease, heart failure, cardiac arrhythmias, hypertension, and hyperthyroidism. Avoid use in acute hemorrhage with unstable CV status and myasthenia gravis.
• Because drug contains benzyl alcohol, do not administer to infants under age 1 month.
• Use cautiously in febrile patients and in those exposed to high temperatures.
• Administer drug carefully to children, especially those under age 2.

• Give carefully to children with brain damage or spastic paralysis.
• Use with caution in Down syndrome and elderly patients.
• Administer cautiously in hyperthyroidism, hypertension, tachyarrhythmias, heart failure, coronary artery disease, hepatic or renal impairment, and COPD.
• Also administer cautiously in esophageal reflux or hiatal hernia, gastric ulcer, known or suspected GI infection, diarrhea, and mild or moderate ulcerative colitis.
• Give drug carefully in autonomic or partial obstructive uropathy and xerostomia.
• Safety and efficacy in children under age 12 in treating peptic ulcer disease have not been established.

SPECIAL CONSIDERATIONS
• Elderly or debilitated patients usually require lower doses.
• Avoid giving drug for 24 hours before gastric acid secretion tests.
• High doses over a prolonged period may cause CNS stimulation, resulting in a curare-like action.
• Monitor intake, output, vital signs, and bowel habits.
• Instruct patient to report signs of urinary frequency or urgency.

granisetron hydrochloride

Kytril
Pregnancy Risk Category: B

INDICATIONS & DOSAGES
Prevention of nausea and vomiting associated with chemotherapy, including high-dose cisplatin therapy—
Adults: 10 mcg/kg IV over 5 minutes, given 30 minutes before chemotherapy.
Children ages 2 to 16: 10 mcg/kg.

PREPARATION & STORAGE
Available as 1 mg/ml strength in a 1-ml single-dose vial. Immediately

before use, dilute with 0.9% NaCl or 5% dextrose injection to a total volume of 20 to 50 ml. Diluted product is stable for up to 24 hours when stored at room temperature under normal lighting conditions. Do not freeze; protect from light.

Incompatibility
Do not mix in solution with other drugs.

ADMINISTRATION
Intermittent injection: Infuse over 5 minutes.

CONTRAINDICATIONS & CAUTIONS
• Contraindicated in patients with previous hypersensitivity to granisetron.

SPECIAL CONSIDERATIONS
• Do not administer solution if discolored or if particulate matter is visible.
• Expect the elderly patient to have a slightly higher incidence of CV adverse effects (hypotension).
• Warn patient against activities requiring alertness until CNS effects are known.

heparin calcium

Calcilean◇, Calciparine◆

heparin sodium

Hepalean◆, Hep-Flush, Hep-Lock, Liquaemin

Pregnancy Risk Category: C

INDICATIONS & DOSAGES
Dosage depends on the patient's weight, disease, hepatorenal function, and APTT. Dosages given below are guidelines.
Venous thrombosis or pulmonary embolism—
Adults: 5,000 U initially, then continuous infusion of 20,000 to

40,000 U in 1,000 ml of 0.9% NaCl over 24 hours; or 10,000 U initially, then 5,000 to 10,000 U q 4 to 6 hours.
Children: 50 U/kg initially, then continuous infusion of 100 U/kg q 4 hours or 20,000 U/m² over 24 hours; or 100 U/kg initially, then 50 to 100 U/kg q 4 hours.
Disseminated intravascular coagulation—
Adults: 50 to 100 U/kg q 4 hours. Discontinue after 4 to 8 hours if no improvement occurs.
Children: 25 to 50 U/kg q 4 hours. Discontinue after 4 to 8 hours if no improvement occurs.
IV flush to maintain indwelling catheter patency—
Adults and children: 10 to 100 U after catheter use or at designated intervals.

PREPARATION & STORAGE
Available in 0.5- to 1-ml ampules, vials, or prefilled syringes and in 1-, 2-, 4-, 5-, 10-, and 30-ml multidose vials, with concentrations ranging from 1,000 to 40,000 U/ml. Heparin flush concentrations range from 10 to 100 U/ml.
    For infusion, dilute with 0.9% NaCl or another compatible solution, such as dextrose and Ringer's combination, dextrose 2.5% in water, D_5W, fructose 10%, Ringer's injection, or lactated Ringer's solution, to achieve the prescribed concentration and volume. When diluting heparin solutions for continuous infusion, invert the container at least six times to ensure adequate mixing and to prevent pooling of heparin in the solution.
    Store commercially available heparin preparations at room temperature. Avoid exposure to excessive heat. Do not freeze heparin solutions.
    Before administration, inspect heparin for particles or discoloration. Discard solution if it contains precipitates or is markedly discolored. Slight discoloration does not affect potency.

Incompatibility

Incompatible with alteplase, amikacin sulfate, amsacrine, amiodarone hydrochloride, ampicillin sodium, atracurium besylate, cephalothin sodium, codeine phosphate, chlorpromazine hydrochloride, ciprofloxacin, cytarabine, dacarbazine, daunorubicin hydrochloride, dextrose 4.3% in NaCl 0.18%, diazepam, diltiazem hydrochloride, dobutamine hydrochloride, doxorubicin hydrochloride, droperidol, ergotamine tartrate, erythromycin gluceptate or lactobionate, fentanyl citrate/droperidol, filgrastim, gentamicin sulfate, haloperidol lactate, hyaluronidase, hydrocortisone sodium succinate, hydroxyzine hydrochloride, idarubicin hydrochloride, kanamycin sulfate, levorphanol tartrate, meperidine hydrochloride, methadone, methicillin sodium, methotrimeprazine, methylprednisolone sodium succinate, morphine sulfate, netilmicin sulfate, penicillin G potassium, penicillin G sodium, pentazocine lactate, phenytoin sodium, polymyxin B sulfate, prochlorperazine edisylate, promethazine hydrochloride, quinidine gluconate, 1/6 M sodium lactate, streptomycin sulfate, tobramycin sulfate, trifluoperazine hydrochloride, triflupromazine hydrochloride, vancomycin hydrochloride, and vinblastine sulfate.

Drug may also be incompatible with solutions containing a phosphate buffer or sodium carbonate.

ADMINISTRATION

Direct injection: Give diluted or undiluted drug through intermittent infusion device or into IV tubing containing a free-flowing, compatible solution.

Intermittent infusion: Give drug undiluted or diluted in 50 to 100 ml of 0.9% NaCl. Using an infusion pump, administer through a peripheral or central venous line over prescribed duration.

Continuous infusion: Using an infusion pump, give diluted solution over 24 hours.

CONTRAINDICATIONS & CAUTIONS

• Contraindicated in heparin hypersensitivity, except in life-threatening situations.

• Also contraindicated in severe thrombocytopenia, in uncontrollable bleeding (except when caused by DIC), and in severe, uncontrolled hypertension.

• In neonates, avoid using commercially available heparin sodium injections and heparin lock flush solutions that contain benzyl alcohol, which has caused death in premature infants. Hep-Lock and Liquaemin contain benzyl alcohol.

• Use with extreme caution in patients with hemorrhage or those at risk for hemorrhage, in patients with history of allergies, during pregnancy and immediately postpartum, in women over age 60, and in patients with mild hepatic disease.

• Give cautiously in hypoaldosteronism or renal insufficiency and in diabetic patients undergoing medical or dental procedures.

SPECIAL CONSIDERATIONS

• Monitor patient for bleeding. Frequently monitor hematocrit and check stools for occult blood to detect asymptomatic bleeding.

• Frequently monitor platelet count and coagulation tests, such as PT, APTT, and activated clotting time.

• If signs of acute adrenal hemorrhage and insufficiency appear, discontinue heparin, give IV corticosteroids, and draw samples for plasma cortisol determinations.

• If white clot syndrome or severe thrombocytopenia occurs, promptly discontinue heparin and substitute a coumarin anticoagulant.

• Observe bleeding precautions. Test all exudates for blood, regularly inspect IV and wound sites and the skin, and promote safety.

hetastarch

HES, Hespan

Pregnancy Risk Category: C

INDICATIONS & DOSAGES
Dosage reflects amount of fluid loss and hemoconcentration.
Plasma volume expansion and fluid replacement—
Adults: 500 to 1,000 ml. Maximum daily infusion is 20 ml/kg, or 1,500 ml. In hemorrhagic shock, maximum hourly infusion is 20 ml/kg. Lower dosages are used in burns and septic shock.

Following the initial dose, subsequent doses should be reduced by 50% to 75% for patients with severe renal impairment (creatinine clearance of less than 10 ml/minute).
Continuous flow centrifugation leukapheresis—
Adults: 250 to 700 ml infused at a fixed ratio of 1 part hetastarch to 8 parts whole blood.

PREPARATION & STORAGE
Available in 500-ml ready-to-use, sterile, and nonpyrogenic bottles. Each bottle contains 6% hetastarch in 0.9% NaCl injection, but no preservative. Store at room temperature; avoid excessive heat or freezing.

Normally a clear, pale yellow to amber color, the solution should not be used if it turns a turbid deep brown or contains a crystalline precipitate. Discard unused solution.

Incompatibility
Incompatible with amikacin sulphate, ampicillin sodium, cefamandole nafate, cefoperazone sodium, cefotaxime sodium, cefoxitin sodium, cephalothin sodium, gentamicin sulfate, ranitidine hydrochloride, theophylline, and tobramycin sulfate.

ADMINISTRATION
Continuous infusion: Infuse at rate determined by patient's condition and therapeutic response.

CONTRAINDICATIONS & CAUTIONS
• Manufacturer warns against use during pregnancy, especially the first trimester, unless the potential benefits outweigh the risks.
• Contraindicated in thrombocytopenia, pulmonary edema, heart failure, or renal impairment and in the elderly.
• Use cautiously in liver disease and in patients allergic to corn.
• Safety and effectiveness in children have not been established.

SPECIAL CONSIDERATIONS
• Continuous flow centrifugation procedures (such as leukapheresis) using hetastarch up to twice weekly for 5 weeks have been reported safe and effective.
• Measure intake and output, and report significant changes in their ratio. Also report oliguria.
• Monitor blood pressure and vital signs frequently, and check for signs of circulatory overload.
• Report dyspnea, wheezing, coughing, crackles, chest pressure, increased pulse and respirations, and elevated central venous pressure.
• Monitor hematocrit, and notify doctor if it drops appreciably.
• Observe patient for bruising or bleeding.

hydralazine hydrochloride

Apresoline♦, Novo-Hylazin◇

Pregnancy Risk Category: C

INDICATIONS & DOSAGES
Emergency treatment of hypertension—
Adults: 10 to 20 mg IV initially and repeated as necessary. May be increased according to response.
Children: 0.1 to 0.2 mg/kg dose q 4 to 6 hours, p.r.n.
Pregnancy-induced hypertension—
Adults: 5 mg initially, then 5 to 20 mg q 20 to 30 minutes, as re-

quired. Consider another agent if therapeutic response is not achieved after 20 mg.

PREPARATION & STORAGE
Available in 1-ml ampules with a concentration of 20 mg/ml. Store ampules at room temperature; do not freeze or refrigerate.

Avoid contact with metal syringe parts because discoloration and change in stability may result. Prepare just before use. Discard unused portion.

Incompatibility
Avoid mixing with other drugs in same container. Incompatible with aminophylline, ampicillin sodium, chlorothiazide, dextrose 10% in lactated Ringer's solution, dextrose 10% in 0.9% NaCl, D_5W, diazoxide, edetate calcium disodium, ethacrynate sodium, fructose 10% in 9% NaCl, fructose 10% in water, furosemide, hydrocortisone sodium succinate, mephentermine sulfate, methohexital, nitroglycerin, phenobarbital sodium, and verapamil.

ADMINISTRATION
Direct injection: Inject undiluted drug directly into vein or as close to IV insertion site as possible. Give at rate of 10 mg/minute.

CONTRAINDICATIONS & CAUTIONS
• Contraindicated in hypersensitivity to drug.
• Also contraindicated in coronary artery disease, dissecting aortic aneurysm, and rheumatic disease affecting the mitral valve.
• Use with caution in patients with CVA or increased intracranial pressure.
• Also administer cautiously and in reduced amounts in renal impairment.

SPECIAL CONSIDERATIONS
• Withdraw drug gradually in patients with marked reduction in blood pressure to avoid rebound hypertension.

• Slow acetylation increases risk of adverse reactions.
• Headache and tachycardia are common; they can be minimized by starting with a small hydralazine dose and gradually increasing dosage.
• Signs of overdose include arrhythmias, headache, hypotension, shock, and tachycardia.
• Check patient's vital signs every 5 to 10 minutes for 1 hour, every hour for the next 2 hours, and then every 4 hours after injection. Continuously monitor ECG.
• Instruct patient to change position slowly to minimize dizziness.

hydrocortisone sodium phosphate

Hydrocortone Phosphate

hydrocortisone sodium succinate

A-hydroCort, Solu-Cortef
Pregnancy Risk Category: C

INDICATIONS & DOSAGES
Severe inflammation, adrenal insufficiency—
Adults: depending on disease, 15 to 240 mg of hydrocortisone sodium phosphate daily; or 100 to 500 mg of hydrocortisone sodium succinate initially, repeated q 2 to 6 hours, p.r.n.
Children: 0.16 to 1 mg/kg or 6 to 30 mg/m^2 of hydrocortisone sodium succinate given 1 to 2 times daily. High-dose therapy should be discontinued within 48 to 72 hours.
Shock—
Adults: 50 mg/kg of hydrocortisone sodium succinate initially, repeated in 4 hours or q 24 hours. Alternatively, 0.5 to 2 g initially, repeated q 2 to 6 hours, as required.

H

PREPARATION & STORAGE

Hydrocortisone sodium phosphate is available in 2- and 10-ml multidose vials, with concentrations of 50 mg/ml.

Hydrocortisone sodium succinate is available in 100-mg vials that require reconstitution with no more than 2 ml of bacteriostatic water for injection or bacteriostatic 0.9% NaCl for injection. Also supplied in 100-, 250-, and 500-mg and 1-g containers that require dilution with D_5W in water, 0.9% NaCl, or D_5W in 0.9% NaCl to a concentration of 0.1 to 1 mg/ml.

Store solutions at 77° F (25° C) or below for up to 3 days. Discard thereafter or if solutions are not clear. Protect from light.

Incompatibility

Incompatible with aminophylline with cephalothin sodium, amobarbital sodium; ampicillin sodium; bleomycin; ciprofloxacin, colistimethate sodium; cytarabine, diazepam; dimenhydrinate; diphenhydramine; doxapram hydrochloride; doxorubicin; ephedrine; ergotamine; furosemide; heparin sodium; hydralazine; idarubicin hydrochloride; kanamycin; metaraminol; methicillin; methylprednisolone sodium succinate; mitoxantrone hydrochloride; nafcillin; pentobarbital sodium; phenobarbital sodium; phenytoin; prochlorperazine edisylate; promethazine hydrochloride; sargramostim; secobarbital sodium; and vitamin B complex with C.

ADMINISTRATION

Direct injection: Inject directly into vein or into an IV line containing a free-flowing, compatible solution to a concentration of 0.1 to 1 mg/ml over 30 seconds to several minutes. *Intermittent infusion:* Give diluted solution over prescribed duration. *Continuous infusion:* Infuse diluted solution over 24 hours.

CONTRAINDICATIONS & CAUTIONS

• Use cautiously in hypothyroidism, cirrhosis, seizure disorders, renal insufficiency, osteoporosis, and history of tuberculosis.
• Give cautiously in recent intestinal anastomosis, diverticulitis, or nonspecific ulcerative colitis if patient is at risk for perforation, abscess, or other pyogenic infection.
• In patients with uncontrolled viral or bacterial infections, give drug carefully.
• Use with caution in children.
• Drug may activate latent amebiasis and may be harmful in chronic active hepatitis positive for hepatitis B surface antigen. Prolonged use may produce posterior subcapsular cataracts or glaucoma. Use cautiously with ocular herpes simplex. Do not use in patients with left ventricular free wall rupture after a recent MI.

SPECIAL CONSIDERATIONS

• Diabetic patients may need an adjustment in antidiabetic drug dosage because of hyperglycemic effects of hydrocortisone.
• Avoid abrupt withdrawal after high-dose therapy.
• Hydrocortone Phosphate contains sulfites. A-hydroCort and Solu-Cortef contain benzyl alcohol.
• Instruct patient to report signs of infection during therapy and for 12 months afterward.
• Avoid exposure to chickenpox or measles and notify doctor immediately if exposure occurs.

hydromorphone hydrochloride

Dilaudid✦, Dilaudid HP✦

Controlled Substance Schedule II

Pregnancy Risk Category: C

INDICATIONS & DOSAGES

Moderate to severe pain—
Adults: 1 to 2 mg SC or IM q 4 to 6 hours p.r.n. for moderate pain; 3

to 4 mg q 4 to 6 hours for severe pain. May be given by slow IV injection over 2 to 5 minutes.

PREPARATION & STORAGE

Available in preservative-containing multidose vials and syringes in concentrations of 1, 2, 3, 4, and 10 mg/ml. Also available in preservative-free ampules in a concentration of 2 mg/ml.

Dilution is not necessary, but most common IV solutions may be used as diluents. Store between 59° and 86° F (15° and 30° C). Protect from freezing and light. Do not refrigerate because of possible precipitation or crystallization. Slight yellowish tint may develop but doesn't indicate loss of potency.

Incompatibility

Incompatible with alkalies, ampicillin sodium, bromides, cefazolin sodium, cloxacillin sodium, dexamethasone, diazepam, gallium nitrate, iodides, minocycline hydrochloride, phenobarbital sodium, phenytoin sodium, prochlorperazine edisylate, sargramostim, sodium bicarbonate, sodium phosphate, and thiopental.

ADMINISTRATION

Rapid administration has been associated with anaphylaxis, respiratory failure, and cardiac arrest.

Direct injection: Inject directly into a vein or into an IV line containing a free-flowing, compatible solution over 2 to 5 minutes, especially if 10 mg/ml preparation is used.

Intermittent infusion: Give diluted drug over prescribed duration.

Continuous infusion: Using an infusion pump, give at the ordered dilution and rate.

CONTRAINDICATIONS & CAUTIONS

• Contraindicated in known hypersensitivity to hydromorphone.
• Also contraindicated in diarrhea caused by poisons or toxins.
• Avoid use in acute respiratory depression, acute bronchial asthma,

upper airway obstruction, status asthmaticus, and obstetric analgesia.
• In patients with head injury and increased intracranial pressure, use only if essential.
• Give drug cautiously in acute abdominal conditions, respiratory impairment, hepatic or renal impairment, gallbladder disease, severe inflammatory bowel disease and history of drug dependence or emotional instability.
• Use cautiously in prostatic hypertrophy or urethral stricture and after recent urinary tract surgery.
• Also use cautiously after recent GI surgery.
• In patients with arrhythmias or history of seizures, give drug carefully.
• Administer carefully to elderly patients and to those with hypothyroidism, Addison's disease, or hypovolemia.
• Safety and efficacy have not been established for children.

SPECIAL CONSIDERATIONS

• Give smallest effective dose. High doses may be required for severe chronic or cancer pain.
• Give drug with patient lying down to minimize hypotensive effects.
• Duration of effects lengthens with repeated doses because of drug accumulation.
• Monitor respiratory status frequently for at least 1 hour after dose. Keep resuscitation equipment and naloxone readily available. If respiratory rate drops below 8 breaths/minute, arouse patient to stimulate breathing. Notify doctor; naloxone or respiratory support may be ordered.
• Monitor shock patient (overdose may occur when circulation is restored).
• Advise patient to avoid using alcoholic beverages or other CNS depressants while taking drug.

H

I-J

ibutilide fumarate

Corvert

Pregnancy Risk Category: C

INDICATIONS & DOSAGES

Rapid conversion of atrial fibrillation or atrial flutter of recent onset to sinus rhythm—

Note: Patients with atrial arrhythmias of longer duration are less likely to respond to ibutilide fumarate. **Adults weighing 132 lb (60 kg) or more:** 1 mg IV over 10 minutes. **Adults weighing below 132 lb:** 0.01 mg/kg IV over 10 minutes.

Stop infusion if arrhythmia is terminated or if ventricular tachycardia or marked prolongation of QT or QTc develops. If arrhythmia is not terminated 10 minutes after infusion ends, another 10-minute infusion of equal strength may be given.

PREPARATION & STORAGE

Single-dose 10-ml clear glass vials (0.1 mg/ml). Store at controlled room temperature 68° to 77° F (20° to 25° C). Store vial in carton until used.

Administer undiluted or diluted in 50 ml of diluent, which forms admixture of about 0.017 mg/ml. Ibutilide may be diluted with 0.9% NaCl injection or 5% D_5W injection before infusion. May be used with polyvinyl chloride plastic bags or polyolefin bags. After dilution, product is stable for 24 hours at room temperature (59° to 86° F [15° to 30° C]) and for 48 hours at refrigerated temperatures (36° to 46° F [2° to 8° C]).

Inspect for particulate matter and discoloration before administration.

Incompatibility
None reported.

ADMINISTRATION

Direct injection: Undiluted solution may be injected over 10 minutes. *Intermittent infusion:* 50 ml infusion bag over 10 minutes.

CONTRAINDICATIONS & CAUTIONS

• Contraindicated in hypersensitivity to drug or its components and in patients with history of polymorphic ventricular tachycardia.
• Use cautiously in patients with hepatic or renal dysfunction.
• Discourage patient from breast-feeding during therapy.
• Safety of drug has not been established in children.

SPECIAL CONSIDERATIONS

• In cases of overdose, stop infusion and provide symptomatic treatment.
• Monitor ECG continuously during administration and for at least 4 hours afterward or until QTc returns to baseline. Drug can worsen ventricular arrhythmias. Longer monitoring is required if ECG shows arrhythmia.
• Cardiac monitor, intracardiac pacing, cardioverter or defibrillator, and medication for sustained ventricular tachycardia must be available.
• Correct hypokalemia and hypomagnesemia before therapy to reduce risk of proarrhythmia.

idarubicin

Idamycin

Pregnancy Risk Category: D

INDICATIONS & DOSAGES

In combination with other approved antileukemic drugs for the treatment of acute myeloid leukemia, including French-American-British classifications M1 through M7—

Adults: 12 mg/m² for 3 days by slow (10 to 15 minutes) IV injection in combination with cytarabine, which may be given as continuous infusion of 100 mg/m² daily for 7 days or as 25 mg/m² bolus followed by continuous infusion of 200 mg/ m² daily for 5 days. A second course may be administered if needed. If patient experiences severe mucositis, delay administration until recovery is complete and reduce dose by 25%.

PREPARATION & STORAGE
Available as a powder for injection in 5-, 10- and 20-mg single-dose vials. Store at room temperature (59° to 86° F [15° to 30° C]) and protect from light. Reconstitute with 0.9% NaCl injection without preservatives. Add 5 ml to 5-mg vial, 10 ml to the 10-mg vial, or 20 ml to the 20-mg vial for a final concentration of 1 mg/ml. *Do not use bacteriostatic saline.* Vial is under negative pressure. Use care when inserting needle; avoid inhalation of any aerosol. Reconstituted solutions are stable for 72 hours at room temperature, 7 days if refrigerated. Discard unused solutions according to guidelines for disposal of chemotherapeutic agents. Use of gloves, goggles, and protective gowns (cytotoxic drug handling precautions) is recommended during preparation and administration.

Incompatibility
Do not mix with other drugs unless specific compatibility data are available. Precipitation occurs with heparin. Drug will degrade with prolonged contact with alkaline solutions.

Incompatible with acyclovir sodium, allopurinol sodium, ampicillin sodium, cefazolin sodium, cefepime hydrochloride, ceftazidime, clindamycin phosphate, dexamethasone sodium phosphate, etoposide, furosemide, gentamycin sulfate, hydrocortisone sodium succinate, lorazepam, meperidine hydrochloride, methotrexate sodium, mezlocillin sodium, piperacillin sodium, sodium carbonate, sulbactam sodium, tazobactam sodium, vancomycin hydrochloride, and vincristine sulfate.

ADMINISTRATION
Direct injection: Administer over 10 to 15 minutes into the tubing of a free-flowing IV solution of 5% dextrose injection or 0.9% NaCl. The tubing should be attached to a winged-tip needle inserted into a large vein.

CONTRAINDICATIONS & CAUTIONS
• Do not use in patients with severe myelosuppression, preexisting cardiac disease, severe hemorrhagic conditions, and overwhelming infection.
• Do not administer drug if bilirubin serum level is above 5 mg/dl.
• Use cautiously in patients with hepatic or renal impairment.

SPECIAL CONSIDERATIONS
• Hyperuricemia due to lysis of leukemic cells may develop.
• Cardiotoxicity may be more frequent in patients over age 60 or in those who have preexisting heart disease or have received a previous course of anthracycline compounds.
• Control systemic infections before starting therapy.
• Give antiemetics to prevent or treat nausea and vomiting.
• Frequent determination of CBC is recommended. Monitor total and differential leukocyte counts; platelet count; hematocrit; and serum hemoglobin, ALT, AST, bilirubin, creatinine, and LD concentrations before and at periodic intervals during therapy. Also monitor hepatic and renal function.
• Examine patient's mouth for ulceration before administrating each dose.
• Tell patient to avoid immunizations. Other members of family household should also avoid immunizations with oral poliovirus vaccine.

ifosfamide

IFEX♦

Pregnancy Risk Category: D

INDICATIONS & DOSAGES
Germ-cell testicular cancers—
Adults: 1,200 mg/m² for 5 consecutive days. Repeat every 3 weeks or

I-J

after recovery from hematologic toxicity (platelets 100,000/mm^3 or more; WBCs above 4,000/mm^3). Administer with mesna, a protective agent used to prevent hemorrhagic cystitis. Extensive hydration required with at least 2 L of oral or IV fluid daily to prevent bladder toxicity.

PREPARATION & STORAGE
Use caution when preparing and giving drug because of mutagenic, teratogenic, and carcinogenic risks. Use a biological containment cabinet; wear gloves and mask. If drug comes in contact with skin or mucosa, immediately wash the area with soap and water. Use syringes with tight fittings (luer-lock) to prevent leakage of solution, and correctly dispose of needles, syringes, vials, and unused drug. Avoid contaminating work surfaces.

Drug is available as an off-white powder in 1- and 3-g vials; also available in Canada in 2-g vials. Intact vials should be stored at room temperature and protected from excessive temperatures above 104° F (40° C). May liquefy at temperatures above 95° F (35° C).

Reconstitute drug with sterile water for injection or bacteriostatic water for injection. Add 20 ml diluent per gram of drug. Final concentration is 50 mg/ml.

For intermittent infusion, drug may be added to D$_5$W, dextrose 2 1/2% in water, 0.45% NaCl injection, 0.9% NaCl injection, or lactated Ringer's injection.

Incompatibility
Incompatible with cefepime hydrochloride.

ADMINISTRATION
Intermittent infusion: Using a 23G or 25G winged-tip needle, infuse solution over at least 30 minutes. Use a new IV site for each infusion, if possible.

CONTRAINDICATIONS & CAUTIONS
• Use cautiously in renal impairment, previous or current radiation therapy, severely depressed bone marrow, or hypersensitivity to drug.

SPECIAL CONSIDERATIONS
• Drug may interfere with wound healing.
• Maintain daily fluid intake of at least 2 L during and for at least 3 days after therapy to reduce risk of urologic toxicity. Along with increased fluids, use of oral ascorbic acid further reduces toxicity risk.
• Tell patient to report immediately hematuria, dysuria, and burning on urination.
• Remind patient to void frequently because this minimizes contact of drug and its metabolites with the bladder mucosa.

imipenem-cilastatin sodium

Primaxin

Pregnancy Risk Category: C

INDICATIONS & DOSAGES
Infections of the lower respiratory tract and urinary tract, intra-abdominal infections, gynecologic infections, bone and joint infections, skin and skin-structure infections, bacterial septicemia, endocarditis, and polymicrobic infections involving susceptible organisms—
Adults and children over age 12 with normal renal function: 250 to 500 mg q 6 hours for mild infections; 500 mg or 1 g q 6 to 8 hours for severe infections. Maximum daily dosage, 4 g or 50 mg/kg, whichever is lower.
Adults and children over age 12 with impaired renal function: dosage based on creatinine clearance. If creatinine clearance is 30 to 70 ml/minute, give 500 mg q 6 to 8 hours; between 20 and 29 ml/minute, 500 mg q 8 to 12 hours;

and if it is less than 20 ml/minute, give 250 to 500 mg q 12 hours.

PREPARATION & STORAGE
Available as a white or yellow powder in 13-ml vials and 120-ml infusion bottles. These contain 250 mg imipenem and 250 mg cilastatin or 500 mg imipenem and 500 mg cilastatin. Reconstitute 13-ml vial with 10 ml of a compatible solution, such as 0.9% NaCl, dextrose 5% or 10% in water, D_5W in 0.9% NaCl, or D_5W with potassium chloride 0.15%. Shake until dissolved. Using a new needle, transfer reconstituted solution into container of remaining 90 ml of solution. Reconstitute 120-ml vial with 100 ml of compatible diluent.

Most solutions are stable for 4 hours at room temperature or 24 hours when refrigerated. Solutions prepared in 0.9% NaCl with a final concentration no greater than 5 mg/ml remain stable for 10 hours at room temperature or 48 hours when refrigerated. Solutions may turn deep yellow; discard if solution turns brown.

Incompatibility
Do not mix drug with other antibiotics. Incompatible with D_5W in lactated Ringer's injection. Manufacturer does not recommend mixing drug in same solution or tubing as other drugs.

ADMINISTRATION
Intermittent infusion: Give diluted solution into an IV line containing a free-flowing, compatible solution. Infuse 125-, 250-, or 500-mg doses over 20 to 30 minutes and 750-mg or 1-g doses over 40 to 60 minutes. Reduce rate if nausea, vomiting, hypotension, dizziness, or sweating occurs.

CONTRAINDICATIONS & CAUTIONS
• Contraindicated in hypersensitivity to either imipenem or cilastatin.

• Use cautiously in patients with hypersensitivity to cephalosporins or penicillins or who have history of seizure disorders or multiple allergies.
• Give cautiously to elderly patients, renally impaired patients, and those with CNS or GI disorders.
• Safety and efficacy in children under age 12 have not been established.

SPECIAL CONSIDERATIONS
• When administering with aminoglycosides, use separate solution containers. However, drug can be infused through same IV line.
• If patient is undergoing hemodialysis, give a supplemental dose after treatment unless the next dose is scheduled within 4 hours.
• Check for previous penicillin or cephalosporin hypersensitivity before first dose.
• If diarrhea persists during therapy, discontinue drug and collect stool specimens for culture to rule out pseudomembranous colitis.
• Monitor BUN and serum creatinine levels to assess renal function.

immune globulin

Gamimune N, Gammagard S/D, Gammar-P IV, Iveegam, Polygam-S/D, Sandoglobulin, Venoglobulin-I, Venoglobulin-S

Pregnancy Risk Category: C

INDICATIONS & DOSAGES
Indications vary by product.
Immunodeficiency diseases, such as congenital agammaglobulinemia, common variable hypogammaglobulinemia, X-linked immunodeficiency with or without hyper-IgM, and combined immunodeficiency; B-cell chronic lymphocytic leukemia, Kawasaki syndrome, bone marrow transplantation, pediatric HIV infections—

I-J

Adults: 200 to 300 mg/kg of Gammagard S/D monthly, with dosage adjusted to ensure adequate serum IgG levels; 100 to 200 mg/kg or 2 to 4 ml/kg of Gamimune N monthly, or up to 400 mg/kg or 8 ml/kg monthly or more frequently to ensure adequate serum IgG levels; Gammar-P IV 100 to 200 mg/kg q 3 or 4 weeks; 200 mg/kg of Sandoglobulin monthly, or up to 300 mg/kg monthly or more frequently to ensure adequate serum IgG levels. *Idiopathic thrombocytopenic purpura—*
Adults and children: 1 g/kg (single dose) Gammagard S/D; up to three separate doses may be given on alternate days, if required. 400 mg/kg of Gamimune N or Sandoglobulin daily for 5 days. Maintenance dosage, 400 mg/kg of Gamimune N once every several weeks, or 1 g/kg as single infusion to maintain platelet count greater than 30,000/mm³.

Venoglobulin-I: start at 0.01 to 0.02 ml/kg/minute for first 30 minutes; then increase as tolerated. Venoglobulin-S: start at 0.01 to 0.02 ml/kg/minute or 0.6 to 1.2 ml/kg/hour for first 30 minutes. If tolerated, rate may be increased to 0.04 ml/kg/minute or 2.4 ml/kg/hour. Venoglobulin 200 mg/kg monthly may be increased to 300 to 400 mg/kg monthly or more frequently.

PREPARATION & STORAGE
Produced by different isolation and purification methods, each immune globulin has a different constitution. After reconstitution, Gammagard S/D contains about 50 mg of protein/ml and no less than 90% IgG. Gamimune N contains 50 mg of protein/ml and no less than 96% IgG; Gammar-P IV contains 50 mg of IgG/ml; and Sandoglobulin contains no less than 96% IgG.

Before use, refrigerate Gamimune N at 36° to 46° F (2° to 8° C). May be diluted in 5% dextrose, but don't use solution that has been frozen.

Before reconstitution, refrigerate Gammagard S/D at 36° to 46° F. Reconstitute with sterile water for injection (make sure the powder and sterile water have been warmed to room temperature). Use the transfer device provided to prepare a solution containing 50 mg of protein/ml. Administer as soon as possible after reconstitution.

Before reconstitution, store Gammar-P IV at room temperature, not to exceed 77° F (25° C). Using the manufacturer's transfer device, reconstitute with the supplied diluent; follow manufacturer's instructions for its proper use. Gently swirl the solution to reconstitute, and use within 3 hours.

Before reconstitution, store Sandoglobulin at room temperature, below 77° F (25° C). Reconstitute with the 0.9% NaCl provided to prepare a solution containing 30 or 60 mg of protein/ml. Use promptly.

Don't administer turbid solutions. Discard unused drug.

Incompatibility
Don't mix with other drugs or fluids. Give in separate infusion line.

ADMINISTRATION
Intermittent infusion: Infuse Gamimune N at a rate of 0.01 to 0.02 ml/kg/minute for 30 minutes. If no adverse reactions occur, increase up to 0.08 ml/kg/minute.

Give Gammagard S/D using the manufacturer's administration set, which contains a 15-micron filter. Start at a rate of 0.5 ml/kg/hour and, if no adverse reactions occur, increase up to 4 ml/kg/hour.

Initially, give Gammar-P IV at a rate of 0.01 ml/kg/minute; after 15 to 30 minutes, increase rate to 0.02 ml/kg/minute. Most patients will tolerate a gradual increase to 0.03 to 0.06 ml/kg/minute.

Infuse initial dose of Sandoglobulin at a rate of 0.5 to 1 ml/minute for 15 to 30 minutes, increasing to 1.5 to 2.5 ml/minute. Give subsequent doses at a rate of 2 to 2.5 ml/minute. If additional high doses are necessary, infuse a 60 mg/ml solution at a rate of 1 to 1.5 ml/ minute for 15 to 30 minutes, increasing up to 2.5 ml/minute.

CONTRAINDICATIONS & CAUTIONS
• Contraindicated in hypersensitivity to immune globulin or thimerosal and in certain IgA deficiencies.
• Use Gamimune N cautiously in patients with compromised acid-base compensatory mechanisms.
• Use with caution in severe thrombocytopenia or bleeding disorders.

SPECIAL CONSIDERATIONS
• Most adverse reactions are related to infusion rate. If patient becomes symptomatic, reduce rate. Use of corticosteroids before infusion may prevent adverse reactions.
• Signs of an allergic reaction may occur 30 to 60 minutes after start of infusion.
• Don't give live virus MMR vaccines for 2 weeks before or 3 months after giving immune globulin.
• Monitor vital signs continuously during infusion.

insulin (regular)

Humulin R, Novolin R, Regular, Velosulin Human BR

Pregnancy Risk Category: B

INDICATIONS & DOSAGES
Diabetic ketoacidosis—
Adults: 6 to 10 U IV, followed by 6 to 10 U/hour by IV infusion. Alternatively, 10 to 20 U of regular insulin initially can be followed by 5 to 10 U/hour IM. During the early stages of treatment, at least 0.1 U/ kg/hour but no more than 0.2 U/ kg/hour.
Children: 0.1 U/kg/hour initially. Maintenance dosage is based on doctor evaluation of blood glucose levels.

Growth hormone secretion test—
Adults: 0.05 to 0.15 U/kg.

PREPARATION & STORAGE
Available in 10-ml vials in concentrations of 100 U/ml. Can be added to most IV and hyperalimentation solutions.

Store insulin at 36° to 46° F (2° to 8° C); avoid freezing. Do not use cloudy, discolored, or unusually viscous preparations. Use only syringes calibrated for the specific insulin concentration being given.

Incompatibility
Incompatible with aminophylline, amobarbital sodium, chlorothiazide sodium, cytarabine, dobutamine, methylprednisolone sodium succinate, pentobarbital sodium, phenobarbital sodium, phenytoin sodium, secobarbital sodium, sodium bicarbonate, and thiopental sodium.

ADMINISTRATION
Buffered insulin human (regular) injection (Velosulin BR) is administered by SC infusion using compatible external controlled infusion devices or conventional syringes only.

The addition of insulin (regular) injection to an IV infusion solution may result in absorption of insulin in the container and tubing. The amount of an insulin dose lost by absorption to an IV infusion system is highly variable and depends on the insulin concentration, the duration of contact time, and the flow rate of the infusion.
Direct injection: Inject directly into vein, through an intermittent infusion device, or into a port close to IV access site at ordered rate.
Continuous infusion: Infuse drug diluted in 0.9% NaCl at a rate sufficient to reverse ketoacidosis.

CONTRAINDICATIONS & CAUTIONS
• Use IV insulin with caution. Prolonged, severe hypoglycemia can result in irreversible brain damage.

I-J

SPECIAL CONSIDERATIONS

• Increased dosages may be required in high fever, hyperthyroidism, severe infections, trauma, or surgery. Reduced dosages may be required in diarrhea, hepatic or renal impairment, hypothyroidism, nausea, and vomiting.

• Insulin (regular) has been added to dextrose infusions to promote intracellular potassium shift in hyperkalemia.

• In cases of overdose, give orange juice, sugar, or candy to conscious patient. In severe hypoglycemia or coma, give 10 to 30 ml of dextrose 50%. Alternatively, give 1 U of glucagon if hepatic glycogen stores are adequate. Severe, untreated hypoglycemia can cause irreversible brain damage.

• Assess patient for signs of hypoglycemia and dehydration.

irinotecan hydrochloride

Camptosar

Pregnancy Risk Category: D

INDICATIONS & DOSAGES

Treatment of metastatic carcinoma of the colon or rectum that has recurred or progressed after fluorouracil therapy—
Adults: initially, 125 mg/m² IV infusion over 90 minutes. Recommended treatment is 125 mg/m² IV once weekly for 4 weeks, followed by 2-week rest period. Additional courses of treatment may be repeated q 6 weeks (4 weeks on and 2 weeks off therapy). Subsequent doses may be adjusted to a low dose of 50 mg/m² or a maximum of 150 mg/m² in 25- to 50-mg/m² increments, depending on patient tolerance.

PREPARATION & STORAGE

Care should be exercised in the handling and preparation of infusion solutions prepared from irinotecan.

Gloves are recommended. Dilute irinotecan for injection (5-ml vial containing 20 mg/ml) with D_5W injection or 0.9% NaCl injection to a final concentration of 0.12 to 1.1 mg/ml. Most commonly, irinotecan has been administered in 500 ml of D_5W. Solution is stable for up to 24 hours at room temperature and in ambient fluorescent lighting. If diluted in D_5W, protected from light, and refrigerated (36° to 46° F [2° to 8° C]), the solution is stable for 48 hours. However, because of possible microbial contamination during dilution, the manufacturer recommends use within 24 hours if refrigerated and 6 hours if at room temperature. Do not freeze. Store the undiluted vial at room temperature (59° to 86° F [15° to 30° C]), protect from light, and leave packaged in backing–plastic blister in the carton.

Incompatibility
Other drugs should not be added to irinotecan infusion.

ADMINISTRATION

Intermittent infusion: Infuse appropriate dose, diluted to a concentration of 0.12 to 1.1 mg over 90 minutes.

CONTRAINDICATIONS & CAUTIONS

• Contraindicated in hypersensitivity to drug.

• Use cautiously in the presence of acute infection.

• Use with caution in the elderly and in patients with renal or hepatic dysfunction, preexisting GI disorders, or diarrhea.

• Exercise caution when administering drug to patients who have previously been treated with pelvic or abdominal irradiation.

• Advise women of childbearing age to avoid pregnancy or breast-feeding during treatment.

• Safety and efficacy in children have not been established.

SPECIAL CONSIDERATIONS
• Drug can induce severe diarrhea.
• Premedicate patient with antiemetic agents on day of treatment, starting at least 30 minutes before administering irinotecan.
• Wear gloves when handling and preparing infusion solutions. If drug contacts skin, wash thoroughly with soap and water. If it contacts mucous membranes, flush thoroughly with water.
• Monitor WBC count with differential, hemoglobin, and platelet count before administration of each dose.

isoproterenol hydrochloride

Isuprel◆

Pregnancy Risk Category: C

INDICATIONS & DOSAGES
Acute asthma unresponsive to inhalation therapy—
Adults: 0.01 to 0.02 mg (0.5 to 1 ml of a 1:50,000 dilution). Repeat as necessary.
Bronchospasm during anesthesia—
Adults: 0.01 to 0.02 mg (0.5 to 1 ml of a 1:50,000 dilution).
Children: individualized.
Arrhythmias—
Adults: bolus of 0.02 to 0.06 mg (1 to 3 ml of a 1:50,000 dilution) initially, then 0.01 to 0.2 mg (0.5 to 10 ml of a 1:50,000 dilution). Alternatively, infuse 2 mg diluted in 500 ml of D_5W at a rate of 0.5 to 5 mcg/minute. Adjust subsequent doses based on patient response.
Children: infuse 2.5 mcg/minute. Adjust subsequent doses based on patient response.
Shock—
Adults: infuse 0.5 to 5 mcg/minute. In advanced shock, give 5 to 30 mcg/minute.

PREPARATION & STORAGE
Available in a dilution of 1:5,000 in 1-ml (0.2-mg) and 5-ml (1-mg) ampules and in 5-ml (1-mg) and 10-ml (2-mg) vials. For direct injection, add 1 ml of isoproterenol to a volume of 10 ml of 0.9% NaCl or D_5W to yield a 1:50,000 dilution (20 mcg/ml). For infusion, dilute 10 ml of isoproterenol with 500 ml of D_5W to yield a dilution of 1:5,000 (2 mg in 500 ml). Drug is also compatible with lactated Ringer's solution and D_5W in lactated Ringer's solution.
   Store in a cool place, protect from light, and keep in an opaque container until used. Do not use if pink or brown or if a precipitate forms.

Incompatibility
Incompatible with alkalies, aminophylline, furosemide, metals, and sodium bicarbonate.

ADMINISTRATION
Direct injection: Inject diluted solution (1:50,000) directly into vein or into an IV line containing a free-flowing, compatible solution. Usual initial dose: 1 to 3 ml (20 to 60 mcg).
Continuous infusion: Using an infusion pump, give appropriate dose and dilution (1:250,000) at ordered rate. Usual initial dose is 5 mcg/minute (1.25 ml/minute).

CONTRAINDICATIONS & CAUTIONS
• Contraindicated in hypersensitivity to sympathomimetics or isoproterenol.
• Also contraindicated in tachyarrhythmias.
• Avoid use in shock patients who have not received fluid replacement and in those with uncorrected hypoxia, acidosis, hypokalemia, hyperkalemia, or hypercapnia.
• Use cautiously in elderly patients and in patients with CV disease, hyperthyroidism, or cardiac glycoside–induced tachycardia.

I-J

• Also use cautiously in sulfite hypersensitivity if isoproterenol preparation contains this element; in Parkinson's disease; and in diabetes mellitus. Dosage adjustment of insulin or hypoglycemic agents may be necessary.

SPECIAL CONSIDERATIONS
• Adjust infusion rate according to heart rate and blood pressure.
• In cardiac arrest, arrhythmias, shock, and heart block, closely observe ECG to help adjust dosage.
• Drug may aggravate ventilation-perfusion abnormalities.
• In cases of overdose, symptoms include severe, persistent chest pain and irregular heartbeat, elevated blood pressure, headache, and dizziness. If these symptoms occur, discontinue drug immediately. Cumulative effects have not been reported.

ketorolac tromethamine

Toradol

Pregnancy Risk Category: C

INDICATIONS & DOSAGES
Short-term management of moderately severe, acute pain for single-dose treatment—
Adults under age 65: 30 mg IV
Adults age 65 or older, renally impaired patients, or those weighing less than 110 lb (50 kg): 15 mg IV
Short-term management of moderately severe, acute pain for multiple-dose treatment—
Adults under age 65: 30 mg IV q 6 hours, not to exceed 120 mg/day.
Adults age 65 or older, renally impaired patients, or those weighing less than 110 lb: 15 mg IV q 6 hours, not to exceed 60 mg/day.

PREPARATION & STORAGE
Ketorolac tromethamine injection is a solution of the drug in sterile water for injection and alcohol, containing 15 or 30 mg/ml. Store at 59° to 86° F (15° to 30° C) and protect from light.

Incompatibility
Incompatible with solutions of drugs such as opiate agonists (meperidine hydrochloride, morphine sulfate) that result in a relatively low pH because precipitation can occur.

ADMINISTRATION
Direct injection: Administer over not less than 15 seconds.

CONTRAINDICATIONS & CAUTIONS
• Contraindicated in hypersensitivity to drug and in patients with advanced renal impairment or at risk for renal impairment due to volume depletion.
• Contraindicated as prophylactic analgesic before major surgery, intraoperatively when hemostasis is critical, for neuraxial administration, in labor and delivery, in breast-feeding patients, and in patients currently receiving aspirin or NSAIDs.
• Contraindicated in patients with confirmed or suspected cerebrovascular bleeding, hemorrhagic diathesis, incomplete hemostasis, high risk of bleeding, history of or active peptic ulcer disease, or history of GI bleeding or perforation.
• Use cautiously in the elderly or patients with heart failure, hepatic or renal dysfunction, history of renal disease, extracellular fluid depletion, or cardiac decompensation, hypertension, or similar conditions associated with fluid retention.
• Use cautiously in patients who may be adversely affected by prolongation of bleeding times or those with history of hepatic impairment.
• Drug is not recommended for use in children.

SPECIAL CONSIDERATIONS
• Drug can mask signs and symptoms of infection.
• Be aware that the maximum combined duration of therapy should be limited to 5 days.

• Monitor renal function (serum creatinine and BUN) closely.
• Monitor bleeding time and observe patients with coagulopathies or those being given anticoagulants.

labetalol hydrochloride

Normodyne, Trandate
Injection

Pregnancy Risk Category: C

INDICATIONS & DOSAGES
Severe hypertension and hypertensive crisis—
Adults: 20 mg initially, then 20 to 80 mg q 10 minutes, up to 300 mg. As an alternative to direct IV injections, drug may be given by continuous infusion at an initial rate of 2 mg/minute, with the rate of infusion adjusted according to blood pressure response.
Hypotension control during halothane anesthesia—
Adults: 10 to 25 mg after induction of anesthesia. Hypotension will then be controlled by inspired halothane.
Hypotension control with use of other anesthetics—
Adults: 30 mg initially, then 5 to 10 mg if needed.

PREPARATION & STORAGE
Available as a clear, colorless to light-yellow solution in 20-, 40-, and 60-ml multidose vials with a concentration of 5 mg/ml. Store at room temperature.
  For infusion, add two 20-ml ampules to 160 ml of D_5W, 0.9% NaCl, dextrose 2.5% in 0.45% NaCl, dextrose 5% in lactated Ringer's solution, or lactated Ringer's solution to yield a concentration of 1 mg/ml. To obtain a concentration of 2 mg/3 ml, add two 20-ml ampules to 250 ml of diluent. Solutions remain stable for at least 24 hours at room temperature or when refrigerated.

Incompatibility
Incompatible with cefoperazone sodium, nafcillin sodium, and sodium bicarbonate.

ADMINISTRATION
Direct injection: Over 2 minutes, inject directly into vein or into an IV line containing a free-flowing, compatible solution.
Continuous infusion: Give 2 mg/minute until satisfactory response is obtained; then stop infusion. May repeat in 6 to 8 hours.

CONTRAINDICATIONS & CAUTIONS
• Contraindicated in patients with second- or third-degree heart block, overt heart failure, cardiac ischemia, cardiogenic shock, or severe bradycardia.
• Also contraindicated in asthma or bronchospastic disease and in children.
• Use cautiously in diabetes mellitus controlled by hypoglycemic agents and in myasthenia gravis, depression, psoriasis, pheochromocytoma, or hepatic impairment.

SPECIAL CONSIDERATIONS
• Administer epinephrine or atropine for treatment of excessive bradycardia.
• Drug masks common signs of shock and hypoglycemia.
• In cases of overdose, for posture-sensitive hypotension, place patient in supine position and elevate legs.
• Monitor blood pressure frequently.
• Advise patient to remain supine for 3 hours after administration to prevent severe orthostatic hypotension.

L

leucovorin calcium (citrovorum factor, folinic acid)

Wellcovorin

Pregnancy Risk Category: C

INDICATIONS & DOSAGES

Treatment of methotrexate overdose—
Adults: up to 75 mg within 12 hours or a dosage sufficient to produce serum levels at least equal to serum methotrexate levels.
Treatment of hematologic toxicity caused by other folic acid antagonists, such as trimethoprim—
Adults and children: 5 to 15 mg/day.
Neutralization of methotrexate's toxic effects (leucovorin rescue)—
Note: Used in various regimens. Specific dosage depends on extent of systemic toxicity.
Adults and children: 10 mg/m² given q 6 hours for ten doses starting 24 hours after the beginning of the methotrexate infusion.
Palliative treatment of advanced colorectal carcinoma—
Adults: 20 mg/m² IV followed by 425 mg/m² of IV fluorouracil, or 200 mg/m² followed by 370 mg/m² of IV fluorouracil, daily for 5 consecutive days. Repeat at 4-week intervals for two additional courses; then repeat at intervals of 4 to 5 weeks if tolerated.

PREPARATION & STORAGE

Available as a yellow-white solution in 3-, 100-, and 350-ml ampules and as a powder in 50-mg vials. Store at room temperature. Reconstitute powder for injection by adding 5 ml of sterile or bacteriostatic water to 50-mg vial, yielding a solution of 10 mg/ml. For intermittent infusion, add 15 to 50 mg of reconstituted drug to 50 ml of a compatible solution, such as lactated Ringer's solution or D₅W or dextrose 10% in water. For continuous infusion, add up to 200 mg of reconstituted drug to 1 L of a compatible solution.

Use solutions containing sterile water immediately. Use those containing bacteriostatic water within 1 week if refrigerated.

When leucovorin is administered by IV infusion, the infusion rate should not exceed 16 ml/minute because of the calcium concentration of the solution.

Incompatibility
Incompatible with droperidol and foscarnet sodium.

ADMINISTRATION

Direct injection: Using a 21G or 23G needle, inject into vein or into IV tubing containing a free-flowing, compatible solution over 5 minutes.
Intermittent infusion: Using a 21G or 23G needle, infuse solution over 15 minutes.
Continuous infusion: Infuse over 24 hours at rate of about 40 ml/hour.

CONTRAINDICATIONS & CAUTIONS
• Contraindicated in leucovorin hypersensitivity and in undiagnosed anemia.
• Use cautiously in pernicious anemia.
• For leucovorin rescue, use cautiously in patients with a urine pH less than 7, ascites, dehydration, pleural or peritoneal effusions, or renal dysfunction.
• Drug may increase seizures in susceptible children.

SPECIAL CONSIDERATIONS
• Begin leucovorin rescue within 24 hours of high-dose methotrexate regimen.
• Do not give drug simultaneously with methotrexate.
• Monitor serum methotrexate and serum creatinine levels, creatinine clearance, and urine pH every 6 to 24 hours during leucovorin rescue.

levofloxacin

Levaquin

Pregnancy Risk Category: C

INDICATIONS & DOSAGES

Indicated for treatment of mild, moderate, and severe infections caused by susceptible microorganisms in adults age 18 and older.
Acute maxillary sinusitis caused by susceptible strains of Streptococcus pneumoniae, Moraxella catarrhalis, *or* Haemophilus influenzae—
Adults: 500 mg IV daily for 10 to 14 days (see note).
Acute bacterial exacerbation of chronic bronchitis caused by Staphylococcus aureus, S. pneumoniae, M. catarrhalis, H. influenzae, *or* Haemophilus parainfluenzae—
Adults: 500 mg IV daily for 7 days (see note).
Community-acquired pneumonia caused by S. aureus, S. pneumoniae, M. catarrhalis, H. influenzae, H. parainfluenzae, Klebsiella pneumoniae, Chlamydia pneumoniae, Legionella pneumophila, *or* Mycoplasma pneumoniae—
Adults: 500 mg IV daily for 7 to 14 days (see note).
Mild to moderate skin and skin structure infections caused by S. aureus *or* Streptococcus pyogenes—
Adults: 500 mg IV daily for 7 to 10 days (see note).
  Note: If creatinine clearance is 20 to 49 ml/minute, subsequent doses are half the initial dose; if it is between 10 and 19 ml/minute, subsequent doses are half the initial dose, and the interval is prolonged to q 48 hours.
Mild to moderate urinary tract infection caused by Enterococcus faecalis, Enterobacter cloacae, Escherichia coli, K. pneumoniae, Proteus mirabilis, *or* Pseudomonas aeruginosa—
Adults: 250 mg IV daily for 10 days (see following note).

Mild to moderate acute pyelonephritis cause by E. coli—
Adults: 250 mg IV daily for 10 days (see following note).
  Note: If creatinine clearance is 10 to 19 ml/minute, dosage interval is increased to every 48 hours.

PREPARATIONS & STORAGE

Supplied in a single-use 20-ml vial containing 500 mg of levofloxacin (25 mg/ml). It must be further diluted to a concentration of 5 mg/ml before IV use. Compatible IV solutions include the following: 0.9% NaCl, D_5W, 5% dextrose in 0.9% NaCl, 5% dextrose in lactated Ringer's solution, Plasma-Lyte 56/5% dextrose, and sodium lactate (1/6 M). Diluted solution is stable for 72 hours when stored below 77° F (25° C) and for 14 days when stored at 41° F (5° C) in plastic IV containers. Solutions frozen in glass bottles or plastic IV containers are stable for 6 months at –4° F (–20° C). If frozen, solutions must be thawed at room temperature. Do not thaw by microwave or water bath and do not refreeze after thawing. Because vials are for single use, unused portion should be discarded. If preparing a 250-mg dose, withdraw entire amount and prepare a second dose for storage. Use careful aseptic technique.

Incompatibility
Do not administer through same IV line with solutions containing multivalent cations (such as magnesium).

ADMINISTRATION
Direct injection: Avoid rapid or bolus IV infusion.
Intermittent infusion: Infuse diluted dose (concentration of 5 mg/ml) slowly over a period of not less than 60 minutes.

CONTRAINDICATIONS & CAUTIONS
• Contraindicated in hypersensitivity to drug, its components, or other fluoroquinolones.

L

• Dosage adjustment is required in patients with impaired renal function.
• Use cautiously in patients with diabetes mellitus or history of seizure disorders or other CNS diseases.
• Safety and efficacy in children under age 18 and in pregnant or breast-feeding women have not been established.

SPECIAL CONSIDERATIONS
• Monitor renal function (serum creatinine and BUN) closely.
• Monitor PT and INR in patients receiving warfarin.
• Monitor blood glucose carefully in patients receiving antidiabetic agents.
• Monitor for increased CNS stimulation and institute seizure precautions as necessary.
• Be aware that levofloxacin can cause pseudomembranous colitis. Notify doctor if diarrhea occurs.

levothyroxine sodium (T_4, L-thyroxine sodium)

Levothroid, Synthroid

Pregnancy Risk Category: A

INDICATIONS & DOSAGES
Hypothyroidism—
Adults: 50 to 100 mcg daily as a single dose.
Children ages 6 to 12: 100 to 150 mcg or 4 to 5 mcg/kg daily.
Children ages 1 to 5: 75 to 100 mcg or 5 to 6 mcg/kg daily.
Infants ages 6 to 12 months: 50 to 75 mcg or 6 to 8 mcg/kg daily.
Healthy infants up to age 6 months: 25 to 50 mcg or 10 to 15 mcg/kg daily.
Premature infants weighing less than 4.4 lb (2 kg) and infants at risk for heart failure: initially, 25 mcg daily, increased to 37.5 mcg daily after 4 to 6 weeks.
Myxedema coma—

Adults: initially, 200 to 500 mcg. Give 100 to 300 mcg on next day to obtain necessary improvement.
Children: see schedule for hypothyroidism.

PREPARATION & STORAGE
Available as a buff-colored, odorless powder in 6-ml vials (concentrations of 200 or 500 mcg) that remain stable at room temperature. Store in light-resistant containers; otherwise, powder may turn light pink.
  Reconstitute Levothroid powder by adding 2 to 5 ml of 0.9% NaCl injection (without preservative) to the 200- or 500-mg vial respectively. Shake until clear. This solution contains 100 mcg/ml.
  To reconstitute Synthroid powder, add 5 ml of 0.9% NaCl injection or bacteriostatic NaCl injection with benzyl alcohol (in infants, avoid diluent containing benzyl alcohol) to the 200- or 500-mcg vial. Shake to dissolve. The solution contains 40 or 100 mcg/ml. Reconstitute drug immediately before use and discard unused portions.

Incompatibility
Do not mix with other solutions for IV infusion.

ADMINISTRATION
Direct injection: Inject into vein over 1 to 2 minutes.

CONTRAINDICATIONS & CAUTIONS
• Use cautiously in angina, coronary artery disease, hypertension, adrenocortical insufficiency, and diabetes.
• Also use cautiously in patients undergoing surgery or emergency treatment and in the elderly.
• In infants, do not reconstitute with diluent containing benzyl alcohol.

SPECIAL CONSIDERATIONS
• In myxedema coma, give levothyroxine with hydrocortisone to prevent adrenal crisis.
• If symptoms of overdose or hyperthyroidism occur, stop drug for 2 to 6 days. Resume at a lower dose.

• Monitor ECG for ventricular arrhythmias. Be alert for tachyarrhythmias and signs of ischemia.
• Monitor vital signs and thyroid function tests.

lidocaine hydrochloride

LidoPen, Xylocaine, Xylocard◇

Pregnancy Risk Category: B

INDICATIONS & DOSAGES
Acute ventricular arrhythmias (PVCs, ventricular tachycardia) associated with acute MI, cardiac glycoside toxicity, cardioversion, cardiac manipulation from trauma or surgery, or drug adverse effects—
Adults: 50 to 100 mg initial bolus, repeated after 5 minutes if arrhythmias continue. For maintenance, infuse 20 to 50 mcg/kg/minute (1 to 4 mg/minute in 70-kg adult). Do not exceed 300 mg within 1 hour. Keep rate below 30 mcg/kg/minute in patients with heart failure or liver disease.
Children: 0.5 to 1 mg/kg initial bolus, repeated as necessary. For maintenance, infuse 10 to 50 mcg/kg/minute. Maximum dosage is 5 mg/kg.
Status epilepticus unresponsive to all other measures—
Adults and children: initial bolus of 1 mg/kg. If seizure doesn't stop after 2 minutes, give 0.5-mg/kg bolus. For maintenance, infuse 30 mcg/kg/minute.

PREPARATION & STORAGE
Available for injection in 5-ml ampules and prefilled syringes with concentrations of 10 and 20 mg/ml.

Available for continuous infusion in 40-mg, 1-g, and 2-g single-use 25- or 50-ml vials and in 5- and 10-ml syringes that require mixing with D_5W in water. Dilute 1 g of drug in 250 ml of D_5W to obtain a 0.4% solution (4 mg/ml). Drug also comes in premixed 250-ml bottles of 0.4% or 0.8% solution or 500 ml bottles of 0.2%, 0.4%, or 0.8% solution.

Store at room temperature. Be sure to use only solutions marked for treating arrhythmias.

Incompatibility
Incompatible with amphotericin B, ampicillin sodium, cefazolin sodium, hydromorphone hydrochloride, methohexital, and phenytoin.

ADMINISTRATION
Direct injection: Inject undiluted drug into large vein or cannula at a rate of 25 to 50 mg/minute.
Continuous infusion: Using an infusion pump and microdrip tubing, titrate dose according to suppression of ventricular ectopy.

CONTRAINDICATIONS & CAUTIONS
• Contraindicated in hypersensitivity to lidocaine or amide-like anesthetics, in Adams-Stokes disease and Wolff-Parkinson-White syndrome, and in second- or third-degree heart block.
• Use cautiously in children, the elderly, and in patients with severe kidney or liver disease, heart failure, or shock.
• Also use cautiously in patients with sinus bradycardia or incomplete heart block who have not received isoproterenol or a pacemaker.
• In children, dosage ranges and drug efficacy have not been determined through controlled studies.

SPECIAL CONSIDERATIONS
• Use smallest lidocaine dose possible to control arrhythmias. Therapeutic level is 1.5 to 5 mcg/ml; toxic level is greater than 5 mcg/ml.
• In case of overdose, stop infusion immediately and notify doctor. Ensure an adequate airway and oxygenation. Give oxygen by nasal cannula if appropriate. Be prepared to initiate cardiopulmonary resuscitation. Continue to monitor ECG for underlying ventricular arrhythmias,

L

and prepare to give an alternate antiarrhythmic, such as procainamide. Monitor respirations and blood pressure every 5 minutes for 20 minutes. If bradycardia develops, give atropine and be alert for tachycardia. If seizures occur, give diazepam and monitor the patient carefully for respiratory depression.
• Monitor ECG continuously during administration. Keep resuscitation equipment nearby.
• Assess often for signs of toxicity.

lorazepam

Ativan

Controlled Substance Schedule IV

Pregnancy Risk Category: D

INDICATIONS & DOSAGES
Short-term symptomatic relief of anxiety in patients who cannot take oral medications—
Adults: 0.044 mg/kg or 2 mg total, whichever is smaller.
Preoperative sedation—
Adults: 2 mg total dose or 0.044 mg/kg, whichever is smaller, 15 to 20 minutes before surgery. In patients age 50 and younger, doses up to 0.05 mg/kg (up to 4 mg total) may be given.
Prevention of nausea and vomiting associated with chemotherapy—
Adults: 2 mg 30 minutes before chemotherapy, followed by 2 mg q 4 hours, p.r.n.

PREPARATION & STORAGE
Available in 1- and 10-ml vials and single-dose prefilled syringes with concentrations of 2 and 4 mg/ml. Refrigerate drug (but do not freeze) and protect from light. Discard if drug becomes discolored or contains precipitate. Immediately before administration, dilute drug with an equal volume of sterile water for injection, 0.9% NaCl, or D_5W in water. Rotate syringe gently to ensure complete mixing.

Incompatibility
Incompatible with idarubicin hydrochloride.

ADMINISTRATION
Direct injection: Inject into vein or into an IV line containing a free-flowing, compatible solution at a maximum rate of 2 mg/minute.

CONTRAINDICATIONS & CAUTIONS
• Contraindicated in hypersensitivity to benzodiazepines, polyethylene glycol, propylene glycol, or benzyl alcohol; in acute angle-closure glaucoma; in shock or coma; in acute alcohol intoxication; and in hepatic or renal failure.
• Avoid use in respiratory depression.
• Give cautiously to psychotic or depressed patients and those with myasthenia gravis or porphyria.
• Use cautiously in patients with renal or hepatic impairment, hypoalbuminemia, or seizures and in addiction-prone patients.
• Also use with caution in elderly or debilitated patients.
• Pediatric safety has not been established.

SPECIAL CONSIDERATIONS
• Overly rapid infusion can cause apnea, hypotension, bradycardia, or cardiac arrest.
• In cases of overdose, maintain a patent airway and adequate ventilation and give IV fluids to enhance drug excretion. Flumazenil (Romazicon) is a benzodiazepine antagonist that may be used to reverse the sedative and respiratory depressant effects of lorazepam. If hypotension occurs, administer norepinephrine or metaraminol.
• Always keep emergency resuscitation equipment nearby. Obtain baseline respiratory rate before administration, and notify doctor if rate falls below 12 breaths/minute. Also obtain baseline blood pressure measurement, and carefully monitor blood pressure during and after administration.

magnesium sulfate

Pregnancy Risk Category: A

INDICATIONS & DOSAGES
Preeclampsia or eclampsia—
Adults: 4 g, followed by either 1 to 2 g/hour given by continuous infusion. Dosage over next 24 hours depends on serum magnesium levels and urine output. Maximum dosage is 30 to 40 g q 24 hours; in renal disease, 20 g q 48 hours.
Prevention and control of seizures in severe preeclampsia or eclampsia, epilepsy, glomerulonephritis, or hypothyroidism—
Adults: 1 to 4 g (8 to 32 mEq of magnesium) of 10% to 20% solution.
Severe hypertension, encephalopathy, and seizures caused by nephritis—
Children: 100 to 200 mg/kg of 1% to 3% solution. Give total dose within 1 hour, half within the first 15 to 20 minutes.
Severe magnesium deficiency—
Adults: 5 g.
Magnesium supplement in total parenteral nutrition—
Adults: 0.5 to 3 g daily (4 to 24 mEq of magnesium).
Infants: 0.25 to 1.25 g daily (2 to 10 mEq of magnesium).
Barium poisoning—
Adults: 1 to 2 g.
Paroxysmal atrial tachycardia—
Adults: 3 to 4 g.

PREPARATION & STORAGE
Available as a 10% concentration in 10- and 20-ml ampules (100 mg/ml) and in 20- and 50-ml vials; 12.5% concentration in 20-ml vials (125 mg/ml); and 50% concentration in 2-ml ampules (500 mg/ml), 2-, 5-, 10-, 30-, and 50-ml vials, and 10-ml syringes. Store at room temperature and avoid freezing.

In seizures, dilute dose in 250 ml of D_5W. In magnesium deficiency, dilute dose in 1 L of D_5W or dextrose 5% in 0.9% NaCl. For all indications, do not use concentrations over 20% (200 mg/ml).

Incompatibility
Incompatible with alcohol, alkali carbonates and bicarbonates, calcium gluceptate, calcium gluconate, cefepime hydrochloride, ciprofloxacin, dobutamine, hydrocortisone sodium succinate, 10% IV fat emulsion, polymyxin B, procaine, sodium bicarbonate, and soluble phosphates.

ADMINISTRATION
Direct injection: Inject directly into vein, not exceeding 150 mg/minute.
Intermittent infusion: Administer diluted drug over 1 to 3 hours.
Continuous infusion: Give by infusion pump, not exceeding 150 mg/minute (1.2 mEq/minute).

CONTRAINDICATIONS & CAUTIONS
• Contraindicated in myocardial damage and heart block.
• Also contraindicated within 2 hours of expected delivery because neonate may show signs of magnesium toxicity.
• Use cautiously in renal impairment.

SPECIAL CONSIDERATIONS
• Keep IV calcium gluconate available; however, use cautiously in patients undergoing digitalization because arrhythmias may develop.
• Disappearance of patellar reflexes signals onset of toxicity. Treat with 5 to 10 mEq of calcium (10 to 20 ml of 10% calcium gluconate), as ordered. In severe overdose, peritoneal dialysis or hemodialysis may be necessary.
• Monitor vital signs every 15 minutes. Be alert for respiratory depression and signs of heart block. Also monitor intake and output.

M

mannitol

Osmitrol✦

Pregnancy Risk Category: C

INDICATIONS & DOSAGES
Prevention of oliguric phase in acute renal failure—

Adults: 50 to 100 g, followed by infusion of a 5% or 10% solution.
Test dose for marked oliguria or suspected inadequate renal function—
Adults and children over age 12: 200 mg/kg, or 12.5 g as a 15% or 20% solution given over 3 to 5 minutes.
Children age 12 and under: 0.2 g/kg given over 3 to 5 minutes, then 2 g/kg.
Treatment of oliguria—
Adults: 100 g of a 15% to 20% solution given over 90 minutes to several hours.
Reduction of intracranial and intraocular pressure—
Adults: 1.5 to 2 g/kg of a 15%, 20%, or 25% solution given over 30 to 60 minutes.
Children age 12 and under: 1 to 2 g/kg of a 15% or 20% solution given over 30 to 60 minutes.
Reduction of nephrotoxic effects of amphotericin B—
Adults: 12.5 g given immediately before and after each dose of amphotericin B.
Promotion of diuresis in drug intoxication (adjunct)—
Adults: 50 to 200 g of a 5% to 25% solution, followed by infusion to maintain urine output at 100 to 500 ml/hour.
Adjunctive treatment of edema and ascites—
Adults: 100 g of a 10% to 20% solution given over 2 to 6 hours.
Children age 12 and under: 2 g/kg of a 15% or 20% solution given over 2 to 6 hours.

PREPARATION & STORAGE
Available in strengths of 5%, 10%, 15%, 20%, and 25% in 150-, 250-, 500-, and 1,000-ml glass and plastic IV containers. Store at room temperature; avoid freezing. Drug may crystallize, especially if chilled. If crystals form, dissolve according to manufacturer's directions. Avoid using solution that contains undissolved crystals.

Incompatibility
Incompatible with imipenem-cilastatin and blood products. If blood must be given with mannitol, add 20 mEq of NaCl to each L of mannitol.

ADMINISTRATION
When giving mannitol solutions with concentrations of 15% or above, make sure the administration set includes a filter. Rapid administration of large doses may lead to drug accumulation and circulatory overload.
    Avoid extravasation to prevent edema and necrosis.
Intermittent infusion: Infuse appropriate dose and concentration at ordered rate.
Continuous infusion: Infuse appropriate dose and concentration at ordered rate.

CONTRAINDICATIONS & CAUTIONS
• Contraindicated in anuria and in intracranial bleeding (except during craniotomy).
• Avoid use in severe dehydration, severe pulmonary congestion, and heart failure.
• Use cautiously in cardiopulmonary impairment, hyperkalemia, hyponatremia, hypovolemia, and severe renal impairment.

SPECIAL CONSIDERATIONS
• Rebound increase in intracranial and intraocular pressure may occur about 12 hours after mannitol administration.
• Large doses may cross the blood-brain barrier and cause CNS damage or death.
• Monitor vital signs frequently during first hour of infusion and hourly thereafter or as needed. Also monitor intake and output, BUN, and serum electrolytes, especially sodium and potassium.
• Advise patient to change positions slowly to avoid dizziness from orthostatic hypotension.

M

---

mechlorethamine hydrochloride (nitrogen mustard)

Mustargen ◆

Pregnancy Risk Category: D

INDICATIONS & DOSAGES
Dosage is based on patient response and degree of toxicity.
Hodgkin's disease—
Adults and children: 6 mg/m² daily on days 1 and 8 of 28-day cycle in combination with other antineoplastics (mechlorethamine-vincristine-procarbazine-prednisone [MOPP] regimen). Dosage repeated for six cycles. Subsequent doses reduced by 50% in MOPP regimen when WBC count is between 3,000 and 3,999/mm³ and by 75% when WBC count is between 1,000 and 2,999/mm³, or platelet count is between 50,000 and 100,000/mm³.
Other neoplastic disorders—
Adults and children: 0.4 mg/kg as single dose or 0.1 to 0.2 mg/kg divided in two or four successive daily doses during each course of therapy.

PREPARATION & STORAGE
Exercise extreme caution when preparing or administering mechlorethamine to avoid mutagenic, teratogenic, and carcinogenic risks. Use a biological containment cabinet, wear gloves and mask, and use syringes with luer-lock fittings to prevent leakage of drug solution. Correctly dispose of needles, vials, and unused drug, and avoid contaminating work surfaces.

Avoid inhalation of mechlorethamine dust or vapors or contact with skin or mucous membranes. If eye contact occurs, irrigate with liberal amounts of water or saline solution and consult an ophthalmologist immediately. If skin contact occurs, irrigate for at least 15 minutes with water and then with 2% sodium thiosulfate solution.

Mechlorethamine is available in 10-mg vials. Store at room temperature. Reconstitute with 10 ml sterile water for injection or 0.9% NaCl for a concentration of 1 mg/ml. Shake vial several times to dissolve. Administer within 15 minutes. Highly unstable, the solution decomposes while standing. Do not use if drug is discolored or if water droplets appear in vial. Discard unused drug.

Incompatibility
Incompatible with methohexital sodium.

ADMINISTRATION
Direct injection: Use one sterile needle to aspirate reconstituted drug from the vial and another for direct injection. Inject reconstituted solution directly into vein or, preferably, into a free-flowing IV solution over a few minutes or according to protocol. After administration, flush tubing and vein with IV solution for 2 to 5 minutes.

CONTRAINDICATIONS & CAUTIONS
• Contraindicated in chickenpox, herpes, or other infections and in acute or chronic suppurative inflammation.
• Use cautiously in concurrent anticoagulant therapy, radiation therapy, or other chemotherapy, and in preexisting myelosuppression or tumor cell infiltration of bone marrow.
• Also use cautiously in patients with gout or history of urate renal stones.

SPECIAL CONSIDERATIONS
• If infiltration occurs, aspirate as much drug as possible from tissues. Then, inject area with sterile isotonic sodium thiosulfate (4.14% of pentahydrate salt, 2.64% of the anhydrous salt, or a 4% solution prepared by diluting 4 ml of sodium thiosulfate 10% injection with 6 ml of sterile water solution) and apply ice compresses for 6 to 12 hours.
• Administer with hydrocortisone, as ordered, to reduce risk of phlebitis or painful administration.

M

• Expect some evidence of toxicity with a therapeutic response. Drug is highly toxic and has a low therapeutic index.

• Give antiemetics to reduce severity of nausea and vomiting, which usually begin 1 to 3 hours after administration.

• Monitor WBC and platelet counts as well as BUN, hematocrit, ALT, AST, bilirubin, creatinine, LD, and uric acid levels.

melphalan hydrochloride

Alkeran

Pregnancy Risk Category: D

INDICATIONS & DOSAGES

Palliative treatment of multiple myeloma—

Adults: 16 mg/m² as a single infusion over 15 to 20 minutes at 2-week intervals for four doses; then, after adequate recovery from toxicity, at 4-week intervals. Adjust dose based on blood cell counts at nadir and on day of treatment.

Note: Dosage reductions of up to 50% are recommended in patients with renal insufficiency (BUN level above 30 mg/dl).

PREPARATION & STORAGE

To avoid mutagenic, teratogenic, and carcinogenic risks, follow institutional guidelines for the safe handling, preparation, administration, and disposal of chemotherapeutic agents.

Available as a 50-mg powder for injection in a single-use vial with a 10-ml vial of sterile diluent (water for injection). Protect from light and dispense in glass.

To prepare, reconstitute with 10 ml of the diluent supplied and shake vigorously until solution is clear. The resultant solution contains 5 mg/ml drug. Immediately dilute the calculated dose in 0.9% NaCl injection. Final concentration should

not exceed 0.45 mg/ml. Complete administration within 60 minutes of reconstitution because both reconstituted and diluted solutions are unstable. Do not refrigerate solutions because precipitate will form.

Incompatibility

Incompatible with amphotericin B, chlorpromazine hydrochloride, D_5W, and lactated Ringer's injection. Compatibility with 0.9% NaCl injection is concentration-dependent; do not prepare solutions with a concentration exceeding 0.45 mg/ml.

ADMINISTRATION

Administer drug under supervision of a doctor experienced in the use of chemotherapeutic agents.

Intermittent infusion: Administer diluted drug over 15 to 20 minutes (within 60 minutes of reconstitution and dilution).

CONTRAINDICATIONS & CAUTIONS

• Contraindicated in hypersensitivity to drug and in patients whose disease is resistant to drug. Patients with hypersensitivity to chlorambucil may exhibit cross-sensitivity to melphalan.

• Drug is not recommended in severe leukopenia, thrombocytopenia, or anemia, or in chronic lymphocytic leukemia.

• Use cautiously in patients who have received cytotoxic drugs or radiation therapy within 3 to 4 weeks.

• Safety and efficacy in children have not been established.

SPECIAL CONSIDERATIONS

• Therapeutic effects are often accompanied by toxicity.

• Anticoagulants and aspirin products should be used cautiously. Watch for signs of bleeding and infection.

• Perform CBCs before starting therapy and before each subsequent dose. If WBC falls below 3,000/mm³, temporarily discontinue drug or decrease dosage. If platelet count

M

falls below 100,000/mm³, do not give IM injections.

meperidine hydrochloride (pethidine hydrochloride)

Demerol Hydrochloride◆

Controlled Substance Schedule II

Pregnancy Risk Category: B (D for prolonged use or high doses at term)

INDICATIONS & DOSAGES
Moderate to severe pain—
Adults: 10 to 50 mg q 2 to 4 hours or 15 to 35 mg/hour by infusion. Dosage reflects patient response and severity of pain.
Adjunct in anesthesia—
Adults: fractional doses of a 10-mg/ml solution, repeated p.r.n., or 1 mg/ml by infusion.

PREPARATION & STORAGE
Available in preservative-free ampules and vials and in preservative-containing syringes with strengths of 10, 25, 50, 75, and 100 mg/ml. Store vials and ampules at room temperature. Single doses in syringes remain stable at room temperature for 24 hours.
    For direct injection, dilute dose with a compatible solution to a concentration of 10 mg/ml. For infusion, dilute with a compatible solution to a concentration of 1 mg/ml.

Incompatibility
Incompatible with aminophylline, amobarbital sodium, ephedrine, heparin, methicillin, morphine, phenobarbital sodium, phenytoin, sodium bicarbonate, sodium iodide, sulfadiazine, and thiopental.

ADMINISTRATION
Direct injection: Inject diluted dose over 3 to 5 minutes. Rapid injection

increases risk of severe adverse reactions.
Continuous infusion: Give at rate of 15 to 35 mg/hour, using an infusion control device. Avoid rapid infusion.

CONTRAINDICATIONS & CAUTIONS
• Contraindicated in sensitivity to drug and in acute respiratory depression.
• Also contraindicated in diarrhea resulting from poisons, toxins, or use of cephalosporins or topical clindamycin until toxic substances clear.
• Use with extreme caution in patients with seizure disorders.
• Use cautiously in patients with altered respiratory function, head injury, increased intracranial pressure (from intracranial lesions), prostatic hypertrophy, urethral stricture, or recent urinary tract surgery.
• Use cautiously in patients with atrial flutter, other supraventricular tachyarrhythmias, gallbladder disease, abdominal disorders, inflammatory bowel disease, recent GI surgery, and hypothyroidism.
• Also administer cautiously in patients with history of drug abuse or emotional instability, or who show evidence of suicide potential.
• Adjust dosage in renal or hepatic impairment or renal failure.

SPECIAL CONSIDERATIONS
• Give drug with patient in supine position to minimize hypotension.
• For improved analgesia, give before patient has intense pain.
• In cases of overdose, maintain airway patency and provide respiratory support. To reverse respiratory depression, give 0.4 mg of naloxone by IV push; repeat as necessary. Maintain blood pressure with IV fluids and vasopressors, as ordered.
• Monitor respirations frequently during infusion and every 15 minutes for 1 hour after infusion. Remember to keep resuscitation equipment and naloxone nearby.
• Assess patient's bowel function, and give a stool softener if necessary.

M

mesna

Mesnex

Pregnancy Risk Category: B

INDICATIONS & DOSAGES

Prevention of ifosfamide-induced hemorrhagic cystitis—
Adults: 60% of ifosfamide dose. Administer in three bolus doses (each 20% of ifosfamide dose), the first given at the time of the ifosfamide dose and subsequent doses given 4 and 8 hours after the ifosfamide dose is administered.

PREPARATION & STORAGE

Available in 2-, 4-, and 10-ml ampules at a concentration of 100 mg/ml. Store ampules at room temperature.

Dilute the appropriate dose in D_5W, 0.9% NaCl injection, or Ringer's lactate to a concentration of 20 mg/ml.

Diluted solutions are stable for 24 hours at 77° F (25° C), but use within 6 hours is recommended. Because mesna becomes oxidized in the presence of oxygen, discard unused drug from open ampules and prepare a new ampule for each administration.

Incompatibility
Incompatible with cisplatin.

ADMINISTRATION

Direct injection: Using a 21G or 23G needle, inject into vein or into IV tubing containing a free-flowing, compatible solution.
Intermittent infusion: Infuse over 15 to 30 minutes.

CONTRAINDICATIONS & CAUTIONS

• Contraindicated in known hypersensitivity to mesna or other thiol compounds.
• Advise breast-feeding patient that it is not known whether mesna is excreted in breast milk.

SPECIAL CONSIDERATIONS

• Mesna does not prevent or alleviate other adverse reactions to ifosfamide.
• Drug has been used to prevent cyclophosphamide-induced hemorrhagic cystitis.
• Tell patient to report adverse reactions promptly.

methicillin sodium

Staphcillin

Pregnancy Risk Category: B

INDICATIONS & DOSAGES

Infections caused by susceptible organisms—
Adults: 1 g q 6 hours.
Children over age 1 month: 100 to 200 mg/kg/day in divided doses q 6 hours.
Endocarditis or acute or chronic osteomyelitis caused by susceptible organisms—
Adults: 1.5 to 2 g q 4 hours.
Children over age 1 month: 200 to 300 mg/kg/day in divided doses q 4 hours.

Note: Adjust dosage in renal impairment. For adults, dosage reflects creatinine clearance. If clearance is 10 ml/minute or less, give 1 g q 8 to 12 hours.

PREPARATION & STORAGE

Available in 1-, 4-, and 6-g vials, in 1-g piggyback units, and 10-g hospital bulk packages. Before reconstitution, store drug at room temperature. Reconstitute by adding 1.5 ml of sterile water for injection or 0.9% NaCl to 1-g vial, 5.7 ml to 4-g vial, or 8.6 ml to 6-g vial.

For direct injection, dilute each gram of drug in 50 ml of 0.9% NaCl.

For infusion, further dilute in 50 to 100 ml of D_5W in 0.9% NaCl, D_5W, fructose 10% in water, fructose 10% in 0.9% NaCl, invert sugar 10% in 0.9% NaCl, or Travert 10% and electrolyte #1, #2, or #3 for a concentration of 2, 10, or 20 mg/ml.

M

Reconstitute glass piggyback unit with volume of diluent specified on the label for IV infusion.

Reconstituted solutions remain stable for 24 hours at room temperature and for 4 days if refrigerated.

Incompatibility
Incompatible with aminoglycosides, chlorpromazine hydrochloride, codeine phosphate, Dextran 40 10% in dextrose 5%, Dextran 40 10% in 0.9% NaCl, 10% fat emulsion, heparin sodium, hydrocortisone sodium succinate, levorphanol tartrate, lincomycin hydrochloride, meperidine, metaraminol bitartrate, methadone hydrochloride, methohexital sodium, morphine sulfate, promethazine hydrochloride, sodium bicarbonate, and vancomycin hydrochloride.

ADMINISTRATION
Direct injection: Inject diluted drug at rate of 10 ml/minute.
Intermittent infusion: Infuse diluted drug into an IV line containing a free-flowing, compatible solution over 20 to 30 minutes.

CONTRAINDICATIONS & CAUTIONS
• Contraindicated in hypersensitivity to penicillins or cephalosporins.
• Use cautiously in patients with GI disorders or impaired renal function.
• Use with caution in breast-feeding women because of potential for adverse reactions in infants.

SPECIAL CONSIDERATIONS
• Hemorrhagic cystitis occurs more commonly when drug is given in large doses to patients with low urine output.
• Elderly patients face a greater risk of thrombophlebitis from methicillin infusion.
• Check for previous penicillin or cephalosporin hypersensitivity before administering first dose.
• Monitor CBC, urinalysis, and BUN, AST, and ALT levels during therapy to detect adverse effects.

• Monitor intake and output, noting hematuria or casts. If patient is on sodium restriction, monitor electrolytes.

methotrexate sodium

Folex, Folex PFS, Mexate, Mexate-AQ
Pregnancy Risk Category: D

INDICATIONS & DOSAGES
Induction of remission in lymphoblastic leukemia—
Adults: 2.5 mg/kg q 14 days. Dosage varies widely.
Psoriasis—
Adults: 10 to 25 mg once weekly. Up to 100 mg may be required; however, manufacturer recommends maximum weekly dose of only 50 mg.
Adjuvant therapy for osteosarcoma—
Adults: 12 g/m². May be increased to 15 g/m² if lower dose proves insufficient to meet a 1×10^{-3} M/L blood level at end of infusion.

PREPARATION & STORAGE
Exercise extreme caution when preparing and administering methotrexate to avoid mutagenic, teratogenic, and carcinogenic risks. Use a biological containment cabinet, wear gloves and mask, and use syringes with luer-lock fittings. Correctly dispose of needles, vials, and unused drug, and avoid contaminating work surfaces.

Available in 20-, 50-, 100-, and 250-mg single-dose vials of lyophilized sterile powder and in 2-, 4-, 8-, and 10-ml vials containing 25 mg/ml solution. Reconstitute with 2 to 10 ml of sterile water for injection, 0.9% NaCl, or D_5W. Reconstituted concentrations range from 2 to 50 mg/ml. Further dilute for injection with 0.9% NaCl or D_5W.

Store drug preparations at room temperature and protect from light.

M

Incompatibility
Incompatible with bleomycin, chlorpromazine, droperidol, fluorouracil, metoclopramide, prednisolone, promethazine, and sodium phosphate.

ADMINISTRATION
Direct injection: Inject directly into vein or into side port of free-flowing IV line over prescribed duration.
Intermittent infusion: May be given as a 4-hour infusion.

CONTRAINDICATIONS & CAUTIONS
• Contraindicated in preexisting or recent exposure to chickenpox or herpes virus.
• Use caution in psoriasis patients with poor nutrition, renal or hepatic impairment, or blood dyscrasias.
• Use cautiously in GI obstruction, ascites, or peritoneal or pleural effusions and in myelosuppression.
• Administer carefully to patients with GI infection, peptic ulcer, ulcerative colitis, oral mucositis, gout, or history of urate stones.
• Use cautiously in nausea and vomiting.
• Advise male patient to use contraceptive measures during therapy and for at least 3 months afterward.
• Advise female to avoid becoming pregnant during therapy and for at least one ovulatory cycle after drug therapy ends.
• Caution women against breastfeeding during therapy.

SPECIAL CONSIDERATIONS
• Expect toxic reactions with therapeutic doses. Drug is highly toxic and has a low therapeutic index.
• If blood cell counts decrease, discontinue drug, as ordered.
• Generic preparations may contain benzyl alcohol.
• In cases of overdose, administer leucovorin calcium as soon as possible, preferably in first hour of overdose. In massive overdose, urine alkalinization and hydration help to prevent precipitation of methotrex-

ate or its metabolites in the renal tubules.
• Do not repeat drug therapy unless WBC increases above $1,500/mm^3$; neutrophil count elevates above $200/mm^3$; platelet count rises above $75,000/mm^3$; serum bilirubin level is less than 1.2 mg/dl; ALT level is less than 450 U/L; serum creatinine level is normal; creatinine clearance is at least 60 ml/minute; and patient shows evidence of healing (if he has mucositis). Also do not repeat therapy if patient experiences pleural effusion.
• Monitor serum creatinine and BUN levels daily during high-dose methotrexate therapy.
• Monitor serum methotrexate levels daily during therapy. Continue monitoring until serum level falls below 5 $\times 10^{-3}$ M/L.
• Notify doctor of changes in breathing patterns or signs of liver dysfunction (jaundice, malaise, nausea).

methyldopate hydrochloride

Aldomet ♦

Pregnancy Risk Category: B

INDICATIONS & DOSAGES
Sustained mild to severe hypertension and, in combination therapy, acute hypertensive emergencies—
Adults: 250 to 500 mg q 6 hours, as necessary. Maximum dosage, 1 g q 6 hours.
Children: 20 to 40 mg/kg q 24 hours or 0.15 to 0.3 g/m^2 q 6 hours. Maximum daily dosage is 65 mg/kg, 2 g/m^2, or 3 g, whichever is least.
Note: Adjust dosage in renal impairment.

PREPARATION & STORAGE
Available in concentrations of 50 mg/ml. For infusion, add the re-

quired dose to 100 ml of D$_5$W for a concentration of 100 mg/10 ml. Drug remains stable for 24 hours in most IV solutions; however, exposure to air may accelerate decomposition. Protect from light and store at room temperature; avoid freezing.

Incompatibility
Incompatible with amphotericin B, methohexital, and some total parenteral nutrition solutions. Mix cautiously with drugs that have poor solubility in acidic media, such as barbiturates and sulfonamides.

ADMINISTRATION
Intermittent infusion: Infuse diluted dose through a patent IV line over 30 to 60 minutes.

CONTRAINDICATIONS & CAUTIONS
• Contraindicated in active hepatitis or cirrhosis and in hypersensitivity to methyldopate hydrochloride.
• Contraindicated in previous methyldopa therapy associated with liver abnormalities or hemolytic anemia (positive direct Coombs' test).
• Administer carefully to dialysis patients and sulfite-sensitive patients.
• Use with caution in pheochromocytoma, coronary insufficiency, Parkinson's disease, or renal impairment and elderly or debilitated patients.

SPECIAL CONSIDERATIONS
• Dialysis may be helpful in removing drug.
• Monitor heart rate, blood pressure, cardiac output, blood volume, electrolyte balance, GI motility, renal function, and cerebral activity. To reverse hypotension, administer IV fluids.
• Monitor hemoglobin level, hematocrit, or CBC before and during therapy. If hemolytic anemia develops, discontinue drug.
• Monitor for signs of drug-induced depression.
• Perform Coombs' test before therapy.

methylergonovine maleate

Methergine
Pregnancy Risk Category: C

INDICATIONS & DOSAGES
Emergency treatment of severe postpartum and postabortion hemorrhage caused by uterine atony or subinvolution—
Adults: 0.2 mg in single dose, repeated q 2 to 4 hours (up to five doses, if necessary).

PREPARATION & STORAGE
Available in 1-ml ampules containing 0.2 mg/ml. Store drug below 46° F (8° C) in light-resistant containers. Avoid freezing. Ready-to-use injections are normally clear and colorless. Discard if solution is discolored or contains a precipitate.
Dilute with 5 ml of 0.9% NaCl, if appropriate.

Incompatibility
None reported.

ADMINISTRATION
Direct injection: Administer directly into vein or into free-flowing, compatible IV solution over at least 60 seconds. If desired, use diluted dosage to facilitate slow injection. Overly rapid administration can cause severe CV effects.

CONTRAINDICATIONS & CAUTIONS
• Contraindicated before placental expulsion and for induction of labor.
• Avoid use in hypersensitivity to ergot preparations.
• Use cautiously in coronary artery disease, hypertension, occlusive peripheral vascular disease, sepsis, and hepatic or renal impairment.

SPECIAL CONSIDERATIONS
• Closely monitor blood pressure and pulse. Give IV hydralazine or chlorpromazine, as ordered, for hypertension.

M

• After administration, closely monitor uterine activity. (Contractions are sustained and uterine tone is high.) If appropriate, give analgesics for discomfort.
• Instruct patient to report dyspnea, headache, numb or cold extremities, or severe abdominal cramping.

methylprednisolone sodium succinate

A-metha-Pred, Solu-Medrol ♦
Pregnancy Risk Category: C

INDICATIONS & DOSAGES
Severe inflammation or immunosuppression—
Adults: 10 mg to 1.5 g daily. Usual dosage, 10 to 250 mg up to q 4 hours.
Severe shock—
Adults: 30 mg/kg initially, repeated q 4 to 6 hours p.r.n.; or 100 to 250 mg initially, repeated q 2 to 6 hours p.r.n. Initial dose may be followed by 30 mg/kg infusion q 12 hours for 24 to 48 hours.
Severe lupus nephritis—
Adults: 1 g (intermittent infusion) for 3 days, followed by oral prednisolone or prednisone.
Children: 30 mg/kg on alternate days for six doses, followed by oral prednisolone or prednisone.
To decrease residual damage following spinal cord trauma—
Adults: 30 mg/kg IV as a bolus injection within 8 hours of injury, followed by cautious infusion of 5.4 mg/kg/hour for next 23 hours.
Adjunctive treatment of Pneumocystis carinii *pneumonia—*
Adults: 30 mg IV b.i.d. for 5 days, then 30 mg daily for 5 days. Finally, give 15 mg IV daily for 11 days or until anti-infective therapy is discontinued.

PREPARATION & STORAGE
Available in container of drug and diluent in the following strengths:

40 mg (1 ml), 125 mg (2 ml), 500 mg (8 ml), 1 g (16 ml), and 2 g (32 ml). Reconstitute with diluent provided and store at room temperature. Avoid freezing. Do not use solution if cloudy, and discard any unused portion after 48 hours. Dilute for infusion with D_5W, 0.9% NaCl, or dextrose 5% in 0.9% NaCl.

Incompatibility
Incompatible with calcium gluconate, cephalothin, cytarabine, filgrastim, glycopyrrolate, metaraminol, nafcillin, and penicillin G sodium.

ADMINISTRATION
Direct injection: Inject diluted drug into vein or free-flowing, compatible IV solution over at least 1 minute. In life-threatening situations, administer initial massive dose over 3 to 15 minutes.
Intermittent infusion: Using appropriately diluted dose, adjust flow rate, depending on disorder and patient's response.
Continuous infusion: Using appropriately diluted dose, adjust flow rate, depending on disorder and patient's response.

CONTRAINDICATIONS & CAUTIONS
• Contraindicated in systemic fungal infection, sepsis syndrome, or septic shock.
• Also contraindicated in viral or bacterial infections uncontrolled by antibiotics (except in life-threatening situations) and peptic ulcer (except in life-threatening situations).
• Avoid use in neonates and in patients with hypersensitivity to drug or its components.
• Use cautiously in hyperthyroidism, hypothyroidism, cirrhosis, seizure disorders, renal insufficiency, diabetes mellitus, osteoporosis, ocular herpes simplex infections, and history of tuberculosis.
• Also use cautiously in psychosis, diverticulitis, nonspecific ulcerative colitis, or recent intestinal anastomosis.

M

• Use carefully in hypoalbuminemia, renal or hepatic dysfunction, and open-angle glaucoma.
• Administer cautiously in children.

SPECIAL CONSIDERATIONS
• Because of risk of anaphylaxis, keep resuscitation equipment nearby.
• Adjust dosage as needed for patients taking insulin, antithyroid drugs, or thyroid hormones.
• In all preparations, diluent contains benzyl alcohol.
• Before therapy, obtain baseline ECG, blood pressure, chest and spinal x-rays, glucose tolerance test, evaluation of hypothalamic-pituitary-adrenal axis function, and results of upper GI series (in patients with predisposition to GI disorders).

metoclopramide hydrochloride

Maxeran◇, Octamide PFS, Reglan♦

Pregnancy Risk Category: B

INDICATIONS & DOSAGES
Nausea and vomiting during chemotherapy—
Adults: 2 mg/kg q 2 hours for three doses, beginning 30 minutes before chemotherapy; then 1 mg/kg q 3 hours for three doses. For less emetogenic regimens, 1 mg/kg/dose may be adequate.
Severe delayed gastric emptying in diabetic gastroparesis (in patients unable to take oral dose)—
Adults: 10 mg q.i.d. 30 minutes before meals and h.s.
Passage of intestinal tubes for diagnostic tests—
Adults: 10 mg.
Children ages 6 to 14: 2.5 to 5 mg.
Children under age 6: 0.1 mg/kg.
Radiologic examination of GI tract (in delayed gastric emptying that interferes with examination of stomach or intestine)—

Adults: 10 mg.
Children ages 6 to 14: 2.5 to 5 mg.
Children under age 6: 0.1 mg/kg.
Note: Adjust dosage in renal impairment. For adults, dosage reflects creatinine clearance. In those patients with creatinine clearance less than 40 ml/minute, decrease dose by 50%.

PREPARATION & STORAGE
Available with a concentration of 5 mg/ml in 2-, 10-, 30-, 50-, and 100-ml vials and in 2- and 10-ml ampules. For infusion, dilute with 50 ml of D_5W, 0.9% NaCl, dextrose 5% in 0.45% NaCl, Ringer's injection, or lactated Ringer's solution.
Solutions remain stable for 48 hours when stored at 39° to 86° F (4° to 30° C) and protected from light. If diluted with 0.9% NaCl, solution may be frozen in polyvinyl chloride bags for up to 4 weeks. (Do not use dextrose 5% diluent with polyvinyl chloride bags if solution will be frozen.)

Incompatibility
Incompatible with allopurinol, ampicillin, calcium gluconate, cefepime hydrochloride, cephalothin, chloramphenicol sodium succinate, cisplatin, erythromycin lactobionate, furosemide, methotrexate sodium, penicillin G potassium, and sodium bicarbonate.

ADMINISTRATION
Direct injection: Inject over 1 to 2 minutes directly into vein or into IV tubing containing a free-flowing, compatible solution. Each 10 mg of drug should be given slowly over 1 to 2 minutes.
Intermittent infusion: Cover solution with a brown paper bag to prevent exposure to light. Infuse over at least 15 minutes. Slow infusion prevents anxiety and restlessness.

CONTRAINDICATIONS & CAUTIONS
• Contraindicated in hypersensitivity or intolerance to metoclopramide or

M

sulfites and when acceleration of GI motility may be hazardous.
• Avoid use in pheochromocytoma and history of seizures.
• Contraindicated in patients taking drugs that may cause extrapyramidal reactions (phenothiazines).
• Use cautiously in renal or hepatic impairment, hypersensitivity to procainamide, and Parkinson's disease.

SPECIAL CONSIDERATIONS
• Adjust insulin dosage, as ordered, in patients with diabetic gastroparesis. Drug affects intestinal food absorption.
• In cases of overdose, to control extrapyramidal symptoms, give antimuscarinic-antiparkinson drugs or antihistamines with antimuscarinic properties.
• Instruct patient to avoid alcohol, OTC sleep remedies, and sedatives during drug therapy.
• Contact doctor if involuntary movements in face, eyes, or limbs occur.

metoprolol tartrate

Betaloc◇, Lopresor◇, Lopressor

Pregnancy Risk Category: C

INDICATIONS & DOSAGES
Early treatment in suspected or definitive acute MI—
Adults: three injections of 5 mg each q 2 minutes, followed by oral maintenance doses if IV doses are tolerated.
  Note: Dosage may need to be reduced in patients with hepatic dysfunction.

PREPARATION & STORAGE
Available in 5-ml ampules or prefilled syringes (1 mg/ml). Store at room temperature and protect from light. Discard solution if discolored or if precipitate forms.

Incompatibility
None reported.

ADMINISTRATION
Direct injection: Rapidly inject bolus into free-flowing IV line.

CONTRAINDICATIONS & CAUTIONS
• Contraindicated in first-degree heart block with PR interval greater than 0.2 second, in second- and third-degree heart block, in bradycardia (under 45 beats/minute), in systolic pressure of less than 100 mm Hg, in moderate to severe heart failure, or in cardiogenic shock.
• Use cautiously in heart failure controlled with cardiac glycosides and diuretics and in the elderly.
• Use with caution in hepatic or renal disease, bronchospastic disease, myasthenia gravis, diabetes mellitus, and hyperthyroidism.
• Administer cautiously in patients with depression and psoriasis.

SPECIAL CONSIDERATIONS
• If bradycardia or hypotension develops before complete dosage is given, notify doctor; injections may be stopped or changed to oral form.
• Do not withdraw drug abruptly. Exacerbation of angina, MI, ventricular arrhythmias, and death have occurred.
• In cases of overdose, administer atropine then prepare for temporary pacemaker insertion for bradycardia if atropine is unsuccessful. Further treatment is symptomatic and supportive.
• Continuously monitor hemodynamic status, blood pressure, heart rate, and ECG during infusion.

metronidazole

metronidazole hydrochloride

Flagyl IV◆, Flagyl IV RTU, Metro IV

Pregnancy Risk Category: B

INDICATIONS & DOSAGES

Severe infections caused by susceptible bacteria—
Adults: 15 mg/kg initially, then 7.5 mg/kg q 6 hours, beginning 6 hours after loading dose. Maximum dosage, 4 g daily.

Surgical prophylaxis—
Adults: 15 mg/kg, completed 1 hour before surgery, then 7.5 mg/kg q 6 hours for two doses at 6 and 12 hours after initial dose.

   Note: Dosage may need to be reduced in patients with severe hepatic dysfunction.

PREPARATION & STORAGE

Flagyl IV is supplied as sterile, off-white, lyophilized powder in single-dose vials containing 500 mg of metronidazole and 415 mg of mannitol. Drug requires reconstitution, dilution, and neutralization.

   Order of mixing is important. Reconstitute drug with 4.4 ml of sterile water for injection, bacteriostatic water for injection, 0.9% NaCl injection, or bacteriostatic 0.9% NaCl injection. Mix thoroughly. Resulting solution provides 5 ml (100 mg/ml).

   Using a glass or plastic container, dilute further with 0.9% NaCl injection, dextrose 5% injection, or lactated Ringer's injection. Concentration should not exceed 8 mg/ml.

   Neutralize final dilution with 5 mEq of sodium bicarbonate injection for each 500 mg of drug. Because this produces carbon dioxide, the container may require venting.

Before reconstitution, store below 86° F (30° C) and protect from light. Reconstituted vials are stable for 96 hours in room light if stored below 86° F. Do not refrigerate when neutralized because a precipitate may form. Use diluted and neutralized solutions within 24 hours.

   Flagyl IV RTU and Metro IV are supplied in 100-ml single-dose plastic containers containing 500 mg of drug. Do not dilute, change pH, or mix any additive with these solutions. Also avoid using aluminum equipment (such as needles or cannulae) that would come in contact with drug. Although drug may cause opacity of plastic containers, needle hubs, or cannulae, this reaction will subside and does not affect solution.

   Flagyl IV RTU and Metro IV need no dilution or neutralization. Store at controlled room temperature, 59° to 86° F (15° to 30° C), and protect from light. Do not refrigerate or freeze.

Incompatibility
Incompatible with aluminum, 10% amino acid, and dopamine. Manufacturer recommends mixing no other drugs with metronidazole.

ADMINISTRATION

Intermittent infusion: Give by slow infusion only, over 1 hour (30 to 60 minutes when used for surgical prophylaxis). Discontinue the primary solution during drug administration.
Continuous infusion: Rarely used. Infuse diluted drug over ordered amount of time.

CONTRAINDICATIONS & CAUTIONS

• Contraindicated in hypersensitivity to metronidazole or other nitroimidazole derivatives.
• Use in pregnancy during the first trimester in patients with trichomoniasis is not recommended.
• Use cautiously in CNS disorders, blood dyscrasias, impaired cardiac function, predisposition to edema, and severe hepatic impairment.

M

• Safety and effectiveness in children have not been established.

SPECIAL CONSIDERATIONS
• RTU form of metronidazole contains 14 mEq (322 mg) of sodium. Neutralized IV solution contains 5 mEq (115 mg) of sodium.
• Symptoms of known or previously undiagnosed candidiasis may become more prominent during therapy, requiring treatment with an antifungal agent.
• Obtain CBC before and after therapy.
• If diarrhea persists during therapy, collect stool specimens for culture to rule out pseudomembranous colitis.

midazolam hydrochloride

Versed◆

Controlled Substance Schedule IV

Pregnancy Risk Category: D

INDICATIONS & DOSAGES
Dosages are highly individualized.
Conscious sedation—
Adults: initially, a maximum of 2.5 mg given over 2 to 3 minutes (some patients may respond to 1 mg), then increased in small increments at intervals of at least 2 minutes (to assess drug effect) until reaching desired effect.
Elderly or debilitated patients: 1 to 1.5 mg initially, given over a longer duration.
Induction of general anesthesia without premedication—
Adults age 55 and over: 300 mcg/kg.
Adults under age 55: 300 to 350 mcg/kg given over 20 to 30 seconds. Increments of 25% of initial dose may be needed to complete induction.
Adults with debilitation or severe systemic disease: 150 to 250 mcg/

kg. Total dose should not exceed 600 mcg/kg.
Induction of anesthesia following premedication with an opioid drug—
Adults age 55 and over: 200 mcg/kg.
Adults under age 55: 250 mcg/kg.
Adults with debilitation or severe systemic disease: 150 mcg/kg.
Clinical experience has shown Versed to be three to four times as potent per milligram as diazepam.

PREPARATION & STORAGE
Available in 1- and 5-mg/ml vials. Drug may be administered undiluted or diluted with D_5W, 0.9% NaCl, or lactated Ringer's solution. Mixtures with D_5W or 0.9% NaCl are stable for 24 hours; those with lactated Ringer's solution, for 4 hours.
Store undiluted solution at room temperature and protect from light. Once diluted, solution no longer requires protection from light.

Incompatibility
Incompatible with dimenhydrinate, pentobarbital sodium, perphenazine, prochlorperazine edisylate, and ranitidine hydrochloride.

ADMINISTRATION
Only staff specially trained in administering anesthetics and managing their adverse reactions should give midazolam. Also, equipment for respiratory and CV support should be readily available.
Direct injection: Inject directly into vein or established IV line containing a compatible solution over 2 to 3 minutes for conscious sedation or over 20 to 30 seconds for anesthesia induction.

CONTRAINDICATIONS & CAUTIONS
• Contraindicated in hypersensitivity to midazolam or other benzodiazepines and in severe shock, coma, or acute alcohol intoxication.
• Contraindicated in acute angle-closure glaucoma.
• Use cautiously in elderly or debilitated patients and in those with

COPD, renal impairment, and myasthenia gravis.
• Give carefully in heart failure and hepatic impairment.
• Safety and efficacy in children have not been established.

SPECIAL CONSIDERATIONS
• Give this potent drug slowly and in divided doses to titrate to effect. Rapid administration can lead to severe apnea, respiratory arrest, and hypotension, especially in elderly or debilitated patients.
• Give flumazenil 0.2 mg IV to reverse sedative effects. Provide general supportive measures.
• Monitor vital signs during administration.

milrinone lactate

Primacor

Pregnancy Risk Category: C

INDICATIONS & DOSAGES
Heart failure—
Adults: initial loading dose of 50 mcg/kg IV over 10 minutes, followed by continuous infusion dose of 0.375 to 0.75 mcg/kg/minute. Adjust dosage to hemodynamic and clinical response, not to exceed 1.13 mg/kg/day.

PREPARATION & STORAGE
Available in 10- and 20-ml vials, 1 mg/ml, and premixed 200 mcg/ ml in 5% dextrose (100 ml). Dilute with 0.45% or 0.9% NaCl or D_5W only. Store at room temperature (59° to 86° F [15° to 30° C]). Drug should not be used if particulate matter or discoloration is evident.

Incompatibility
Furosemide added to a line that contains this drug will form a precipitate.

ADMINISTRATION
Direct injection: A loading dose may be given undiluted, but diluting to a total volume of 10 to 20 ml aids with visualization of the injection rate.
Continuous infusion: Maintenance dosage should be adjusted according to patient response of increased cardiac output and reductions in pulmonary artery wedge pressure.

CONTRAINDICATIONS & CAUTIONS
• Contraindicated in hypersensitivity to drug and during acute phase of MI.
• Contraindicated in severe aortic or pulmonic valvular disease in place of surgical correction.
• Use cautiously in patients with atrial fibrillation or flutter.
• Safety and effectiveness in children have not been established.
• Caution women against breastfeeding during therapy.

SPECIAL CONSIDERATIONS
• Correct hypokalemia with potassium supplements before or during use of drug.
• Monitor renal function and fluid and electrolyte changes.
• Monitor blood pressure, heart rate, and clinical symptoms.

mitomycin

Mutamycin◆

Pregnancy Risk Category: NR

INDICATIONS & DOSAGES
Neoplasms, including adenocarcinomas of the stomach, pancreas, and colon, head and neck cancers, chronic myelogenous leukemia, advanced biliary, ovarian, and lung cancers, cervical squamous cell carcinomas, and transitional cell carcinoma of the urinary bladder—
Adults: dosage based on clinical and hematologic response and on concurrent myelosuppressant therapy. Twenty mg/m² can be given in sin-

M

gle dose and repeated q 6 to 8 weeks.

PREPARATION & STORAGE

Exercise extreme caution when preparing and administering mitomycin to avoid carcinogenic, teratogenic, and mutagenic risks. Use a biological containment cabinet, wear gloves and mask, and use syringes with luer-lock fittings. Dispose of vials, needles, syringes, and unused drug carefully.

Supplied in 5-, 20-, and 40-mg vials. Before reconstitution, store at room temperature. Reconstitute 5-mg vial with 10 ml (20 mg vial with 40 ml, 40 mg vial with 80 ml) of sterile water for injection. Shake to dissolve; do not use until completely dissolved.

Reconstituted solutions remain stable for 7 days at room temperature or for 14 days if refrigerated. Solutions further diluted in D_5W are stable for 3 hours at room temperature; in 0.9% NaCl, 12 hours; and in sodium lactate, 24 hours. If not used within 24 hours, protect from light.

Incompatibility
Incompatible with bleomycin sulfate.

ADMINISTRATION

Direct injection: Administer through a new IV site, preferably using a 23G or 25G winged-tip needle or an IV catheter. Use distal rather than major veins to allow for repeated venipunctures.
Intermittent infusion: Infuse diluted drug through a newly started IV line.

CONTRAINDICATIONS & CAUTIONS

• Contraindicated in existing or recent chickenpox or herpes zoster infection.
• Also contraindicated if patient's platelet count is below 75,000/mm^3, WBC count is below 3,000/mm^3, or serum creatinine exceeds 1.7 mg/dl.

• Administer cautiously in hypersensitivity to drug and in coagulation disorders, prolonged PT or bleeding time, or increased bleeding from other causes.
• Also use with caution in renal impairment, bone marrow depression, and infection.

SPECIAL CONSIDERATIONS

• Expect toxic effects with therapeutic doses. Evaluate patient before each course of therapy.
• Assess patient for renal dysfunction.
• Because of cumulative myelosuppression, monitor hematologic studies weekly during treatment and for at least 8 weeks afterward.
• Monitor pulmonary function during therapy.

mitoxantrone hydrochloride

Novantrone✦

Pregnancy Risk Category: D

INDICATIONS & DOSAGES

Combination therapy (with cytosine arabinoside) for acute nonlymphocytic leukemia—
Adults: initial therapy, 12 mg/m^2 on days 1 to 3 (combined with continuous IV infusion therapy with cytosine arabinoside given on days 1 to 7); consolidation therapy, 12 mg/m^2 on days 1 and 2 and cytosine arabinoside given as continuous infusion on days 1 to 5.

PREPARATION & STORAGE

Exercise extreme caution when preparing or administering drug to avoid mutagenic, teratogenic, and carcinogenic risks. Use a biological containment cabinet, wear gloves and mask, and use syringes with luerlock fittings to prevent leakage of drug solution. Be careful to correctly dispose of needles, vials, and unused drug, and avoid contaminating work

M

surfaces. Avoid inhalation of dust or vapors or contact with skin or mucous membranes.

Available as an aqueous solution of 2 mg/ml in volumes of 10, 12.5, and 15 ml. Store undiluted solution at room temperature. Avoid freezing.

Dilute dose in at least 50 ml of 0.9% NaCl injection or dextrose 5% injection. May be further diluted in D_5W, 0.9% NaCl, or dextrose 5% and 0.9% NaCl. Use immediately and discard unused solution.

Incompatibility
Incompatible with heparin sodium. Manufacturer recommends against mixing drug with any other drugs because not all incompatibilities are known.

ADMINISTRATION
Intermittent infusion: Infuse diluted solution slowly into a free-flowing IV line of 0.9% NaCl or D_5W over at least 3 minutes.

CONTRAINDICATIONS & CAUTIONS
• Contraindicated in hypersensitivity to drug.
• Also contraindicated in significant myelosuppression, unless benefits outweigh the risks.
• Use cautiously in patients with previous exposure to anthracyclines or other cardiotoxic drugs and in those with severe hepatic dysfunction.

SPECIAL CONSIDERATIONS
• Monitor hematology and chemistry laboratory parameters and liver function tests closely.
• Monitor left ventricular ejection fraction during administration.
• Monitor serum uric acid levels during therapy. Keeping patient well hydrated, alkalinizing urine, and administering allopurinol may prevent uric acid nephropathy.
• Inform patient that urine may appear blue-green within 24 hours after administration. Some bluish discoloration of the sclera may also occur.

mivacurium chloride

Mivacron

Pregnancy Risk Category: C

INDICATIONS & DOSAGES
As an adjunct to anesthesia, to facilitate endotracheal intubation, and to relax skeletal muscles during surgery or mechanical ventilation—
Adults: dosage is individualized; 0.15 mg/kg IV push over 5 to 15 seconds, 2.5 minutes prior to intubation. Supplemental doses of 0.1 mg/kg IV q 15 minutes. Continuous infusion of 4 mcg/kg/minute begun simultaneously with initial dose maintains neuromuscular blockade. Or, 9 to 10 mcg/kg/minute started after spontaneous recovery is noted from initial dose. Dosage is reduced up to 40% when used with isoflurane or enflurane anesthesia.
Children ages 2 to 12: 0.20 mg/kg IV push administered over 5 to 15 seconds. Maintenance doses are usually required more frequently in children. Neuromuscular blockade can be maintained with a continuous infusion titrated to effect. Most children respond to 5 to 31 mcg/kg/minute (average, 14 mcg/kg/minute).

PREPARATION & STORAGE
Available as 2 mg/ml in 5-ml single use and 10-ml multidose vials, and as an infusion of 0.5 mg/ml in 50- and 100-ml D_5W. Protect from ultraviolet light and from freezing, use within 24 hours.

Incompatibility
Drug should not be mixed with other medications.

ADMINISTRATION
Direct injection: Rapid IV bolus, 5 to 15 seconds.
Continuous infusion: Titrate drip to peripheral nerve stimulation and clinical criteria.

M

CONTRAINDICATIONS & CAUTIONS
• Contraindicated in hypersensitivity to drug. Multiple-dose vials contain benzyl alcohol as a preservative.
• Use cautiously in patients with significant CV disease and in those who may be adversely affected by release of histamine (asthmatics).
• Use cautiously in debilitated or breast-feeding patients and in those with metastatic cancer, severe electrolyte disturbances, or neuromuscular diseases.
• Use cautiously in patients in whom potentiation or difficulty in reversal of neuromuscular blockade is anticipated. Patients with myasthenia gravis or myasthenic syndrome are particularly sensitive.
• Use very cautiously, if at all, in patients who are homozygous for the atypical plasma pseudocholinesterase gene.

SPECIAL CONSIDERATIONS
• To avoid patient distress, do not administer until patient's consciousness is obtunded by general anesthetic because drug has no effect on consciousness or pain threshold.
• Dosage requirements for children are higher on a mg/kg basis than for adults. Onset and recovery occur more rapidly in children.
• Maintain airway and control ventilation until recovery of normal neuromuscular function is ensured.
• Monitor respirations closely until patient is fully recovered, as evidenced by tests of muscle strength (hand grip, head lift, and ability to cough).

morphine sulfate

Astramorph PF, Duramorph, Epimorph◇, Morphine H.P.◇

Controlled Substance Schedule II

Pregnancy Risk Category: C

INDICATIONS & DOSAGES
Severe pain—

Adults: 2.5 to 15 mg q 4 hours p.r.n.
Children: 50 to 100 mcg/kg; maximum single dose, 10 mg.
Pain associated with MI—
Adults: 2 to 15 mg, followed by smaller doses q 3 to 4 hours p.r.n.
Severe chronic pain—
Adults: 1 to 10 mg/hour by continuous infusion. Maintenance dosage, 20 to 150 mg/hour.
Children: 0.025 to 2.6 mg/kg/hour.

PREPARATION & STORAGE
Available with preservative in concentrations of 1, 2, 4, 5, 8, 10, 15, 25, and 50 mg/ml in the United States; 1-mg/ml solutions are available in Canada only. Available without preservatives in concentrations of 0.5, 1, and 15 mg/ml in the United States; 50-mg/ml solutions are available in Canada only.

For direct injection, dilute with 4 or 5 ml of D_5W. Dilute with larger volumes for slow infusion. Morphine is compatible with most common IV solutions. Store below 104° F (40° C), and protect from light and freezing.

Incompatibility
Incompatible with aminophylline, amobarbital sodium, soluble barbiturates, cefepime hydrochloride, chlorothiazide, heparin sodium, meperidine, methicillin, phenobarbital sodium, phenytoin sodium, promethazine hydrochloride, sodium bicarbonate, sodium iodide, and thiopental sodium.

ADMINISTRATION
Direct injection: Inject diluted drug over 4 to 5 minutes through IV tubing containing a free-flowing, compatible solution. Monitor vital signs and respiratory status for at least 1 hour after injection.
Continuous infusion: Infuse diluted drug at 1 to 10 mg/hour initially, increasing rate until reaching effective dosage. Monitor vital signs and respiratory status.

CONTRAINDICATIONS & CAUTIONS
• Contraindicated in hypersensitivity to morphine.
• Also contraindicated in acute respiratory depression or diarrhea resulting from pseudomembranous colitis or poisoning.
• Drug should not be used in pulmonary edema caused by a chemical respiratory irritant.
• Use with caution in altered respiratory function and in arrhythmias.
• Use cautiously in patients with history of drug dependence or emotional instability, or in those who show evidence of suicidal ideation.
• Administer carefully in seizure disorders, hypothyroidism, acute abdominal conditions, gallbladder disease, inflammatory bowel disease, and after recent GI surgery.
• Also use cautiously in head injury and increased intracranial pressure (from intracranial lesions).
• Also give cautiously to patients with hepatic or renal impairment, prostatic hypertrophy, urethral stricture, or recent urinary tract surgery.

SPECIAL CONSIDERATIONS
• Administer drug with patient in supine position to minimize hypotension.
• Rapid infusion can cause life-threatening adverse reactions. Ambulatory patients and patients who are not experiencing severe pain have a higher incidence of adverse reactions.
• Dose may need to be extended in patients with severe chronic pain who have become tolerant to analgesic effects of opioids.
• Generic preparations may contain sulfites.
• Keep a narcotic antagonist available.
• Monitor respirations frequently during infusion and every 15 minutes for 1 hour after infusion.

muromonab-CD3

Orthoclone OKT3 ✦

Pregnancy Risk Category: C

INDICATIONS & DOSAGES
Acute allograft rejection in heart, liver, or kidney transplant—
Adults: 5 mg daily for 10 to 14 days.

PREPARATION & STORAGE
Available in 1-mg/ml ampules. Store in refrigerator unless otherwise specified by the manufacturer. Protect from freezing. Do not shake ampule. Draw solution into syringe through a low-protein-binding 0.2 or 0.22 micrometer filter, then discard filter and attach appropriate needle. Appearance of fine, translucent particles in solution does not indicate loss of potency.

Incompatibility
None reported.

ADMINISTRATION
Direct injection: Give by IV push directly into vein over less than 1 minute. Do not administer with IV fluids.

CONTRAINDICATIONS & CAUTIONS
• Contraindicated in existing or recent chickenpox and herpes zoster infection or if patient's temperature exceeds 100°F (37.8° C).
• Also contraindicated in patients with fluid overload.
• Use cautiously in infection, hypersensitivity to drug, or a predisposition to or history of seizures.
• Use with caution in breast-feeding patients. Advise women to avoid becoming pregnant during therapy.
• Safe use in children has not been established.

SPECIAL CONSIDERATIONS
• Keep equipment and medication for advanced life support readily available during first dose.

- Give an antipyretic and antihistamine before therapy to reduce expected pyrexia and chills. Keep cooling blanket available.
- Usually, muromonab-CD3 is used with azathioprine, corticosteroids, or both.
- Monitor temperature, CBC, and tests for circulating T cells expressing the CD3 antigen.

nafcillin sodium

Nafcil, Nallpen, Unipen◆

Pregnancy Risk Category: B

INDICATIONS & DOSAGES
Severe systemic infections caused by susceptible organisms—
Adults: 0.5 to 1 g q 4 hours (depending on severity of infection) for 14 days.
Children over age 1 month: 50 to 100 mg/kg/day in equally divided doses q 6 hours for 14 days.
Osteomyelitis and endocarditis—
Adults: 1 to 2 g q 4 hours for 4 to 8 weeks.
Children over age 1 month: 100 to 200 mg/kg/day in equally divided doses q 4 to 6 hours for 4 to 8 weeks.
Meningitis—
Adults: 100 to 200 mg/kg/day in equally divided doses q 4 to 6 hours for at least 14 days.

PREPARATION & STORAGE
Available as a white to yellow-white powder in 500-mg and 1-, 2-, and 10-g vials. Store at room temperature. To reconstitute, add 1.7 ml, 3.4 ml, or 6.8 ml of sterile water for injection, bacteriostatic water for injection, or 0.9% NaCl to 500-mg, 1-g, or 2-g vials, respectively. For larger doses, follow manufacturer's directions.

For direct injection, further dilute with 15 to 30 ml of sterile water for injection or 0.45% or 0.9% NaCl for injection. For intermittent infusion, further dilute to a concentration of 2 to 40 mg/ml or according to manufacturer's directions (Nallpen). Drug is compatible with D_5W, lactated Ringer's, or 0.9% NaCl.

After reconstitution with sterile water or 0.9% NaCl, solution of 250 mg/ml is stable for 3 days at 77° F (25° C), for 7 days if refrigerated, or for 3 months if frozen. At concentrations of 10 to 40 mg/ml, drug begins to lose potency in 24 hours at room temperature or in 4 days if refrigerated.

Incompatibility
Incompatible with aminoglycosides, aminophylline, ascorbic acid, aztreonam, bleomycin sulfate, cytarabine, droperidol, fentanyl, hydrocortisone sodium succinate, insulin (regular), labetalol hydrochloride, metaraminol bitartrate, meperidine hydrochloride, methylprednisolone sodium succinate, nalbuphine hydrochloride, pentazocine lactate, promazine hydrochloride, verapamil hydrochloride, and vitamin B complex with C.

ADMINISTRATION
Direct injection: Inject dose directly into vein or into IV line containing a free-flowing, compatible solution. Administer over 5 to 10 minutes.
Intermittent infusion: Infuse dose over at least 30 to 60 minutes.
Continuous infusion: Add daily amount of nafcillin (only in concentrations of 2 to 40 mg/ml) to solution to be administered over 24 hours. Regulate accordingly.

CONTRAINDICATIONS & CAUTIONS
- Contraindicated in hypersensitivity to penicillins, cephalosporins, or imipenem.
- Use with caution in hepatic impairment, eosinophilia or hemolytic anemia, GI disorders, and history of an allergy.
- Use cautiously in patients with sodium restrictions.
- Advise patient using oral contraceptives to use alternative method of birth control while taking drug.

◆Also available in Canada. ◇Available in Canada only.

SPECIAL CONSIDERATIONS
• Before giving first dose, ask patient about previous allergic reactions to penicillins or cephalosporins. Negative history does not rule out future hypersensitivity reaction.
• Obtain WBC count and differential before therapy and one to three times weekly during therapy.
• If diarrhea persists during therapy, collect stool specimens for culture to rule out pseudomembranous colitis.

nalbuphine hydrochloride

Nubain♦

Pregnancy Risk Category: B (D for prolonged use or in high doses given at term)

INDICATIONS & DOSAGES
Moderate to severe pain and preoperative analgesia; supplement to obstetric analgesia—
Adults: 10 mg (or 0.14 mg/kg) q 3 to 6 hours. Maximum single dose, 20 mg; maximum daily dose, 160 mg.
Supplement to balanced anesthesia—
Adults: 0.3 to 3 mg/kg over 10 to 15 minutes. Maintenance dosage, 0.25 to 0.5 mg/kg p.r.n.

PREPARATION & STORAGE
Supplied in 1-ml ampules, 10-ml vials, and 1-ml disposable syringes in 10-mg/ml or 20-mg/ml concentration. Protect from freezing, excessive light, and heat. Store at room temperature. Nalbuphine is compatible with D_5W, lactated Ringer's, and 0.9% NaCl.

Incompatibility
Incompatible with allopurinol sodium, cefepime hydrochloride, diazepam, ketorolac, nafcillin sodium, pentobarbital sodium, piperacillin-tazobactam sodium, promethazine hydrochloride, sargramostim, thiethylperazine maleate, and tromethamine.

ADMINISTRATION
Direct injection: Inject drug directly into vein or into an IV line containing a compatible, free-flowing IV solution over 2 to 3 minutes or longer. Avoid rapid injection, which can precipitate anaphylaxis, peripheral circulatory collapse, or cardiac arrest.

CONTRAINDICATIONS & CAUTIONS
• Contraindicated in hypersensitivity to nalbuphine and in diarrhea associated with pseudomembranous colitis or poisoning.
• Avoid use in severely altered respiratory function.
• Use with extreme caution in head injury and increased intracranial pressure.
• Use cautiously in patients with MI who experience nausea and vomiting.
• Use cautiously in patients receiving chronic opioid therapy.
• Administer carefully to patients about to undergo biliary tract surgery or to those with gallbladder disease, acute abdominal conditions, or inflammatory bowel disease, and after recent GI surgery.
• Also administer carefully to patients with sulfite sensitivity, asthma, chronic respiratory disease, or hypothyroidism, sulfite sensitivity, or history of seizures.
• Use carefully in the elderly and in prostatic hyperplasia, urinary tract obstruction, urethral stricture, recent urinary tract surgery, renal dysfunction, and hepatic or renal impairment.

SPECIAL CONSIDERATIONS
• Administer drug with patient in supine position to minimize hypotensive effects.
• In long-term use of other opioid agonists, give only 25% of initial nalbuphine dose, as ordered. Monitor for withdrawal symptoms. If necessary, give slowly in small increments. If withdrawal symptoms fail to occur, increase dose progressively until reaching desired level of analgesia.
• Drug may contain sulfites.

N

• In cases of overdose, provide airway and respiratory support. Give naloxone, as needed, to reverse respiratory depression. Also administer IV fluids and vasopressors to maintain blood pressure.

naloxone hydrochloride

Narcan♦

Pregnancy Risk Category: B

INDICATIONS & DOSAGES
Opioid toxicity—
Adults: 0.4 mg to 2 mg initially, repeated q 2 to 3 minutes p.r.n.; or 0.4 mg followed by continuous infusion of 0.4 mg/hour, titrated to patient's response.
Children: 0.01 mg/kg initially, then 0.1 mg/kg repeated q 2 to 3 minutes for up to two more doses; or 0.4 mg/hour by continuous infusion, titrated to patient's response.
Neonates: 0.01 mg/kg initially, repeated q 2 to 3 minutes until desired response is obtained.
Postoperative opioid depression—
Adults: 0.1 to 0.2 mg q 2 to 3 minutes until ventilation is adequate; may be repeated at 1- to 2-hour intervals.
Children: 0.005 to 0.01 mg q 2 to 3 minutes until ventilation is adequate and child is alert; may be repeated at 1- to 2-hour intervals.

PREPARATION & STORAGE
Available in 0.02-, 0.4-, and 1-mg vials, ampules, and syringes. Store at 59° to 86° F (15° to 30° C) and protect from light. Avoid freezing. For a concentration of 0.004 mg/ml, mix 2 mg of drug in 500 ml of D_5W or 0.9% NaCl. Solution is stable for 24 hours. Discard unused portion after 24 hours. For a concentration of 0.02 mg/ml, dilute 0.5 ml of adult dose (0.4 mg/ml) with 9.5 ml of sterile water or 0.9% NaCl for injection.

Incompatibility
None reported. However, manufacturer recommends that naloxone not be mixed with any other drug, especially preparations containing bisulfite, metabisulfite, long-chain or high-molecular-weight anions, or alkaline solutions.

ADMINISTRATION
Direct injection: Inject drug directly into vein or into an established IV line containing a free-flowing, compatible solution.
Continuous infusion: Infuse at rate titrated to patient's needs. Pediatric rate may range from 0.024 to 0.16 mg/kg/hour.

CONTRAINDICATIONS & CAUTIONS
• Contraindicated in hypersensitivity to naloxone.
• Use cautiously in patients physically dependent on opioids.
• Also use cautiously in postoperative patients with cardiac dysfunction or in those receiving cardiotoxic drugs.

SPECIAL CONSIDERATIONS
• In the detoxified opioid addict, give naloxone challenge test, as ordered, before initiating therapy.
• Closely monitor respiratory, cardiac, and hemodynamic status for at least 24 hours. Duration of action of some narcotics may be longer than that of naloxone. Also, respiratory rate may suddenly exceed patient's normal rate.
• Monitor for signs of withdrawal.
• Lack of response indicates condition is not caused by opioid CNS depressant.

neostigmine methylsulfate

Prostigmin♦

Pregnancy Risk Category: C

INDICATIONS & DOSAGES
Myasthenia gravis—

Dosage varies widely, depending on patient needs and response.
Adults: 0.5 to 2.5 mg p.r.n.
Antidote for nondepolarizing neuro-muscular blocking agents—
Adults: 0.5 to 2 mg, repeated p.r.n. to maximum total dose of 5 mg.
Children: 0.025 to 0.8 mg/kg.

PREPARATION & STORAGE
Available in 1-ml ampules of 1:2,000 (0.5 mg/ml) and 1:4,000 (0.25 mg/ ml). Also available in multidose vials of 1:1,000 (1 mg/ml) and 1:2,000 (0.5 mg/ml). Protect solution from light and avoid freezing. Neostig-mine needs no further dilution.

Incompatibility
None reported.

ADMINISTRATION
Direct injection: Inject drug slowly into tubing of patent, free-flowing IV line containing D_5W, 0.9% NaCl, or another compatible IV solution.

CONTRAINDICATIONS & CAUTIONS
• Contraindicated in hypersensitivity to neostigmine.
• Also contraindicated in peritonitis or mechanical obstruction of intesti-nal or urinary tract.
• Use with caution in patients with asthma, bradycardia, arrhythmias, peptic ulcer disease, epilepsy, and hy-perthyroidism.
• Give carefully after surgery because respiratory difficulty may be aggra-vated.

SPECIAL CONSIDERATIONS
• When drug is used to reverse the effects of nondepolarizing neuro-muscular blockers, keep patient on assisted ventilation.
• IV dose will be much smaller than an oral dose. In critically ill patients, exact dose may be titrated with the use of peripheral nerve stimulators.
• In cases of overdose, maintain ade-quate ventilation, discontinue neo-stigmine and administer 1 to 4 mg of atropine sulfate. Additional doses

of atropine may be given every 5 to 30 minutes, as needed.
• Establish baseline respiratory rate and maintain a patent airway using suctioning, oxygen, and assisted ven-tilation, as necessary.
• Instruct patient to report excessive salivation, muscle weakness, severe abdominal pain, irregular heartbeat, or difficulty breathing.

nitroglycerin

Nitro-Bid IV◆, Nitrol, Nitrostat◆, Tridil◆
Pregnancy Risk Category: C

INDICATIONS & DOSAGES
Heart failure and chest pain associat-ed with MI; acute angina pectoris; blood pressure reduction during surgery—
Adults: 5 mcg/minute initially, then increased by 5 mcg/minute q 3 to 5 minutes until desired response is achieved. If response is inadequate at 20 mcg/minute, increase dose by 10 to 20 mcg/minute and give q 3 to 5 minutes if necessary. Once partial re-sponse is obtained, increases in dosage increments should be re-duced and interval between dosage increases should be lengthened. Maximum dose is not established.

PREPARATION & STORAGE
Several preparations of nitroglycerin for IV injection are available in vari-ous concentrations. Each comes with diluent instruction and dosage.
    Nitro-Bid IV is supplied in 1-, 5-, and 10-ml vials of 5 mg/ml. Dilute with D_5W or 0.9% NaCl. For a con-centration of 50 mcg/ml, mix 1 ml of drug in 100 ml of solution; for 100 mcg/ml, mix 1 ml of drug in 50 ml of solution; for 200 mcg/ml, mix 2 ml of drug in 50 ml of solu-tion.
    Nitrol concentrate is available in a 10-ml ampule containing 5 mg/ml. Dilute initially by adding one 10-ml

N

ampule (50 mg) to 500 ml of D_5W or 0.9% NaCl to yield 100 mcg/ml. For maintenance infusion, dilute two ampules in 500 ml of solution for a concentration of 200 mcg/ml, or four ampules in 500 ml of solution for 400 mcg/ml.

Nitrostat comes in a kit with a 10-ml ampule containing 0.8 mg/ml and a disposable IV infusion set. Mix contents of ampule with 250 ml of D_5W or 0.9% NaCl for 32 mcg/ml.

Tridil is available as a 5-mg/ml concentration in 5-, 10-, and 20-ml ampules and vials. It is also available as a 0.5-mg/ml concentration in 10-ml ampules. Mix a 25-mg or 50-mg ampule with 500 ml of D_5W or 0.9% NaCl for 50 or 100 mcg/ml, respectively. Diluting 5 mg of drug in 100 ml of solution yields 50 mcg/ml.

Store nitroglycerin preparations at room temperature and protect from light. Avoid freezing. After reconstitution, drug is stable for 48 hours at room temperature. Mix and store in glass bottle, which is usually supplied (along with tubing) with most products.

Know that the type of infusion set affects the amount of drug delivered. Use only nonabsorbent tubing; polyvinyl chloride tubing may absorb up to 80% of diluted drug from solution. Using polyvinyl chloride extension tubing for the infusion pump may negate advantages of the nonpolyvinyl chloride set supplied with the drug.

Incompatibility
Avoid mixing with other drugs. Incompatible with alteplase, hydralazine hydrochloride, and phenytoin sodium.

ADMINISTRATION
Continuous infusion: Infuse diluted drug at the rate required for therapeutic effect. Always use a volume-control device and a microdrip regulator. Closely monitor the patient's response to nitroglycerin.

CONTRAINDICATIONS & CAUTIONS
• Contraindicated in hypersensitivity to nitroglycerin or nitrates.
• Also contraindicated in hypotension, uncorrected hypovolemia, and increased intracranial pressure.
• Avoid use in constrictive pericarditis, pericardial tamponade, and hypertrophic cardiomyopathy.
• Use cautiously in glaucoma, hyperthyroidism, hypotension, tachycardia, and severe hepatic or renal impairment.

SPECIAL CONSIDERATIONS
• In cases of overdose, elevate patient's legs and reduce infusion rate or temporarily stop infusion. If severe hypotension persists, give an alpha-adrenergic agonist (phenylephrine) IV, as ordered.
• During therapy, monitor blood pressure and heart rate and rhythm continuously; response to drug varies greatly.
• Assist patient with sitting up and standing until he can tolerate orthostatic hypotension.
• Instruct patient to report chest pain or angina.

nitroprusside sodium

Nipride◇, Nitropress
Pregnancy Risk Category: C

INDICATIONS & DOSAGES
Rapid blood pressure reduction in hypertensive emergencies, control of hypertension during anesthesia, reduction of preload and afterload in cardiac pump failure or cardiogenic shock—
Adults and children who are not receiving other hypotensive drugs: 0.3 to 10 mcg/kg/minute; average dose, 3 mcg/kg/minute. Monitor blood pressure closely and titrate drug to patient's response. Maximum dose is 10 mcg/kg/minute.

PREPARATION & STORAGE

Available as a powder in 50-mg vial. Reconstitute with 2 to 3 ml of D_5W or sterile water for injection *without* preservatives. Then dilute in 250 to 1,000 ml of D_5W to desired concentration. Store at room temperature and protect from light, heat, and moisture. Reconstituted solution is stable for 24 hours. Discard solution if discolored (blue, green, or dark red), which indicates a reaction with another substance. After reconstitution, protect solution from light by covering with aluminum foil or other opaque material. It is unnecessary to cover tubing or drip chamber.

Incompatibility

Incompatible with bacteriostatic water for injection. Do not add any other drug or preservative to nitroprusside solution.

ADMINISTRATION

Use nitroprusside only if adequate staff and equipment are available for arterial blood pressure monitoring. *Continuous infusion:* Using an infusion pump, administer diluted solution at a rate that maintains desired hypotensive effect.

CONTRAINDICATIONS & CAUTIONS

• Contraindicated in inadequate cerebral circulation or coronary artery insufficiency; in compensatory hypertension; and during emergency surgery for patients near death.
• Use with extreme caution in patients who are poor surgical risks.
• Use with caution in severe renal impairment, hepatic insufficiency, hypothyroidism, anemia, hypovolemia, Leber's hereditary optic atrophy, or tobacco amblyopia.
• Also give cautiously in the elderly and in pulmonary impairment and low serum vitamin B_{12} levels.

SPECIAL CONSIDERATIONS

• Avoid extravasation.
• If metabolic acidosis occurs, discontinue drug and expect to try alternative therapy.

• In cases of overdose, give nitrites to promote methemoglobin formation. In massive overdose, discontinue nitroprusside and administer amyl nitrate by inhalation for 15 to 30 seconds each minute until a 3% sodium nitrite solution can be prepared.
• Monitor blood pressure frequently.

norepinephrine bitartrate

Levophed ♦

Pregnancy Risk Category: C

INDICATIONS & DOSAGES

Control of acute hypotensive states and as an adjunct in the treatment of cardiac arrest—
Adults: 8 to 12 mcg/minute initially, then adjusted (usually 2 to 4 mcg/minute) to maintain desired blood pressure range.
Children: 0.1 mcg/kg/minute initially, then adjusted (usually 2 mcg/minute) to maintain desired blood pressure range.

PREPARATION & STORAGE

Available in 4-ml ampules containing 1 mg/ml. Store ampules at room temperature. For infusion, mix one ampule (4 mg) of norepinephrine in 1,000 ml of D_5W or dextrose 5% in 0.9% NaCl for a concentration of 4 mcg/ml. Alter concentration, as necessary, to reflect patient's drug and fluid volume requirements. Discard diluted solution after 24 hours. Discard if solution contains precipitate or if it is brown, pink, or yellow.

Incompatibility

Incompatible with aminophylline, amobarbital sodium, cephalothin sodium, cephapirin sodium, chlorothiazide sodium, chlorpheniramine maleate, lidocaine hydrochloride, pentobarbital sodium, phenobarbital sodium, phenytoin sodium,

N

secobarbital sodium, sodium bicarbonate, sodium iodide, streptomycin sulfate, thiopental sodium, and whole blood. Also, manufacturer recommends that drug not be mixed in 0.9% NaCl.

ADMINISTRATION
Continuous injection: Insert a plastic IV catheter deeply into large vein. Do not use leg veins in the elderly or in patients with peripheral vascular disease. Use microdrip tubing and an infusion pump to carefully regulate flow rate. Infuse drug at a rate that maintains blood pressure at a low normal, usually 80 to 100 mm Hg systolic or, for previously hypertensive patients, maximum of 40 mm Hg below previous systolic pressure.

CONTRAINDICATIONS & CAUTIONS
• Contraindicated in hypersensitivity to norepinephrine, other sympathomimetics, or sulfite content in preparation.
• Also contraindicated in patients with hypotension from blood loss.
• Avoid use in mesenteric or peripheral vascular thrombosis or other occlusive vascular disorders; in patients receiving cyclopropane or halothane anesthetics; or in hypoxia or hypercarbia.
• Give drug cautiously to patients with hyperthyroidism, hypertension, or severe cardiac disease, and to the elderly.

SPECIAL CONSIDERATIONS
• Avoid prolonged use, when possible, to prevent ischemia of vital organs.
• Drug may contain sulfites.
• During infusion, check blood pressure every 2 minutes until stable, then every 5 to 15 minutes, using intra-arterial monitoring.
• Also monitor the patient's mental status, skin temperature, and color of extremities (especially earlobes, lips, and nail beds).

octreotide acetate

Sandostatin
Pregnancy Risk Category: B

INDICATIONS & DOSAGES
Symptomatic treatment of flushing and diarrhea associated with carcinoid tumors—
Adults: initially, 100 to 600 mcg daily in two to four divided doses for first 2 weeks (usual daily dosage, 300 mcg). Subsequent dosage based on individual response.
Symptomatic treatment of watery diarrhea associated with vasoactive intestinal peptide-secreting tumors—
Adults: 200 to 300 mcg daily in two to four divided doses for first 2 weeks of therapy. Subsequent dosage based on individual response, but usually does not exceed 450 mcg daily.
Acromegaly—
Adults: initially, 50 mcg t.i.d. Subsequent dosage based on individual response. Usual dosage is 100 mcg t.i.d. but some patients require up to 500 mcg t.i.d. for maximum effectiveness.

PREPARATION & STORAGE
Available in 50-, 100-, and 500-mcg/ml ampules and 200- and 1,000-mcg/ml multidose vials. Store vials and ampules in refrigerator at 36° to 46° F (2° to 8° C) and protect from light. Stable at room temperature for 14 days if protected from light. Do not warm solution artificially. Solution is stable in sterile isotonic saline solution or D_5W for 24 hours. After initial use, multidose vials should be discarded after 14 days. Discard unused portion of ampules. Do not use if particulates or discoloration, or both, are noted.
Dilute in volumes of 50 to 200 ml and infuse IV or by IV push.

Incompatibility
Incompatible with total parenteral nutrition.

ADMINISTRATION
Direct injection: Inject directly into vein or compatible IV solution over 3 minutes.
Intermittent infusion: Administer diluted solution over 15 to 30 minutes.

CONTRAINDICATIONS & CAUTIONS
• Contraindicated in hypersensitivity to drug or its components.
• Use with caution when giving to breast-feeding women because it is not known whether drug is excreted into breast milk.
• Half-life of drug may be altered in patients undergoing dialysis for end-stage renal failure.

SPECIAL CONSIDERATIONS
• Monitor fluid and electrolyte balance during therapy.
• Perform baseline and periodic testing of thyroid function because drug suppresses thyroid-stimulating hormone secretion.
• Mild, transient high or low blood sugar may occur during therapy.
• Instruct patient to notify doctor if abdominal discomfort occurs because drug may cause gallstones.

ofloxacin

Floxin IV

Pregnancy Risk Category: C

INDICATIONS & DOSAGES
Acute bacterial exacerbations of bronchitis or pneumonia caused by susceptible organisms—
Adults: 400 mg infused over 60 minutes q 12 hours for 10 days.
Endocervical and urethral chlamydial infection with or without concurrent gonorrhea—
Adults: 300 mg infused over 60 minutes q 12 hours for 7 days.
Uncomplicated gonorrhea—
Adults: 400 mg infused over 60 minutes as a single dose.
Prostatitis caused by Escherichia coli—

Adults: 300 mg infused over 60 minutes q 12 hours for 6 weeks (can switch to oral route after 10 days).
Skin and soft-tissue infections—
Adults: 400 mg infused over 60 minutes q 12 hours for 10 days.
Cystitis caused by E. coli *or* Klebsiella pneumoniae—
Adults: 200 mg infused over 60 minutes q 12 hours for 3 days.
Urinary tract infections caused by susceptible strains of Citrobacter diversus, Enterobacter aerogenes, E. coli, Proteus mirabilis, *or* Pseudomonas aeruginosa—
Adults: 200 mg infused over 60 minutes q 12 hours for 7 days. Complicated infections may require therapy for 10 days.
    Note: Adjust dosage in patients with creatinine clearance of 50 ml/minute or less.

PREPARATION & STORAGE
Available premixed in 100-ml glass bottles or 50- and 100-ml plastic bags with 4 mg/ml of drug in dextrose 5% injection. Premixed solutions do not require further dilution. Also supplied in 10- and 20-ml single-use vials with 400 mg of drug in water for injection. Store below 86° F (30° C) and protect from freezing or light. Use immediately after opening. Discard unused portions.
    To dilute, withdraw the appropriate dose from vial and add to 50 or 100 ml of 0.9% NaCl, D_5W, or other compatible IV fluid to yield a concentration of 4 mg/ml. Resultant solution is stable for 72 hours when stored at or below 75° F (24° C), and for 14 days when refrigerated at 41° F (5° C) in glass bottles or plastic IV containers. Solutions that are diluted and frozen are stable for 6 months at –4° F (–20° C). Thaw frozen solution at room temperature or in the refrigerator; do not microwave or immerse in hot water. Once thawed, solution is stable for up to 14 days under refrigeration. Do not refreeze after

O

initial thawing. Do not use a discolored or precipitated solution.

Incompatibility
Do not mix with other drugs or infuse simultaneously through the same line.

ADMINISTRATION
Intermittent infusion: Infuse over 60 minutes.

CONTRAINDICATIONS & CAUTIONS
• Contraindicated in hypersensitivity to drug or other quinolones and in children or breast-feeding women.
• Use cautiously in patients with history of seizure disorders or other CNS diseases.
• Use during pregnancy only when benefits outweigh fetal risks.

SPECIAL CONSIDERATIONS
• Perform regular blood studies and hepatic and renal function tests during prolonged therapy.
• Patients treated for gonorrhea should have a serologic test for syphilis. Drug is not effective against syphilis, and treatment of gonorrhea may mask or delay symptoms of syphilis.
• If rash or other signs of hypersensitivity develop, discontinue drug and notify doctor.

ondansetron hydrochloride

Zofran

Pregnancy Risk Category: B

INDICATIONS & DOSAGES
Prevention of nausea and vomiting associated with emetogenic chemotherapy—
Adults and children age 4 and over: three doses of 0.15 mg/kg. Give first dose 30 minutes before chemotherapy; subsequent doses at 4 and 8 hours after first dose. Alternatively, adults and children age 12 and over may receive 32-mg infusion over 15 minutes beginning 30 minutes before chemotherapy.
Prevention of postoperative nausea and vomiting—
Adults: 4 mg (undiluted) over 2 to 5 minutes.

PREPARATION & STORAGE
Available in 2-mg/ml and 20-ml multiple-dose vials containing 2 mg/ml. Solution has pH of 3.3 to 4. Before administration, dilute drug in 50 ml of compatible solution (such as D_5W for injection, 0.9% NaCl for injection, dextrose 5% in 0.9% NaCl for injection, dextrose 5% in 0.45% NaCl for injection, and 3% NaCl for injection). Drug is stable for up to 48 hours in polyvinyl chloride bags after dilution when refrigerated at 39° F (4° C) or kept at room temperature 77° F (25° C). Store at room temperature and protect from light. It is not necessary to protect drug from light during administration.

Incompatibility
Incompatible with acyclovir sodium, allopurinol, aminophylline, amphotericin B, ampicillin sodium, ampicillin sodium and sulbactam sodium, amsacrine, cefepime hydrochloride, cefoperazone sodium, fluorouracil, furosemide, ganciclovir sodium, lorazepam, methylprednisolone sodium succinate, mezlocillin sodium, piperacillin sodium, sargramostim, and sodium bicarbonate.

ADMINISTRATION
Direct injection: Give undiluted over 2 to 5 minutes. (For postoperative nausea and vomiting only.)
Intermittent infusion: Dilute drug in 50 ml of compatible solution and infuse over 15 minutes.

CONTRAINDICATIONS & CAUTIONS
• Contraindicated in hypersensitivity to drug.
• Use cautiously in patients with compromised liver function.

• Drug is not currently indicated for use in patients receiving multiple-day courses of antineoplastic therapy or for prophylaxis of chemotherapy-induced delayed nausea and vomiting.

SPECIAL CONSIDERATIONS
• In clinical trials, use of dexamethasone combined with ondansetron provided significantly better control of emesis than ondansetron alone.
• Monitor liver function tests for hepatotoxicity.
• Instruct patient to alert nurse immediately if difficulty in breathing occurs after drug administration.
• Tell patient to immediately report discomfort at IV site.

oxacillin sodium

Bactocill, Prostaphlin
Pregnancy Risk Category: B

INDICATIONS & DOSAGES
Severe infections caused by susceptible organisms—
Adults: 1 g q 4 to 6 hours.
Children weighing less than 88 lb (40 kg): 100 to 200 mg/kg/day in equal doses q 4 to 6 hours.
Mild to moderate infections caused by susceptible organisms—
Adults: 250 to 500 mg q 4 to 6 hours.
Children weighing less than 88 lb: 50 mg/kg/day in equal doses q 6 hours.
Endocarditis or chronic osteomyelitis caused by susceptible organisms—
Adults: 1.5 to 2 g q 4 hours.
   Note: Adjust dosage in renal impairment. For adults, dosage reflects creatinine clearance. If clearance is less than 10 ml/minute, dosage is 1 g q 4 to 6 hours.

PREPARATION & STORAGE
Available in powder form in 250- and 500-mg and 1-, 2-, and 4-g vials. Reconstitute with sterile water for injection or 0.9% NaCl. For di-

rect injection, add 5 ml of sterile water for injection or 0.9% NaCl to 250- or 500-mg vial; 10 ml to 1-g vial; 20 ml to 2-g vial; and 40 ml to 4-g vial. For intermittent infusion, mix 50 to 100 ml of diluent with 1- or 2-g vial and 93 ml with 4-g vial. Solutions are stable for 3 days at room temperature and for 1 week if refrigerated. Compatible solutions include dextrose 5% in lactated Ringer's, dextrose 5% in 0.9% NaCl, D_5W or dextrose 10% in water, lactated Ringer's, and 0.9% NaCl.

Incompatibility
Incompatible with acidic drugs, aminoglycosides, cytarabine, and verapamil hydrochloride.

ADMINISTRATION
Direct injection: Inject drug over 10 minutes through an intermittent infusion device or into an IV line containing a free-flowing, compatible solution.
Intermittent infusion: Infuse diluted solution through an intermittent infusion device or using an IV line containing a free-flowing, compatible solution over the ordered duration.

CONTRAINDICATIONS & CAUTIONS
• Contraindicated in penicillin, cephalosporin, or imipenem hypersensitivity.
• Use with caution in interstitial nephritis and history of GI disease.

SPECIAL CONSIDERATIONS
• Drug contains about 3.1 mEq of sodium per gram.
• Monitor WBC count before therapy and once to three times weekly during therapy.
• Assess renal and hepatic function before therapy and periodically during therapy. Closely monitor neonates for hepatotoxicity and nephrotoxicity.
• If diarrhea persists during therapy, obtain stool specimen for culture.
• Instruct patient to notify doctor if sore throat, fever, mucosal ulcera-

O

tions, rash, or unusual bleeding or bruising occurs.
• Inform patient that discomfort at injection site is a typical reaction.

oxymorphone hydrochloride

Numorphan ♦

Controlled Substance Schedule II

Pregnancy Risk Category: C

INDICATIONS & DOSAGES
Moderate to severe pain—
Adults: initially, 0.5 mg q 3 to 4 hours. Dose may be increased cautiously up to 1 mg in nondebilitated patients.

PREPARATION & STORAGE
Supplied in 1- and 1.5-mg/ml ampules and in 1.5-mg/ml vials. Protect from freezing, light, and excessive heat. Store between 59° and 86° F (15° and 30° C). No further dilution is needed for direct injection. Compatible solutions include D_5W, dextrose 5% in 0.9% NaCl, and lactated Ringer's.

Incompatibility
None reported.

ADMINISTRATION
Direct injection: Inject dose directly into a vein or into an IV line containing a free-flowing, compatible solution. Administer over 2 to 3 minutes.

CONTRAINDICATIONS & CAUTIONS
• Contraindicated in hypersensitivity to drug and in children under age 12.
• Also contraindicated in patients with diarrhea related to pseudomembranous colitis or poisoning.
• Avoid use in acute respiratory depression.
• Use with extreme caution in altered respiratory function, head in-

jury, or increased intracranial pressure.
• Use cautiously and in lower doses in hepatic or renal impairment.
• Administer carefully to elderly or debilitated patients and in those with hypothyroidism or history of arrhythmias or seizures.
• Also use cautiously in acute abdominal conditions, gallbladder disease, recent GI surgery, inflammatory bowel disease, prostatic hyperplasia or obstruction, urethral stricture, or recent urinary tract surgery.
• Administer cautiously to patients with history of substance abuse, emotional instability, or suicidal ideation.

SPECIAL CONSIDERATIONS
• To minimize hypotension, keep patient in supine position when administering drug.
• Do not administer drug if respirations are below 12 breaths/minute. Monitor respirations for at least 1 hour after giving dose. Keep resuscitation equipment available.
• For improved analgesia, give before patient has intense pain.
• In cases of overdose, support airway and respirations. As ordered, give naloxone, repeating as needed to reverse respiratory depression. Administer IV fluids and vasopressors to maintain blood pressure.

oxytocin, synthetic injection

Pitocin, Syntocinon ♦

Pregnancy Risk Category: NR

INDICATIONS & DOSAGES
Induction and stimulation of labor—
Adults: usually 0.5 to 2 milliunits/minute. Dosage is determined by uterine response. May be increased q 30 to 60 minutes in increments of 1 to 2 milliunits/minute until contraction pattern simulates

that of normal labor. Maximum dosage is 10 milliunits/minute.
Incomplete or inevitable abortion—
Adults: 10 to 20 milliunits/minute. After abortion, 20 to 100 milliunits/minute.
Control of postpartum uterine bleeding—
Adults: 20 to 40 milliunits/minute to total of 10 U.
Evaluation of fetal distress after 31 weeks—
Adults: initially, 0.5 milliunits/ minute, increased q 15 to 30 minutes to maximum dosage of 20 milliunits/minute. Stop infusion when three moderate contractions occur within 10 minutes.

PREPARATION & STORAGE
Available in a concentration of 10 U/ml in 10-ml vials, 0.5- and 1-ml ampules, and 1-ml disposable syringes. Store below 77° F (25° C). If stored correctly, drug reportedly remains stable for 5 years.

For infusion to initiate labor, add 1 ml of drug to 1,000 ml of D_5W, 0.9% NaCl, or lactated Ringer's. For infusion to control postpartum bleeding, add 1 to 4 ml to 1,000 ml of D_5W or 0.9% NaCl. For use after abortion, thoroughly mix 1 ml of drug with 500 ml of dextrose 5% in 0.9% NaCl or with 0.9% NaCl. For evaluation of fetal distress, dilute 0.5 to 1 ml in 1,000 ml of D_5W.

Incompatibility
Incompatible with fibrinolysin or Normosol-M with dextrose 5%.

ADMINISTRATION
Continuous infusion: Use an infusion pump. Start IV line with 0.9% NaCl, adding oxytocin-containing solution as a secondary line to port as close to infusion needle as possible. Discontinue infusion at first sign of uterine hyperactivity or fetal distress. Do not administer drug for more than 8 hours.

CONTRAINDICATIONS & CAUTIONS
• Contraindicated in hypersensitivity to drug and in patients who have had cervical or uterine surgery.
• Also contraindicated during labor in significant cephalopelvic disproportion, cord presentation or prolapse, total placenta previa, uterine inertia, severe toxemia, hypertonic uterine contractions, and fetal distress when delivery is not imminent.
• Avoid use when vaginal delivery is contraindicated.
• Except in unusual circumstances, do not give drug in abruptio placentae, borderline cephalopelvic disproportion, or grand multiparity; in patients over age 35; or in those with history of sepsis, difficult or traumatic delivery, partial placenta previa, unengaged fetal head, and prematurity.
• Contraindicated when adequate uterine activity fails to achieve satisfactory progress and fetal position is unfavorable, requiring predelivery rotations.
• Use cautiously in abortion using hypertonic saline and in patients with cardiac disease.

SPECIAL CONSIDERATIONS
• Do not administer drug simultaneously by more than one route.
• Keep magnesium sulfate (20% solution) available to relax myometrium.
• Continuously monitor frequency, duration, and force of uterine contractions; resting uterine tone; fetal heart rate; maternal blood pressure; and intrauterine pressure.
• Stop infusion if contractions occur less than 2 minutes apart, exceed 50 mm Hg, or last longer than 90 seconds. Turn patient on her side and notify doctor.
• Instruct patient to inform doctor promptly if palpitations or other adverse reactions occur.

O

paclitaxel

Taxol
Pregnancy Risk Category: D

INDICATIONS & DOSAGES
Manufacturer suggests premedicating all patients with corticosteroids (dexamethasone 20 mg PO or IV) approximately 12 and 6 hours before therapy, diphenhydramine 50 mg IV 30 to 60 minutes before therapy, and cimetidine 300 mg IV 30 to 60 minutes before therapy (or ranitidine 50 mg IV or famotidine 20 mg IV) to prevent hypersensitivity reactions.
Ovarian cancer after failure of first-line or subsequent chemotherapy—
Adults: 135 mg/m² given over 3 hours, repeated q 21 days (optimal dosages have not been established).
Breast cancer after failure of combination chemotherapy for metastatic disease—
Adults: 175 mg/m² given over 3 hours, repeated q 21 days (optimal dosages have not been established).

PREPARATION & STORAGE
To avoid mutagenic, teratogenic, and carcinogenic risks, follow institutional guidelines for the safe handling, preparation, administration, and disposal of chemotherapeutic agents.

Available in a 5-ml single-dose vial containing 30 mg/5 ml. Unopened vials are stable until expiration date on label when stored under refrigeration at 36° to 46° F (2° to 8° C). Retain product in original package to protect from light.

To prepare, calculate dose and dilute in 0.9% NaCl, D₅W, dextrose 5% in 0.9% NaCl, or dextrose 5% in lactated Ringer's solution to a final concentration of 0.3 to 1.2 mg/ml. Diluted solutions are physically and chemically stable for up to 27 hours at ambient room temperature and room lighting conditions. Diluted solutions may show haziness attributable to the formulation vehicle. Avoid contact of undiluted concentrate with polyvinyl chloride equipment or devices. Store diluted solutions in glass or polypropylene bottles or polypropylene, polyolefin bags and administer through polyethylene-lined administration sets.

Incompatibility
Incompatible with amphotericin B, chlorpromazine hydrochloride, hydroxyzine hydrochloride, methylprednisolone sodium succinate, and mitoxantrone hydrochloride.

ADMINISTRATION
Intermittent infusion: Infuse over 3 hours through a 0.22 micron in-line filter. Changing the filter every 12 hours may be necessary due to clogging. Do not use polyvinyl chloride containers of administration sets.

CONTRAINDICATIONS & CAUTIONS
• Contraindicated in known hypersensitivity to paclitaxel or other drugs formulated in polyoxyethylated castor oil and in baseline neutropenia of less than 1,500 cells/mm³.
• Use cautiously in patients with cardiac conduction abnormalities, hepatic dysfunction, or previous treatment with other cytotoxic agents or radiation.
• Safety and efficacy in children have not been established.

SPECIAL CONSIDERATIONS
• Position needle carefully in vein to avoid extravasation.
• Monitor hematocrit, hemoglobin, WBC, and platelet count before and at periodic intervals during treatment. Monitor vital signs frequently, especially during first hour.
• Monitor patient continuously, particularly during first 30 minutes of infusion. Have epinephrine, oxygen, and other medications and equipment for treatment of anaphylaxis available during administration.
• Watch patients in whom neutropenia develops for signs of infection; antibiotics may be required.

• Advise patient to report signs and symptoms of peripheral neuropathy (such as tingling, burning sensation, or numbness in the extremities).

pamidronate disodium

Aredia

Pregnancy Risk Category: C

INDICATIONS & DOSAGES

Moderate to severe hypercalcemia associated with cancer with or without bone metastases—
Adults: dosage depends on severity and symptoms of hypercalcemia. Recommended dose in moderate hypercalcemia (corrected calcium of 12 to 13.5 mg/dl) is 60 to 90 mg as a single dose infused over 4 and 24 hours, respectively. In severe hypercalcemia (corrected calcium of above 13.5 mg/dl), the recommended dose is 90 mg as a single dose infused over 24 hours. Allow a minimum of 7 days to elapse before retreatment if hypercalcemia recurs.
Osteolytic bone lesions of multiple myeloma—
Adults: 90 mg over 4 hours on monthly basis.
Paget's disease—
Adults: 30 mg daily over 4 hours for 3 consecutive days.

PREPARATION & STORAGE
Available as 30-, 60-, and 90-mg lyophilized powder in single-dose vials. Store at 59° to 86° F (15° to 30° C). Do not freeze.
To prepare, reconstitute with 10 ml sterile water for injection. Allow drug to dissolve completely. Reconstituted solution is stable for up to 24 hours when refrigerated at 36° to 46° F (2° to 8° C). Withdraw daily dose and dilute in 1,000 ml of 0.45% or 0.9% NaCl or D_5W. Diluted product is stable for up to 24 hours.

In Paget's disease and osteolytic bone lesions of multiple myeloma, dilute in 500 ml of 0.9% NaCl or D_5W.

Incompatibility
Do not mix with calcium-containing infusion solutions such as Ringer's injection or lactated Ringer's solution.

ADMINISTRATION
Continuous infusion: Infuse as directed for specific indication and dosage.

CONTRAINDICATIONS & CAUTIONS
• Contraindicated in hypersensitivity to biphosphonates.
• Use cautiously in cardiac failure or renal impairment.

SPECIAL CONSIDERATIONS
• Vigorously hydrate patient with saline prior to use (if not contraindicated). In patients with mild to moderate hypercalcemia, hydration alone may be sufficient.
• Use of corticosteroids may be helpful in hypercalcemia associated with hematologic cancers.
• Periodically monitor alkaline phosphatase, a disease marker for Paget's disease, during therapy.
• Monitor electrolytes, including serum calcium, potassium, magnesium, phosphate. Monitor hemoglobin, hematocrit, CBC with differential, and serum creatinine periodically during therapy.
• Avoid overhydration in patients with potential for cardiac failure.

pancuronium bromide

Pavulon ◆

Pregnancy Risk Category: C

INDICATIONS & DOSAGES
Adjunct to anesthesia—

Adults and children over age 1 month: 0.04 to 0.1 mg/kg. Additional doses of 0.01 mg/kg may be given at 25- to 60-minute intervals. **Neonates:** carefully individualized. A test dose of 0.02 mg/kg should be given to assess responsiveness.
Facilitate management of mechanically ventilated patients and to facilitate endotracheal intubation—
Adults and children over age 1 month: 0.015 mg/kg.
Neonates: carefully individualized. A test dose of 0.02 mg/kg should be given to assess responsiveness.
Note: Large doses may increase frequency and severity of tachycardia.

PREPARATION & STORAGE
Available in 2- and 5-ml ampules, in vials and syringes containing 2 mg/ ml, and in 10-ml vials containing 1 mg/ml. Store at 36° to 46° F (2° to 8° C). Drug remains potent for 6 months at room temperature. Do not store in plastic containers. (However, may give drug in plastic syringes.) For infusion, dilute pancuronium with ordered amount of D_5W, 0.9% NaCl, or lactated Ringer's.

Incompatibility
Incompatible with barbiturates or diazepam.

ADMINISTRATION
Direct injection: Slowly inject into an established IV line containing a compatible, free-flowing solution.
Intermittent infusion: Infuse diluted drug at ordered rate.

CONTRAINDICATIONS & CAUTIONS
• Contraindicated in hypersensitivity to pancuronium or bromides and in patients with tachycardia or for whom an increase in heart rate is undesirable.
• Use cautiously in bronchogenic carcinoma, myasthenia gravis, Eaton-Lambert syndrome, renal impairment, and electrolyte imbalance.
• Also use cautiously in hepatic impairment, hyperthermia, pulmonary impairment, respiratory depression, severe obesity, or neuromuscular disease.
• Use with caution in breast-feeding women and neonates.

SPECIAL CONSIDERATIONS
• Adequate anesthesia is necessary when using pancuronium; drug has no effect on consciousness, pain threshold, or cerebration.
• Drug may contain benzyl alcohol.
• A nerve stimulator and train-of-four monitoring are recommended to assess recovery of muscle strength. Before attempting pharmacologic reversal with neostigmine, some evidence of spontaneous recovery should appear.
• Be prepared to give mechanical ventilation or airway support because apnea will follow administration. Keep antagonists, such as neostigmine and edrophonium, and resuscitation equipment available.

pegaspargase

Oncaspar

Pregnancy Risk Category: C

INDICATIONS & DOSAGES
Acute lymphoblastic leukemia in patients who require L-asparaginase but in whom hypersensitivity to the native forms of L-asparaginase has developed—
Adults and children with body surface area (BSA) of at least 0.6 m²: 2,500 IU/m² q 14 days.
Children with BSA less than 0.6 m²: 82.5 IU/kg q 14 days.

PREPARATION & STORAGE
Available in a preservative-free, single-use, 5-ml vial containing 750 IU/ml. Excessive heat should be avoided. Do not shake the vials. Keep vials refrigerated at 36° to 46° F (2° to 8° C). Do not freeze. Do not use if cloudy or if precipitate is present. Drug is stable at room temperature for 48 hours. Discard unused portions.

Incompatibility
None reported. Should not be mixed with other drugs.

ADMINISTRATION
Intermittent infusion: Desired dose should be diluted in 100 ml of 0.9% NaCl or dextrose 5%. The diluted solution should be administered into tubing of a free-flowing compatible IV solution over 1 to 2 hours.

CONTRAINDICATIONS & CAUTIONS
• Contraindicated in patients with pancreatitis or history of pancreatitis, in those who have had significant hemorrhagic events with prior L-asparaginase, and in patients with previous serious allergic reactions.
• Give to pregnant women only when clearly indicated.
• Use cautiously in liver dysfunction.

SPECIAL CONSIDERATIONS
• Take preventive measures (including adequate hydration) before starting treatment. Allopurinol may be ordered.
• Avoid excessive agitation; do not shake.
• Drug may be a contact irritant; solution must be handled and administered with care.
• Monitor patient closely for hypersensitivity reactions. Hypersensitivity reactions, including anaphylaxis, may occur during therapy. Keep patient under observation for 1 hour and have resuscitation equipment and other agents necessary to treat anaphylaxis readily available.
• Monitor patient's peripheral blood count and bone marrow, as ordered.
• Monitor serum amylase levels, and glucose levels.
• Monitor patient for liver dysfunction when drug is used in conjunction with hepatotoxic chemotherapeutic agents.
• Monitor fibrinogen, PT, and PTT.

penicillin G potassium
Pfizerpen

penicillin G sodium

Pregnancy Risk Category: B

INDICATIONS & DOSAGES
Both drugs are given in the same dosages.
Anthrax—
Adults and children over age 12: 5 to 20 million U daily in equally divided doses until cured.
Clostridium *infection—*
Adults and children over age 12: 20 million U daily.
Disseminated gonorrhea—
Adults and children weighing at least 99 lb (45 kg): 10 million U daily for 7 to 14 days.
Children weighing under 99 lb: 150,000 to 250,000 U/kg daily for 7 to 10 days.
Children with meningitis weighing under 99 lb: 250,000 U/kg daily in six divided doses for 10 days.
Neonates: 25,000 U/kg b.i.d. for week 1, then 75,000 U/kg daily in three to four divided doses for weeks 2 to 4.
Neonates with meningitis: 100,000 U/kg daily in three to four divided doses for 10 days.
Endocarditis from enterococci—
Adults and children over age 12: 20 to 40 million U daily in equally divided doses q 4 hours or by continuous infusion for 4 to 6 weeks.
Endocarditis from Streptococcus viridans *nonenterococcal group D streptococci—*
Adults and children over age 12: 10 to 20 million U daily in equally divided doses q 4 hours or by continuous infusion for 2 to 4 weeks.
Erysipelothrix *endocarditis—*
Adults and children over age 12: 2 to 20 million U daily for 4 to 6 weeks.

P

Fusobacterium *infection*—
Adults and children over age 12: 5 to 10 million U daily.
Gonococcal arthritis and septicemia—
Neonates: 75,000 to 100,000 U/kg daily in four divided doses for 7 to 14 days.
Gonococcal ophthalmia—
Adults and children over age 12: 10 million U daily for 5 days.
Neonates: 100,000 U/kg daily in four divided doses for 7 days.
Listeria *infection*—
Adults and children over age 12: 15 to 20 million U daily in equally divided doses for 2 to 4 weeks.
Neonates: 500,000 to 1 million U daily.
Neisseria meningitidis *infection*—
Adults and children over age 12: 20 to 30 million U daily by continuous infusion for at least 10 to 14 days.
Prophylaxis for infective endocarditis—
Adults and children over age 12: 2 million U 30 minutes to 1 hour before procedure, then 1 million U 6 hours after procedure.
Children: 50,000 U/kg 30 minutes to 1 hour before procedure, then 25,000 to 50,000 U/kg 6 hours after procedure.
Pasteurella multocida *infection*—
Adults and children over age 12: 4 to 6 million U daily for 2 weeks.
Pulmonary or abdominal actinomycosis—
Adults and children over age 12: 10 to 20 million U daily for 4 to 6 weeks followed by oral penicillin or tetracycline for an additional 6 to 12 months.
Severe infections caused by susceptible streptococci or nonpenicillinase-producing staphylococci—
Adults and children over age 12: 5 to 14 million U daily in equally divided doses q 4 hours.
Syphilis—
Adults and children over age 12: 2 to 4 million U q 4 hours for 10 to 14 days, then given IM
Note: In adults with renal or hepatic impairment, dosage reflects degree of impairment, severity of infection, and susceptible causative organism.

PREPARATION & STORAGE
Available in a variety of vial sizes containing 200,000 or 500,000 U and 1, 5, 10, or 20 million U of penicillin G potassium and 5 million U of penicillin G sodium. Reconstitute with sterile water for injection, 0.9% NaCl, or D_5W, as manufacturer directs. For intermittent infusion, dilute in 50 to 100 ml of 0.9% NaCl or D_5W. For continuous infusion, dilute daily dose in 1 to 2 L of compatible IV solution.

To prepare, first loosen powder in vial, then hold vial horizontally while rotating it and slowly directing stream of diluent against vial wall. Shake vigorously. Diluted solution is stable for 24 hours at room temperature and for 7 days at 36° to 46° F (2° to 8° C).

Also available in premixed frozen IV bags containing 1, 2, and 3 million U in 50 ml dextrose 5%. Frozen container should be thawed at room temperature. Thawed solution is stable for 24 hours at room temperature and 14 days if refrigerated.

Incompatibility
Penicillin G potassium is incompatible with alcohol 5%, amikacin, aminophylline, amphotericin B sodium, cephalothin sodium, chlorpromazine hydrochloride, dextran, dopamine hydrochloride, heparin sodium, hydroxyzine hydrochloride, lincomycin hydrochloride, metaraminol bitartrate, metoclopramide, pentobarbital sodium, phenytoin sodium, prochlorperazine mesylate, promazine hydrochloride, promethazine hydrochloride, sodium bicarbonate, thiopental, vancomycin, and vitamin B complex with C.

Penicillin G sodium is incompatible with 10% fat emulsions, 10% invert sugar, amphotericin B, bleomycin, cephalothin sodium, chlorpromazine hydrochloride, heparin sodium, hydroxyzine hydrochloride, lincomycin hydrochloride, methylprednisolone sodium succinate, potassium chloride, prochlorperazine mesylate, and promethazine hydrochloride.

ADMINISTRATION
Intermittent infusion: Infuse diluted drug over 1 to 2 hours.
Continuous infusion: Infuse diluted solution over 24 hours.

CONTRAINDICATIONS & CAUTIONS
• Contraindicated in hypersensitivity to penicillin, cephalosporins, and imipenem.
• Use cautiously in atopic patient, in GI disorders, and in renal impairment.

SPECIAL CONSIDERATIONS
• Patients with poor renal function are at risk for seizures.
• Ask patient about penicillin, cephalosporin, or imipenem allergy before giving first dose.
• Administer penicillin and aminoglycosides separately at different sites.
• Take special care to prevent infusion near major peripheral nerves or blood vessels; severe or permanent neurovascular damage may occur.
• Treat anaphylaxis by discontinuing drug and treating symptoms. Anaphylaxis may occur within 30 minutes of infusion.
• Obtain specimens for culture and sensitivity tests before giving first dose. Start therapy immediately.
• Monitor vital signs, CBC, PT, PTT, BUN, AST, and serum electrolyte and creatinine levels. Monitor intake and output and give fluids.
• Watch for signs of bleeding or hypersensitivity. Monitor for bacterial or fungal superinfection, especially when using indwelling IV catheters.

pentamidine isethionate

Pentam

Pregnancy Risk Category: C

INDICATIONS & DOSAGES
Pneumocystis. carinii pneumonia—
Adults and children: 3 to 4 mg/kg once daily for 14 to 21 days.
Alternative children's dosage:
150 mg/m² once daily for 5 days followed by 100 mg/m² once daily for 9 days. Adults and children with AIDS who do not respond in 14 days may receive drug for 7 more days.
Leishmaniasis (visceral) caused by Leishmania donovani—
Adults and children: 2 to 4 mg/kg once daily or every other day up to 15 doses, or 4 mg/kg three times weekly for 5 to 25 weeks or longer, based on response.
Trypanosomiasis—
Adults and children: 4 mg/kg once daily for 10 days, or 3 to 4 mg/kg once daily or every other day for 7 to 10 doses.
Note: Adjust dosage in renal impairment. Dosage for adults reflects creatinine clearance. If clearance is less than 10 ml/minute, give usual dose q 48 hours.

PREPARATION & STORAGE
Available as a powder in 300-mg vials. Before reconstituting, store at 59° to 86° F (15° to 30° C). Protect both dry powder and reconstituted solution from light. Drug contains no preservatives.
Reconstitute with 3 to 5 ml of sterile water for injection or D₅W. For infusion, dilute further in 50 to 250 ml of D₅W.
Solutions of 1 to 2.5 mg/ml prepared in dextrose 5% remain potent for up to 24 hours at room temperature. Discard unused portion.

Incompatibility
Incompatible with fluconazole or foscarnet sodium.

P

ADMINISTRATION
Intermittent infusion: Infuse diluted drug over 60 minutes.

CONTRAINDICATIONS & CAUTIONS
• Contraindicated in patients with history of allergy to pentamidine or diamidine compounds.
• Use cautiously in patients with history of bleeding disorders and in those with anemia, cardiac disease, and hepatic or renal impairment.
• Also use cautiously in diabetes mellitus, hypoglycemia, or hypotension to avoid exacerbation.

SPECIAL CONSIDERATIONS
• Because drug can cause severe hypotension, keep patient supine during administration and for several hours afterward. Monitor blood pressure, and keep resuscitation equipment available.
• Monitor fluid status to ensure adequate hydration and minimize possible nephrotoxicity.
• Before, during, and after therapy, monitor CBC, platelets, ECG, and AST, ALT, BUN, serum alkaline phosphatase, bilirubin, calcium, creatinine, and glucose levels.

pentobarbital sodium

Nembutal♦

Controlled Substance Schedule II

Pregnancy Risk Category: D

INDICATIONS & DOSAGES
Insomnia, anesthesia (adjunct), and seizures—
Adults: 100 mg initially, then smaller doses, p.r.n. at 1-minute intervals, to maximum of 200 to 500 mg. Dose is lower in elderly.
Children: 50 mg initially, then smaller doses at 1-minute intervals until desired effect is reached.

PREPARATION & STORAGE
Available in concentrations of 50 mg/ml in 2-ml vials, in 1- and 2-ml prefilled syringes, and in 20- and 50-ml multidose vials. Store at room temperature. Drug is compatible with most common solutions, such as D_5W and 0.9% NaCl. Pentobarbital should not be added to acidic solutions because precipitation may occur.

Incompatibility
Incompatible with benzquinamide, butorphanol, chlorpheniramine, chlorpromazine hydrochloride, cimetidine, codeine phosphate, dimenhydrinate hydrochloride, diphenhydramine hydrochloride, droperidol, ephedrine sulfate, fentanyl citrate, glycopyrrolate, hydrocortisone sodium succinate, hydroxyzine hydrochloride, insulin (regular), meperidine hydrochloride, methadone hydrochloride, midazolam hydrochloride, morphine sulfate, nalbuphine hydrochloride, norepinephrine bitartrate, opium alkaloids, penicillin G potassium, pentazocine lactate, perphenazine, phenytoin sodium, prochlorperazine edisylate, promazine, promethazine hydrochloride, ranitidine hydrochloride, sodium bicarbonate, streptomycin, succinylcholine, triflupromazine hydrochloride, and vancomycin hydrochloride.

ADMINISTRATION
Direct injection: Inject drug into IV tubing of free-flowing, compatible solution at a rate not exceeding 50 mg/minute. Avoid extravasation; solution is alkaline and may cause local tissue damage and necrosis. Guard against inadvertent intra-arterial injection, which may cause arterial spasm, severe pain, and possibly gangrene.

CONTRAINDICATIONS & CAUTIONS
• Contraindicated in hypersensitivity to barbiturates and in patients with intermittent or variegate porphyria.
• Use cautiously in severe anemia, hyperkinesis, hyperthyroidism, asthma, and respiratory dysfunction.
• Also administer with caution in borderline hyperadrenalism, pain,

P

hepatic or renal impairment and history of substance abuse or emotional instability.
• Also administer cautiously to depressed patient because drug may worsen suicidal tendencies.

SPECIAL CONSIDERATIONS
• Keep emergency resuscitation equipment available.
• Monitor vital signs, blood pressure, and cardiac function.
• Monitor EEG and blood levels when used for barbiturate coma. Patient will require mechanical ventilation.
• Advise patient to change positions and rise slowly secondary to possible loss of equilibrium and hangover effect.

pentostatin (2'-deoxycoformycin; DCF)

Nipent

Pregnancy Risk Category: D

INDICATIONS & DOSAGES
Treatment of alpha-interferon-refractory hairy cell leukemia—
Adults with creatinine clearance of 60 ml/minute or greater:
4 mg/m² every other week by IV bolus or diluted in a larger volume and administered over 20 to 30 minutes. Treat until complete response is achieved. Hydrate patient with 500 to 1,000 ml of dextrose 5% in 0.45% NaCl before treatment and with 500 ml after treatment to minimize to risk of adverse renal effects.

PREPARATION & STORAGE
To avoid mutagenic, teratogenic, and carcinogenic risks, follow facility guidelines for the safe handling, preparation, administration, and disposal of chemotherapeutic agents. Use 5% sodium hypochlorite to treat spills and wastes.

Available as 10-mg/vial powder for injection, in single-dose vials. Store refrigerated at 36° to 46° F (2° to 8° C). To prepare, add 5 ml sterile water for injection to vial and mix to obtain complete dissolution. Resultant solution contains 2 mg/ ml of pentostatin. Administer as IV bolus or further dilute using 25 or 50 ml D₅W or 0.9% NaCl and infuse. Use reconstituted vials and diluted infusions within 8 hours if stored at room temperature (contains no preservatives).

Incompatibility
Do not mix with other drugs unless specific compatibility data are available.

ADMINISTRATION
Direct injection: Give by rapid (over 5 minutes) IV bolus.
Intermittent infusion: Infuse diluted solution over 20 to 30 minutes.

CONTRAINDICATIONS & CAUTIONS
• Contraindicated in patients with renal damage and hypersensitivity to drug.
• Use cautiously in patients with renal impairment, CV disease, bone marrow depression, or previous cytotoxic drug therapy or radiation.
• Use cautiously and only under supervision of doctor qualified and experienced in use of chemotherapeutic agents.
• Patient with infections should be treated only when potential benefit of treatment justifies potential risk.
• Safety and efficacy in children have not been established.

SPECIAL CONSIDERATIONS
• Withhold or discontinue drug in patients with evidence of CNS toxicity, severe rash, or active infection.
• Temporarily withhold drug, as ordered, if absolute neutrophil count falls below 200 cells/mm³.
• Monitor creatinine, hematocrit, hemoglobin, WBC, platelet count, and uric acid concentrations.

P

phenobarbital sodium

Luminal◆

Controlled Substance Schedule IV

Pregnancy Risk Category: D

INDICATIONS & DOSAGES

Status epilepticus and acute seizure disorders—

Adults: 200 to 600 mg, or 40 to 120 mg at 5- to 10-minute intervals. Total dosage is 20 mg/kg.

Children: 100 to 400 mg, or 20 to 80 mg at 5- to 10-minute intervals. Total dosage is 20 mg/kg.

PREPARATION & STORAGE

Available in single-dose vials, ampules, and prefilled syringes in concentrations of 30, 60, 65, 120, and 130 mg/ml. Discard if solution contains precipitate. Drug is compatible with commonly used IV solutions including 0.45% and 0.9% NaCl, dextrose 5% and lactated Ringer's.

Incompatibility

Incompatible with alcohol-dextrose solutions, cephalothin sodium, chlorpromazine hydrochloride, codeine phosphate, ephedrine hydrochloride, hydralazine, hydrocortisone sodium succinate, insulin (regular), levorphanol, meperidine, morphine, norepinephrine, pentazocine lactate, prochlorperazine mesylate, promazine, promethazine hydrochloride, ranitidine hydrochloride, streptomycin, and vancomycin.

ADMINISTRATION

Direct injection: Inject dose slowly, not exceeding 60 mg/minute, into vein or IV tubing containing a free-flowing, compatible solution. Observe injection site for signs of thrombophlebitis. If patient reports local pain, stop injection and check cannula placement. Avoid extravasation; high alkalinity of drug causes tissue necrosis.

CONTRAINDICATIONS & CAUTIONS

• Contraindicated in hypersensitivity to barbiturates and in those with severe pulmonary disease and history of acute intermittent or variegate porphyria.

• Use cautiously in hepatic or renal impairment, elevated serum ammonia levels, CV disease or unstable blood pressure, diabetes mellitus, hyperthyroidism, hypothyroidism, or acute or chronic pain and in the elderly or children.

• Be cautious when giving drug to patient with a history of drug abuse, depression, or suicidal tendencies.

SPECIAL CONSIDERATIONS

• Drug dependence and severe withdrawal symptoms may follow long-term therapy. When discontinuing drug, withdraw single dose over 5 to 6 days to prevent withdrawal symptoms and rebound rapid-eye-movement stage of sleep.

• Signs of overdose include clammy skin, coma, cyanosis, hypotension, and pupillary constriction. Treatment is chiefly supportive. Maintain a patent airway, using oxygen and assisted ventilation as necessary. Keep patient well hydrated with IV fluids, and give sodium bicarbonate to alkalinize urine and increase drug excretion. In severe overdose, peritoneal dialysis and hemodialysis are helpful. Keep resuscitation equipment readily available.

• Establish baseline blood pressure, and continuously monitor for hypotension.

• Obtain baseline respiratory rate and continuously monitor.

• Discontinue drug immediately if a skin reaction occurs; it may indicate a possibly fatal reaction.

• For full anticonvulsant effect, wait 30 minutes after initial dose before giving additional doses. Maintain serum level at 15 to 40 mcg/ml. Halt injections when seizures stop or when total dosage is reached.

phentolamine mesylate

Regitine, Rogitine◇

Pregnancy Risk Category: C

INDICATIONS & DOSAGES

Diagnosis of pheochromocytoma—
Adults: 5 mg.
Children: 1 mg or 0.1 mg/kg or
3 mg/m².
*Hypertension in pheochromocytoma
before surgical removal of tumor—*
Adults: 5 mg 1 to 2 hours before
surgery.
Children: 1 mg or 0.1 mg/kg or
3 mg/m² 1 to 2 hours before
surgery, repeated if needed.
*Left-sided heart failure secondary to
acute MI—*
Adults: 0.17 to 0.4 mg/minute by
continuous infusion.
Norepinephrine extravasation—
Adults: 5 to 10 mg in 10 ml of 0.9%
NaCl into affected tissues within 12
hours of extravasation.
*Prevention of severe tissue sloughing
in norepinephrine infusion—*
Adults: 10 mg added to each
1,000 ml norepinephrine infusion.
*Hypertensive crisis from interaction
between MAO inhibitor and sympath-
omimetic amines—*
Adults: 5 to 10 mg.

PREPARATION & STORAGE

Supplied in 5-mg vials with 1 ml ampule of sterile water for injection as
diluent. Store unreconstituted powder at room temperature. Reconstitute with diluent to 5 mg/ml. Reconstituted product remains stable
for 48 hours at room temperature or
for 7 days at 36° to 46° F (2° to
8° C). Manufacturer recommends
that solution be used immediately after reconstitution. For infusion, dilute 5 to 10 mg of drug in 500 ml of
0.9% NaCl.

Incompatibility
None known.

ADMINISTRATION

Direct injection: Delay injection until
venipuncture effect subsides, then
rapidly inject desired dose.
Continuous infusion: Infuse at rate
ordered for norepinephrine solution;
to treat left-sided heart failure, infuse
at rate necessary to control symptoms, using infusion pump.

CONTRAINDICATIONS & CAUTIONS

• Contraindicated in sensitivity to
phentolamine or related drugs and
possibly in acute MI.
• Use cautiously in coronary artery
disease, angina, previous MI, gastri-
tis, or peptic ulcer disease.

SPECIAL CONSIDERATIONS

• Before performing pheochromocytoma test, make sure that patient's
blood pressure has returned to pretreatment level. Give drug rapidly,
recording blood pressure immediately after injection, every 30 seconds
for 3 minutes, then every 60 seconds
for 7 more minutes. Severe hypotension after test dose indicates pheochromocytoma
• In cases of overdose with severe
hypotension or other signs of shock,
treat with norepinephrine and supportive measures. For arrhythmias,
administer cardiac glycosides. Do
not use epinephrine.
• When treating left-sided heart failure, continuously monitor ECG and
left ventricular function.

phenylephrine hydrochloride

Neo-Synephrine Injection✦

Pregnancy Risk Category: C

INDICATIONS & DOSAGES

Shock or severe hypotension—
Adults: initially, 0.1 to 0.18 mg/
minute; then, after blood pressure
stabilizes, 0.04 to 0.06 mg/minute.
Mild to moderate hypotension—

P

Adults: 0.1 to 0.5 mg (usual dose, 0.2 mg). Subsequent doses given at intervals of 10 to 15 minutes.
Paroxysmal supraventricular tachycardia—
Adults: initial dose not to exceed 0.5 mg. Administer subsequent doses in 0.1- to 0.2-mg increments, depending on blood pressure (systolic not to exceed 160 mm Hg), with no single dose exceeding 1 mg.
Hypotensive emergencies during spinal anesthesia—
Adults: initial dose, 0.2 mg. Give later doses in 0.1- to 0.2-mg increments, with no single dose exceeding 0.5 mg.

PREPARATION & STORAGE
Available in 1-ml ampules and disposable cartridge U (10 mg/ml or 1% solution). Store at room temperature. Discard brown or precipitate-containing solutions. For infusion, dilute 10 mg in 500 ml of D_5W or 0.9% NaCl. Discard diluted solutions after 48 hours. Drug is compatible with most IV solutions.

Incompatibility
Incompatible with alkaline solutions and iron salts.

ADMINISTRATION
Direct injection: Inject dose over 1 minute to treat mild to moderate hypotension or hypotensive emergencies during spinal anesthesia. Inject dose over 20 to 30 seconds for paroxysmal supraventricular tachycardia; rapid injection may cause short paroxysms of ventricular tachycardia, ventricular extrasystoles, or a sensation of fullness in the head.
Continuous infusion: Infuse diluted drug at rate required to maintain adequate blood pressure and tissue perfusion. Regulate rate with microdrip tubing and infusion pump. Administer through a patent IV line into large vein in the antecubital fossa to prevent extravasation. Closely monitor infusion site.

CONTRAINDICATIONS & CAUTIONS
• Contraindicated in ventricular tachycardia, severe hypertension, MI, and hypersensitivity to phenylephrine or sulfites.
• Also contraindicated in mesenteric or peripheral vascular thrombosis, acute pancreatitis, or hepatitis.
• Give cautiously in hyperthyroidism, incomplete heart block, severe arteriosclerosis, and myocardial disease.
• Use with caution in the elderly because of diminished cerebral and coronary circulation.
• IV use is not recommended in children.

SPECIAL CONSIDERATIONS
• Correct hypovolemia either before or during drug administration.
• Drug may contain sulfites.
• In cases of overdose, treat hypertension with phentolamine and cardiac arrhythmias with propranolol, as ordered.
• If extravasation occurs, discontinue infusion and restart at another site. Infiltrate area with 5 to 10 mg of phentolamine in 10 to 15 ml of 0.9% NaCl, using syringe with a fine needle. For best results, treat within 12 hours.
• During infusion, check blood pressure every 2 minutes until stable, then every 5 to 15 minutes via intra-arterial monitoring. Discontinue slowly to avoid severe hypotension.
• Continuously monitor ECG. Notify doctor of arrhythmias.
• Monitor vital signs hourly until stable after stopping infusion. Watch for severe hypotension. Restart infusion if systolic pressure drops below 70 mm Hg. Maintain blood pressure slightly below patient's usual blood pressure.

phenytoin sodium

Dilantin◆

Pregnancy Risk Category: D

INDICATIONS & DOSAGES
Status epilepticus—

P

Adults: initially, 10 to 15 mg/kg by direct injection; then 100 to 150 mg after 30 minutes if necessary, or 8 to 18 mg/kg, at a rate not to exceed 50 mg/minute. Maximum total daily dose is 1.5 g.
Children: 15 to 20 mg/kg at 0.5 to 1.5 mg/kg/minute. Maximum total daily dose is 20 mg/kg.
Ventricular tachycardia, paroxysmal atrial tachycardia, or arrhythmias caused by digitalis toxicity—
Adults: 50 to 100 mg at 5-minute intervals, p.r.n., to terminate arrhythmias, not to exceed a total dose of 15 mg/kg.

PREPARATION & STORAGE
Available in 100- and 250-mg ampules containing 50 mg/ml. Store at room temperature; avoid freezing. Solution should be clear. If refrigerated, discard if slight yellowing does not clear after slow warming.

Manufacturer warns against using drug with other drugs or IV infusion solutions. However, researchers note that drug may be diluted for intermittent infusion with 0.9% NaCl injection. Add no more than 100 ml (preferably 25 or 50 ml) 0.9% NaCl injection to 100 mg drug. Prepare immediately before use, always use an in-line filter, and infuse within 1 hour.

Incompatibility
Incompatible with amikacin sulfate, aminophylline, bretylium tosylate, cephapirin sodium, clindamycin phosphate, codeine phosphate, D_5W, dobutamine hydrochloride, fat emulsions, insulin (regular), levorphanol hydrochloride, lidocaine hydrochloride, lincomycin hydrochloride, meperidine hydrochloride, metaraminol bitartrate, methadone hydrochloride, morphine sulfate, norepinephrine bitartrate, nitroglycerin, pentobarbital sodium, procaine hydrochloride, secobarbital sodium, and streptomycin sulfate.

ADMINISTRATION
Direct injection: Avoid injecting drug into dorsal hand veins to prevent extravasation. Inject dose directly into vein using a 0.22-micron in-line filter. Or, inject into IV line containing a compatible solution, infusing at a rate of less than 50 mg/minute. In elderly or debilitated patients, give at rate of 17 to 25 mg/minute.
Intermittent infusion: Infuse prescribed dose at ordered rate.

CONTRAINDICATIONS & CAUTIONS
• Contraindicated in hypersensitivity to hydantoins.
• Avoid use in sinus bradycardia, SA block, second- or third-degree AV block, and Adams-Stokes syndrome.
• Use cautiously in myocardial insufficiency, heart failure, respiratory depression, hepatic impairment, renal disease, hypoglycemia-induced seizures, diabetes mellitus, or other hyperglycemic states.
• Administer carefully in hypotension, impaired thyroid function, blood dyscrasias, and fever lasting for over 24 hours.

SPECIAL CONSIDERATIONS
• Flush IV tubing before and after use with 0.9% NaCl to remove drug and reduce venous irritation.
• In cases of overdose, immediately discontinue drug. Therapeutic serum level is 10 to 20 mcg/ml; toxic level, above 20 mcg/ml; lethal level, 100 mcg/ml. No known antidote exists.
• Drug may decrease effectiveness of oral contraceptives.
• Monitor ECG, blood pressure, and respiratory status.
• Frequently check IV site because phenytoin extravasation causes severe tissue damage.
• Closely monitor serum levels.
• Closely monitor for seizures. Keep intubation and aspiration equipment as well as padded side rails available.
• If measles-like rash appears, immediately discontinue drug.
• Monitor intake and output; hydration affects seizure threshold.

P

phytonadione (vitamin K₁)

AquaMEPHYTON

Pregnancy Risk Category: C

INDICATIONS & DOSAGES
Drug-induced hypoprothrombinemia with existing or imminent bleeding—
Adults: 10 to 50 mg q 4 hours p.r.n. Dosage guided by coagulation studies.
Infants and children: 1 to 2 mg IM or SC Further dosage guided by coagulation studies.

PREPARATION & STORAGE
Available in 0.5- and 1-ml ampules and 2.5- and 5-ml multidose vials containing 2 and 10 mg/ml. Protect drug from light, even after dilution. For direct injection, dilute with 10 ml of preservative-free D_5W, 0.9% NaCl, or dextrose 5% in 0.9% NaCl. For infusion, dilute with 50 to 100 ml of any of these solutions. Administer immediately after dilution. Discard unused drug.

Incompatibility
Incompatible with dobutamine hydrochloride and phenytoin sodium.

ADMINISTRATION
Direct injection: Using a 21G or 23G needle, inject diluted drug directly into vein or into IV tubing containing a free-flowing, compatible solution at a maximum rate of 1 mg/minute.
Intermittent infusion: Infuse diluted drug at a maximum rate of 1 mg/minute.

CONTRAINDICATIONS & CAUTIONS
• Contraindicated in hypersensitivity to vitamin K_1 or ingredient in preparation.
• Use cautiously in hepatic impairment.

SPECIAL CONSIDERATIONS
• Even dilution and slow infusion may not prevent severe reactions. To reverse vitamin K effects, administer heparin or warfarin, as ordered.
• Vitamin K_1 is used in hypoprothrombinemia caused by vitamin K deficiency or in moderate to severe bleeding caused by coumadin or indanedione derivatives. It does not antagonize the action of heparin.
• Drug may contain benzyl alcohol.
• Monitor coagulation studies 12 hours after administration and repeat as needed.

piperacillin sodium

Pipracil♦

Pregnancy Risk Category: B

INDICATIONS & DOSAGES
Severe systemic infections caused by susceptible organisms—
Adults: 200 to 300 mg/kg or 12 to 18 g daily in divided doses q 4 to 6 hours.
Complicated urinary tract infection (UTI)—
Adults: 125 to 200 mg/kg or 8 to 16 g daily in divided doses q 6 to 8 hours.
Uncomplicated UTI—
Adults: 100 to 125 mg/kg or 6 to 8 g daily in divided doses q 6 to 12 hours.
Acute Pseudomonas aeruginosa *infection in cystic fibrosis (in conjunction with aminoglycosides)—*
Adults: 300 to 600 mg/kg daily.
Prophylaxis for abdominal surgery—
Adults: 2 g before surgery, during surgery, and q 6 hours after surgery for up to 24 hours.
Note: Maximum daily adult dose for any indication, 24 g. Adjust dosage in renal failure: For adults, dosage reflects creatinine clearance. In uncomplicated UTI, give 3 g q 12 hours if creatinine clearance is below 20 ml/minute; if it is above 20 ml/minute, give usual adult dose. In complicated UTI, give 3 g q 12 hours if creatinine clearance is below 20 ml/minute; if it is between 20 and 40 ml/minute, give 3 g q 8

hours; and if it is above 40 ml/minute, give usual adult dose. In serious systemic infections, give 4 g q 12 hours if creatinine clearance is below 20 ml/minute; if it is between 20 and 40 ml/minute, give 4 g q 8 hours; and if it is above 40 ml/minute, give usual adult dose.

PREPARATION & STORAGE
Available in powder form in 2-, 3-, 4-, and 40-g vials. Store at room temperature. Reconstitute each gram of drug with 5 ml of sterile bacteriostatic water for injection or bacteriostatic NaCl injection. Shake vigorously to dissolve. For infusion, dilute reconstituted solution with at least 50 ml of D_5W, 0.9% NaCl, dextrose 5% in 0.9% NaCl, or lactated Ringer's. After reconstitution, drug remains stable for 24 hours at room temperature or for 7 days when refrigerated at 36° to 46° F (2° to 8° C).

Incompatibility
Incompatible with fluconazole.

ADMINISTRATION
Direct injection: Inject reconstituted drug directly into vein over 3 to 5 minutes.
Intermittent infusion: Infuse reconstituted and diluted solution over 30 minutes.
Continuous infusion: Inject reconstituted 24-hour dose into required daily IV volume. Infuse at rate needed for delivery of required fluid volume.

CONTRAINDICATIONS & CAUTIONS
• Contraindicated in hypersensitivity to penicillins or cephalosporins and in children under age 12.
• Use cautiously in ulcerative colitis and hepatic or renal dysfunction and in those with sodium-restricted diets.
• Use cautiously in breast-feeding patients.

SPECIAL CONSIDERATIONS
• Before giving drug, ask patient if he has had allergic reactions to penicillin.
• Treat anaphylaxis symptomatically. Keep emergency equipment available.
• Obtain specimens for culture and sensitivity tests before giving first dose.
• Closely monitor for possible hypersensitivity for at least 30 minutes after administration.
• Check CBC frequently and monitor serum potassium level. Monitor PT and bleeding times. Assess patient for possible bleeding.
• Establish baseline renal function, then periodically monitor renal, hepatic, and CV status in patients on prolonged therapy.

piperacillin sodium and tazobactam sodium

Zosyn

Pregnancy Risk Category: B

INDICATIONS & DOSAGES
Appendicitis (complicated by rupture or abscess), peritonitis, uncomplicated and complicated skin and skin structure infections, postpartum endometritis, pelvic inflammatory disease, and community-acquired pneumonia caused by piperacillin-resistant organisms—
Adults: 12 g piperacillin and 1.5 g tazobactam, given as 3.375 g (3 g piperacillin and 0.375 g tazobactam) q 6 hours by IV infusion over 30 minutes.
Note: Adjust dosage in patients with creatinine clearance of 40 ml/minute or less. If creatinine clearance is 20 to 40 ml/minute, give 8 g piperacillin and 1 g tazobactam daily in divided doses of 2.25 g q 6 hours; if it is below 20 ml/minute, give 6 g piperacillin and 0.75 g

P

tazobactam daily in divided doses of 2.25 g q 8 hours.

PREPARATION & STORAGE
Available as powder for injection in single-dose vials containing 2 g piperacillin and 0.25 g tazobactam, 3 g piperacillin and 0.375 g tazobactam, 4 g piperacillin and 0.5 g tazobactam.

Reconstitute drug with 5 ml of suitable diluent for each 1 g of piperacillin. Shake well until dissolved. May further dilute to the desired volume (at least 50 ml). Drug is compatible with 0.9% NaCl, sterile water for injection, 6% dextrose in 0.9% NaCl, D_5W, potassium chloride 40 mEq, bacteriostatic saline with parabens, bacteriostatic water with parabens, bacteriostatic water with benzyl alcohol, or bacteriostatic saline with benzyl alcohol.

Use reconstituted single-dose vials immediately. Discard unused portion after 24 hours if stored at room temperature or 48 hours if refrigerated. After reconstitution, product is stable in glass and plastic containers for up to 24 hours at room temperature and up to 1 week if refrigerated. Also stable in ambulatory IV infusion pump for 12 hours at room temperature.

Incompatibility
Do not reconstitute with lactated Ringer's because drug degrades over time (8 hours), decreasing its potency. Incompatible with acyclovir sodium, amphotericin B, chlorpromazine hydrochloride, dacarbazine, daunorubicin hydrochloride, dobutamine hydrochloride, doxorubicin hydrochloride, doxycycline hyclate, droperidol, famotidine, ganciclovir sodium, haloperidol lactate, hydroxyzine hydrochloride, idarubicin hydrochloride, miconazole, minocycline, mitomycin, mitoxantrone hydrochloride, nalbuphine hydrochloride, prochlorperazine edisylate, promethazine hydrochloride, streptozocin, and vancomycin hydrochloride.

ADMINISTRATION
Intermittent infusion: Infuse over 30 minutes.

CONTRAINDICATIONS & CAUTIONS
• Contraindicated in hypersensitivity to penicillins, cephalosporins, or beta-lactam inhibitors.
• Use cautiously in patients with renal impairment, bleeding tendencies, uremia, or hypokalemia.
• Use cautiously in patients who require sodium restriction.

SPECIAL CONSIDERATIONS
• Monitor CBC, differential blood count, platelet count, and electrolytes (especially potassium). Observe for occult bleeding.
• Monitor neurologic status.
• Instruct patient to inform doctor if sore throat, fever, rash, or easy bruising or bleeding occurs.

plicamycin (mithramycin)

Mithracin
Pregnancy Risk Category: X

INDICATIONS & DOSAGES
Testicular cancer—
Adults: 25 to 30 mcg/kg daily for 8 to 10 days or until toxicity occurs. Maximum dosage is 10 daily doses or a total of 30 mcg/kg daily. May repeat monthly.
Hypercalcemia and hypercalciuria (related to cancer)—
Adults: 25 mcg/kg daily for 3 or 4 days. May repeat at intervals of 1 week or more.

PREPARATION & STORAGE
Use extreme caution when preparing or administering plicamycin to avoid mutagenic, teratogenic, and carcinogenic risks. Use a biological containment cabinet, wear gloves and mask, and use syringes with luer-lock tips to prevent drug leakage. Correctly

P

dispose of vials, needles, syringes, and unused drug.

Available in 2,500-mcg vials. Refrigerate unreconstituted vials. Reconstitute drug with 4.9 ml of sterile water for injection for a concentration of 500 mcg/ml. For infusion, dilute appropriate dose in 1,000 ml of D$_5$W or 0.9% NaCl. Discard unused solution. Reconstituted solution remains stable for 24 hours at room temperature and for 48 hours when refrigerated.

Incompatibility
None reported. However, drug may form a complex with metal ions such as iron and readily hydrolyzes in acidic solutions (pH below 4).

ADMINISTRATION
Intermittent infusion: Infuse diluted drug over 4 to 6 hours. (Rapid infusion increases incidence and severity of GI disease.)

CONTRAINDICATIONS & CAUTIONS
• Contraindicated in blood dyscrasias, impaired bone marrow function, coagulation disorders, thrombocytopathy, or thrombocytopenia.
• Administer cautiously in severe renal or hepatic impairment and electrolyte imbalance, especially hypocalcemia, hypokalemia, and hypophosphatemia.
• Use only in hospitalized patients who are under constant supervision.

SPECIAL CONSIDERATIONS
• Administer antiemetics before and during treatment to help reduce nausea.
• If extravasation occurs, stop infusion and restart in another area. Apply cold to reduce pain and prevent swelling. However, if swelling develops, apply moderate heat to reduce discomfort and irritation.
• Frequently obtain platelet counts and PT and bleeding times during therapy and for several days after last dose.

• Monitor liver and kidney function daily in patients with preexisting impairment.
• Instruct patient to inform doctor if sore throat, fever, mucosal ulcerations, or easy bruising or bleeding occurs.

potassium chloride

Potassium Chloride Injection
Pregnancy Risk Category: C

INDICATIONS & DOSAGES
Hypokalemia—
Dosage reflects patient needs and response.
Adults: if serum potassium exceeds 2.5 mEq/L, up to 200 mEq daily (concentration below 40 mEq/L), not to exceed 10 mEq/hour. If serum potassium is below 2 mEq/L, up to 400 mEq daily, not to exceed 20 mEq/hour.
Children: 2 to 3 mEq/kg or 40 mEq/m^2 daily. Maximum daily dose, 3 mEq/kg, not to exceed 0.5 mEq/kg/hour.

PREPARATION & STORAGE
Supplied in 5-, 10-, 15-, 20-, 30-, and 60-ml ampules and vials containing 10, 20, 30, 40, 60, 90, and 120 mEq potassium. Store at room temperature. Always dilute before use. Dilution varies widely, but potassium concentration usually should not exceed 40 mEq/L. In emergencies, maximum concentration of 80 mEq/L may be temporarily exceeded.

Incompatibility
Incompatible with amikacin, amphotericin B, diazepam, ergotamine, fat emulsion (10%), mannitol (20% or 25%), penicillin G sodium, phenytoin sodium, promethazine hydrochloride, and streptomycin.

ADMINISTRATION
Intermittent infusion: Infuse diluted solution slowly, not to exceed 10 to

P

20 mEq/hour. Overly rapid infusion can cause fatal hyperkalemia. Infusion rate should not exceed 1 mEq/minute for adults or 0.02 mEq/kg/minute for children.
Continuous infusion: Same as intermittent infusion.

CONTRAINDICATIONS & CAUTIONS
• Contraindicated in severe renal impairment, untreated Addison's disease, hyperkalemia, acute dehydration, heat cramps, and burns.
• Use cautiously in patients with cardiac disorders who require cardiac glycosides and in those with renal impairment or myotonia congenita.
• Use cautiously in breast-feeding patients.

SPECIAL CONSIDERATIONS
• Never administer potassium chloride undiluted.
• In dehydrated patients, administer 1 L of potassium-free fluid before potassium therapy.
• Adding concentrated potassium chloride solutions to a hanging flexible plastic container can cause hyperkalemia because of inadequate mixing. When adding potassium solutions, invert the plastic container to avoid pooling of concentrated potassium at its base. Then knead the container to mix contents.
• Do not administer potassium chloride postoperatively until urine flow is established.
• In cases of overdose, discontinue potassium-containing foods and drugs. Give insulin IV, as ordered, in 10% to 25% dextrose solution (10 U insulin/20 g dextrose) at 300 to 500 ml/hour. Also give sodium bicarbonate by infusion to correct acidosis. May use exchange resins, hemodialysis, or peritoneal dialysis.
• Monitor ECG, serum potassium, BUN, and serum creatinine, pH, and intake and output.
• In digitalized patients, treat hyperkalemia with caution; rapid reduction of serum potassium levels may result in digitalis toxicity.

potassium phosphate

Potassium Phosphate Injection

Pregnancy Risk Category: C

INDICATIONS & DOSAGES
Electrolyte imbalance—
Adults: equivalent of 10 mmol or 310 mg of phosphorus daily.
Children: equivalent of 1.5 to 2 mmol or 46.5 to 62 mg of phosphorus daily. Dose must be individualized.

PREPARATION & STORAGE
Supplied in 5- and 15-ml flip-top vials, 5-ml pin-top vial, and 50-ml bulk additive vial. Available strength is equivalent to 3 mmol or 93 mg/ml of phosphorus. For infusion, dilute and thoroughly mix in a larger volume of compatible fluid. Store at room temperature.

Incompatibility
Incompatible with dobutamine and solutions that contain calcium and magnesium, such as lactated Ringer's, Ringer's injection, dextrose and Ringer's injection, dextrose 10% in 0.9% NaCl, and Ionosol solutions.

ADMINISTRATION
Intermittent infusion: Infuse diluted solution slowly over the ordered time to avoid phosphate intoxication and severe hyperkalemia. Rate must be individualized.
Continuous infusion: Same as intermittent infusion.

CONTRAINDICATIONS & CAUTIONS
• Contraindicated in hyperkalemia, hyperphosphatemia, infected urolithiasis caused by magnesium ammonium phosphate stones, and severe renal dysfunction.
• Use cautiously in hypoparathyroidism, osteomalacia, acute pancreatitis, chronic renal disease, and vitamin D deficiency.

P

• Use cautiously in patients with cardiac disorders, especially those taking cardiac glycosides.
• Also give carefully in severe Addison's disease, acute dehydration, myotonia congenita, severe renal insufficiency, and extensive tissue necrosis resulting from severe burns.

SPECIAL CONSIDERATIONS
• Never administer potassium phosphate undiluted.
• Do not administer postoperatively until urine flow is established.
• IV infusion of phosphates in high concentrations can cause hypocalcemia.
• Frequently monitor serum electrolyte levels and renal function. Also monitor ECG for signs of conduction disturbances.

procainamide hydrochloride

Pronestyl♦

Pregnancy Risk Category: C

INDICATIONS & DOSAGES
Arrhythmias (paroxysmal atrial tachycardia, PVCs, ventricular tachycardia, and, in some cases, atrial fibrillation)—
Adults: initially, 50 to 100 mg given slowly (not exceeding 50 mg/minute), then repeated q 5 minutes until arrhythmias are controlled or a total of 500 mg has been given. If necessary, continue giving 100 mg slowly q 10 minutes until arrhythmias are controlled, adverse reactions occur, or maximum loading dose of 1 g has been given. Maintenance dose is 1 to 6 mg/minute titrated to maintain control of arrhythmias.
Children: dosage not established. Recommendations include 2 to 5 mg/kg (not exceeding 100 mg) repeated p.r.n. at 10- to 30-minute intervals (not exceeding 30 mg/kg in 24 hours), or 3 to 6 mg/kg over 5 minutes, followed by maintenance

infusion of 0.02 to 0.08 mg/kg/minute.
Malignant hyperthermia—
Adults: 200 to 900 mg, then maintenance infusion of 0.02 to 0.08 mg/kg/minute.
Note: In all indications, lowered doses may be required in heart failure or renal impairment.

PREPARATION & STORAGE
Supplied in 10-ml (100 mg/ml) and 2-ml (500 mg/ml) vials. Store at room temperature. Protect from light and freezing. Do not use if markedly discolored or if precipitate has formed. For injection or loading infusion, dilute 1 g with 50 ml of D_5W to yield 20 mg/ml. For continuous infusion, dilute 1 g with 500 ml of D_5W to yield 2 mg/ml. In patients with fluid restrictions, dilute 1 g with 250 ml of D_5W to yield 4 mg/ml. Note that drug may form a complex with dextrose, causing gradual loss of potency.

Incompatibility
Incompatible with bretylium, esmolol hydrochloride, ethacrynate sodium, milrinone, and phenytoin sodium.

ADMINISTRATION
Direct injection: Inject dose over 2 minutes or longer directly into vein or into IV tubing containing a free-flowing, compatible solution.
Intermittent infusion: Give loading infusion at 1 ml/minute for 25 to 30 minutes. Therapeutic effects usually occur after infusion of 100 to 200 mg. If no effect occurs after infusing 500 mg, wait at least 10 minutes to allow for drug distribution, then continue administration.
Continuous infusion: Using an infusion pump, give diluted solution at ordered rate, usually 2 to 6 mg/minute.

CONTRAINDICATIONS & CAUTIONS
• Contraindicated in hypersensitivity to procaine or other local anesthetics.
• Also contraindicated in second- or third-degree or complete AV heart

P

block, and in atypical ventricular tachycardia.
• Use cautiously in digitalis toxicity, severe first-degree AV block, or bundle-branch heart block.
• Also use cautiously in heart failure, hepatic or renal impairment, bronchial asthma, myasthenia gravis, and systemic lupus erythematosus.

SPECIAL CONSIDERATIONS
• Drug may contain benzyl alcohol and sulfites.
• Keep phenylephrine or norepinephrine available to treat severe hypotension.
• Signs of overdose include severe hypotension, confusion, dizziness or fainting, drowsiness, nausea, vomiting, oliguria, and unusually rapid or irregular heartbeat. If these signs or symptoms develop, stop drug immediately. Replace fluids, then give norepinephrine or phenylephrine, as ordered. Maintain airway patency and ventilate the patient as necessary. Infusion of 1/6 M sodium lactate injection may reverse cardiotoxic effects of procainamide. Hemodialysis reduces serum half-life of procainamide, removing both procainamide and NAPA.
• During administration, continuously monitor blood pressure and cardiac function (including ECG). Place patient in a supine position for blood pressure monitoring.
• In ventricular tachycardia, discontinue infusion if ventricular rate declines significantly without attaining regular AV conduction.

prochlorperazine edisylate

Compazine

Pregnancy Risk Category: C

INDICATIONS & DOSAGES
Dosage reflects patient's needs and response to drug.

Severe nausea and vomiting resulting from surgery or toxins, radiation, or cytotoxic drugs—
Adults: 2.5 to 10 mg (0.5 to 2 ml). May repeat q 3 to 4 hours.
Prevention of nausea and vomiting during surgery—
Adults: 5 to 10 mg by direct injection 15 to 30 minutes before induction of anesthesia. Repeat once before surgery, if necessary. Or 20 mg/L by infusion 15 to 30 minutes before induction of anesthesia. Maximum dosage, 40 mg daily.

PREPARATION & STORAGE
Available as a 5 mg/ml concentration in 2-ml ampules, 10-ml vials, 2-ml disposable syringes, and 1- and 2-ml prefilled cartridges. Store at room temperature and protect from light and freezing. Don't use if markedly discolored or a precipitate is present. Dilute for continuous infusion with at least 1 L of a compatible isotonic solution, such as 0.9% NaCl, to yield 20 mg/L.

Incompatibility
Incompatible with aminophylline, amphotericin B, ampicillin sodium, calcium gluceptate and gluconate, cephalothin sodium, chloramphenicol sodium succinate, chlorothiazide, dexamethasone sodium phosphate, dimenhydrinate, heparin sodium, hydrocortisone sodium succinate, hydromorphone, methicillin, methotrexate sodium, midazolam hydrochloride, penicillin G potassium and sodium, phenobarbital sodium, phenytoin sodium, prednisolone sodium phosphate, thiopental, and vitamin B complex with C. Also incompatible with solutions containing methylparaben or propylparaben.
Don't mix prochlorperazine in the same syringe with other drugs.

ADMINISTRATION
Direct injection: Slowly inject undiluted drug at a rate of 5 mg/minute. Never give as bolus injection.

P

Continuous infusion: Infuse diluted drug at ordered rate over prescribed duration.

CONTRAINDICATIONS & CAUTIONS
• Contraindicated in hypersensitivity to drug or other phenothiazines.
• Also contraindicated in severe CNS depression, coma, and severe CV disease because drug may worsen these conditions.
• Avoid use of IV prochlorperazine in children.
• Use cautiously in Parkinson's disease, myelosuppression, CV disease, hepatic impairment, seizure disorders, and alcoholism.
• Use carefully in patients with peptic ulcer, chronic respiratory disorders, symptomatic prostatic hyperplasia, or urine retention.
• Also use cautiously in patients exposed to extreme heat or in those with glaucoma or a predisposition to it.
• Use with lower doses in debilitated patients.
• Use cautiously in breast-feeding patients.
• Avoid use in pregnancy unless nausea is severe and benefits of drug therapy outweigh the risks.

SPECIAL CONSIDERATIONS
• Because of risk of hypotension, use IV route only for closely monitored patients.
• Initially, administer low doses to the elderly and increase gradually.
• Antiemetic effect may mask signs of drug toxicity or obscure diagnosis of conditions having nausea as a primary symptom.
• Anticholinergic antiparkinson drugs may help to control extrapyramidal reactions.
• Monitor blood pressure closely.

promethazine hydrochloride

Phenergan◆
Pregnancy Risk Category: C

INDICATIONS & DOSAGES
Allergic reactions—
Adults: 25 mg, repeated in 2 hours if necessary.
Nausea and vomiting—
Adults: 12.5 to 25 mg q 4 hours p.r.n.
Children: 0.25 to 0.5 mg/kg four to six times daily.
Obstetric sedation—
Adults: 50 mg during early labor stage; then 25 to 75 mg in established labor (given with an opioid agonist). If necessary, 25 to 50 mg dose may be repeated once or twice at 4-hour intervals. Maximum dose is 100 mg in 24 hours.
Sedation and relief of apprehension, postoperative pain (anesthesia and analgesia adjunct)—
Adults: 25 to 50 mg p.r.n.; maximum dosage, 150 mg daily.

PREPARATION & STORAGE
Available as a 25 mg/ml concentration in 1- and 10-ml ampules, 1- and 10-ml vials, and 1-ml prefilled cartridges. Store at room temperature, and protect from light and freezing. Do not use if solution is discolored or if a precipitate is present.

Incompatibility
Incompatible with aminophylline, chloramphenicol sodium succinate, chlorothiazide, diatrizoate meglumine (34.3%) and diatrizoate sodium (35%), diatrizoate meglumine (52%) and diatrizoate sodium (8%), diatrizoate sodium (75%), dimenhydrinate, heparin sodium, hydrocortisone sodium succinate, iodipamide meglumine (52%), iothalamate meglumine (60%), iothalamate sodium (80%), methicillin, methohexital, morphine, penicillin G potassium and sodium, pentobarbital sodium, phenobarbital

P

sodium, phenytoin sodium, prednisolone sodium phosphate, thiopental, and vitamin B complex.

ADMINISTRATION
Direct injection: Inject at a rate not exceeding 25 mg/minute into an IV line containing a free-flowing, compatible solution. Rapid administration may reduce blood pressure temporarily.

Concentration should not exceed 25 mg/ml. Be sure IV line is patent before injection, and avoid extravasation or inadvertent intra-arterial injection because of possible gangrene or severe arteriospasm.

CONTRAINDICATIONS & CAUTIONS
• Contraindicated in hypersensitivity to drug and in breast-feeding patients.
• Avoid use in coma.
• Use cautiously in acute asthma, respiratory disorders, severe obesity, bladder neck obstruction, symptomatic prostatic hyperplasia, or predisposition to urine retention.
• Give cautiously in epilepsy, hepatic impairment, jaundice, myelosuppression, CV disease, hypertension, and angle-closure glaucoma or predisposition to this condition.
• Give drug cautiously in patients with stenosis caused by peptic ulcer or with history of peptic ulcer.
• Also give cautiously to elderly patients.

SPECIAL CONSIDERATIONS
• Be aware that antiemetic effects may obscure signs of intestinal obstruction, brain tumor, or promethazine overdose.
• In cases of overdose, give oxygen and IV fluids as needed to maintain cardiopulmonary function. Give phenylephrine or norepinephrine to treat hypotension. Do not use epinephrine, which may further lower blood pressure. Also administer anticholinergic antiparkinson drugs, diphenhydramine, or barbiturates, as ordered, to treat extrapyramidal symptoms.

• Watch for extrapyramidal reactions, especially in the elderly.
• Monitor blood pressure closely.

propofol
Diprivan
Pregnancy Risk Category: B

INDICATIONS & DOSAGES
Induction of anesthesia—
Adults: doses must be individualized according to patient's condition and age. Most patients classified as American Society of Anesthesiologists (ASA) Physical Status category (PS) I or II under age 55 require 2 to 2.5 mg/kg. Drug is usually administered in 40-mg boluses q 10 seconds until desired response is obtained. Elderly, debilitated, or hypovolemic patients or those in ASA PS III or IV should receive half of usual induction dose (20-mg boluses q 10 seconds).
Maintenance of anesthesia—
Adults: may be given as a variable rate infusion, titrated to clinical effect. Most patients may be maintained with 0.1 to 0.2 mg/kg/minute (6 to 12 mg/ kg/hour). Elderly, debilitated, or hypovolemic patients or those in ASA PS III or IV should receive half of usual maintenance dose (0.05 to 0.1 mg/kg/minute or 3 to 6 mg/kg/hour).
Monitored anesthesia care—
Adults: initially, most patients require 100 to 150 mcg/kg/minute (6 to 9 mg/kg/hour) for 3 to 5 minutes or a slow injection of 0.5 mg/kg over 3 to 5 minutes. Maintenance, most patients require an infusion of 25 to 75 mcg/kg/minute (1.5 to 4.5 mg/kg/hour) or incremental bolus doses of 10 or 20 mg. Elderly, debilitated or ASA PS III or IV patients require 80% of usual adult maintenance dose. Rapid bolus should not be used.
Sedation of intubated intensive care unit patients—

P

Adults: initial infusion is 5 mcg/kg/minute (0.3 mg/kg/hour) for 5 minutes. Increments of 5 to 10 mcg/kg/minute (0.3 to 0.6 mg/kg/hour) over 5 to 10 minutes may be used until desired sedation is achieved. Maintenance rate, 5 to 50 mcg/kg/minute (0.3 to 3 mg/kg/hour).

PREPARATION & STORAGE
Supplied in 20-ml ampules containing 10 mg/ml. If drug is to be diluted before infusion, use only D_5W, and do not dilute to a concentration less than 2 mg/ml. After dilution, drug is probably more stable in glass containers than in plastic ones.

When administered into a running IV line, propofol emulsion is compatible with D_5W, lactated Ringer's injection, lactated Ringer's and 5% dextrose injection, 5% dextrose and 0.45% NaCl injection, and 5% dextrose and 0.2% NaCl injection. Store unopened ampules above 40° F (4° C) and below 72° F (22° C). Do not refrigerate.

Note: Strict aseptic technique must always be maintained during handling. Propofol injectable emulsion is a single-use parenteral product, which contains 0.005% disodium edetate to retard the rate of growth of microorganisms in the event of accidental extrinsic contamination. However, propofol can still support the growth of microorganisms in that it is not an antimicrobially preserved product.

Incompatibility
Do not mix with other drugs.

ADMINISTRATION
Direct injection: For induction in adults, administer 40 mg every 10 seconds until desired response is obtained. For maintenance of anesthesia in adults, 25 to 50 mg (2.5 to 5 ml) boluses administered as needed based on patient's change in vital signs.

Continuous infusion: For maintenance of anesthesia in adults, give 0.1 to 0.2 mg/kg/minute.

CONTRAINDICATIONS & CAUTIONS
• Contraindicated in hypersensitivity to drug or components of the emulsion, including soybean oil, egg lecithin, and glycerol.
• Avoid using drug for obstetric anesthesia and in increased intracranial pressure or impaired cerebral circulation.
• Use with caution in patients with history of epilepsy or lipid metabolism disorders and in those with diabetic hyperlipidemia or circulatory disorders.
• Use cautiously in elderly or debilitated patients.
• Drug is not recommended for use in children and in breast-feeding patients.

SPECIAL CONSIDERATIONS
• Avoid abrupt discontinuation of drug before weaning. This may result in sudden awakening with anxiety, agitation, and resistance to mechanical ventilation.
• Treatment of significant hypotension or bradycardia includes increased rate of fluid administration, pressor agents, elevation of lower extremities, or atropine. Apnea commonly occurs during induction and may persist for longer than 60 seconds. Ventilatory support may be required.
• Daily monitoring of lipids is recommended.

propranolol hydrochloride

Inderal◆

Pregnancy Risk Category: C

INDICATIONS & DOSAGES
Life-threatening arrhythmias or those occurring under anesthesia—

Adults: 0.5 to 3 mg repeated after 2 minutes and again after 4 hours if necessary.
Children: 0.01 to 0.02 mg/kg.
Substitute for oral administration during surgery—
Adults: 10% of oral dose.

PREPARATION & STORAGE
Available in 1-ml ampules containing 1 mg/ml. Compatible with 0.9% NaCl solution and D_5W. Store at room temperature and protect from light and freezing.

Incompatibility
Incompatible with diazoxide.

ADMINISTRATION
Direct injection: Inject drug at a maximum rate of 1 mg/minute through an IV line containing a free-flowing, compatible solution.
Intermittent infusion: In children, infuse over 10 minutes.

CONTRAINDICATIONS & CAUTIONS
• Contraindicated in Raynaud's syndrome, malignant hypertension, and bronchial asthma, sinus bradycardia, heart block greater than first degree, MI (systolic pressure below 100 mm Hg), heart failure (unless caused by tachyarrhythmia treatable with propranolol), and cardiogenic shock.
• Avoid use in myasthenia gravis.
• Use cautiously in cardiac impairment, hyperthyroidism, nonallergic bronchospastic disease, depression, hepatic or renal failure, and in breast-feeding patients.
• Also use with caution in patients with diabetes mellitus who receive oral hypoglycemic drugs.
• Safety and efficacy in children have not been established.

SPECIAL CONSIDERATIONS
• Keep in mind that IV doses are appreciably smaller than oral ones.
• In cases of overdose, correct severe bradycardia with atropine by infusion and, if necessary, give isoproterenol. For PVCs, administer IV lidocaine or phenytoin. For cardiac

failure, give oxygen, diuretics, and cardiac glycosides. A transvenous pacemaker may be used if drug therapy is unsuccessful.
For hypotension, place patient in the Trendelenburg position and administer IV fluids (unless pulmonary edema is present) and an IV vasopressor, such as epinephrine. If seizures occur, give IV diazepam (or, if necessary, phenytoin). For bronchospasm, give isoproterenol or a theophylline derivative. Glucagon may be used to counter CV effects of propranolol overdose.
• Carefully monitor ECG, blood pressure, and central venous pressure during administration.
• Inform diabetic patient that normal signs of hypoglycemia may be masked.

protamine sulfate

Pregnancy Risk Category: C

INDICATIONS & DOSAGES
Severe heparin overdose—
Adults: dosage reflects heparin dose, route, and time elapsed since administration. Typically, 1 mg of protamine sulfate neutralizes about 90 U heparin sodium derived from bovine lung tissue, 100 U of heparin calcium derived from porcine intestinal mucosa, or 115 U of heparin sodium derived from porcine intestinal mucosa.
Dosage guidelines: 1 to 1.5 mg/100 U heparin when given a few minutes after IV heparin injection; 0.5 to 0.75 mg/100 U heparin when given 30 to 60 minutes after IV heparin injection; 0.25 to 0.375 mg/100 U heparin when given more than 2 hours after IV heparin injection; 25 to 50 mg after continuous infusion of heparin; 1 to 1.5 mg/100 U heparin after deep SC heparin injection, or 25 to 50 mg by slow IV injection and the rest of calculated dose given by continuous IV infusion over 8 to 16

P

hours or expected duration of heparin absorption.
Neutralization of heparin administered during extracorporeal circulation in arterial and cardiac surgery or dialysis procedures—
Adults and children: usually 1.5 mg/100 U heparin.

PREPARATION & STORAGE
Available in a concentration of 10 mg/ml as liquid in 5- and 25-ml vials or supplied as powder in 50- and 250-mg vials. Store liquid in refrigerator and powder at room temperature. Avoid freezing.

Reconstitute powder with sterile water for injection or bacteriostatic water for injection containing 0.9% benzyl alcohol (5 ml for 50 mg vial or 25 ml for 250 mg vial) to yield 10 mg/ml. Shake vigorously. If reconstituted with sterile water, use immediately and discard unused portions. If reconstituted with bacteriostatic water and benzyl alcohol, solution remains stable for 72 hours at room temperature.

Reconstituted solutions are not intended for further dilution, but if desired, may be diluted in D_5W or 0.9% NaCl. Do not store diluted solutions; they contain no preservatives.

Incompatibility
Incompatible with cephalosporins, diatrizoate meglumine, diatrizoate sodium, ioxaglate meglumine, ioxaglate sodium, and penicillins.

ADMINISTRATION
Direct injection: Inject reconstituted drug slowly over 1 to 3 minutes. Do not give more than 50 mg in 10 minutes. Overly rapid administration can cause severe hypotension and anaphylactoid reactions.

CONTRAINDICATIONS & CAUTIONS
• Contraindicated in hypersensitivity to drug and in neonates if drug is reconstituted with bacteriostatic water containing benzyl alcohol.

• Use cautiously in patients with allergies to fish; drug is derived from fish sperm.
• Use cautiously in patients with diabetes who receive protamine zinc insulin and in infertile or vasectomized men. Also use cautiously in patients who have received high doses of drug in the past.

SPECIAL CONSIDERATIONS
• Carefully titrate drug dose, especially if patient received a large heparin dose.
• Do not give more than 100 mg over 2 hours (drug's duration of action) unless coagulation studies indicate need for higher dosage.
• Drug is used to treat severe heparin overdose only. Mild overdose can be corrected by discontinuing heparin.
• Keep epinephrine 1:1,000 available to treat hypersensitivity.
• Check vital signs frequently.
• Monitor coagulation studies, such as activated clotting time, APTT, or thrombin time. These should be performed 5 to 15 minutes after therapy and repeated as necessary.
• Closely observe patient who has undergone extracorporeal circulation during arterial and cardiac surgery or hemodialysis. Heparin rebound with bleeding can occur 30 minutes to 18 hours later despite heparin neutralization by protamine sulfate.

quinidine gluconate

Quinidine Gluconate Injection

Pregnancy Risk Category: C

INDICATIONS & DOSAGES
Arrhythmias (atrial fibrillation or flutter, paroxysmal atrial or junctional tachycardia, ventricular or atrial premature contractions, ventricular tachycardia)—
Adults: initially, up to 0.25 mg/kg/minute, then adjusted to control arrhythmias. Usual dose required to

control ventricular arrhythmias is 300 mg or less. Maximum dosage is 4 g daily. Dosage may need to be reduced in patient with heart failure or hepatic disease.

Children: 30 mg/kg daily or 900 mg/m² daily in five divided doses.

Severe malaria caused by Plasmodium falciparum *(when IV quinine dihydrochloride is not available)—*

Adults: Centers for Disease Control and Prevention recommends 10 mg/kg diluted in 250 ml of 0.9% NaCl solution given over 1 to 2 hours followed by a continuous infusion of 0.02 mg/kg/minute for 72 hours or until parasitemia is reduced to less than 1%.

Note: Dosage may need adjustment in hemodialysis patient.

PREPARATION & STORAGE
Available in 10-ml vials (80 mg/ml). Store at room temperature, and protect from light and freezing. For intermittent infusion, dilute with D$_5$W to ordered concentration. For continuous infusion, dilute 800 mg (one vial) with 40 ml of D$_5$W to yield 16 mg/ml. Do not use solution if brown. Discard diluted solutions after 24 hours.

Incompatibility
Incompatible with alkalies, amiodarone, furosemide, heparin sodium, and iodides.

ADMINISTRATION
Intermittent infusion: Infuse solution through IV line over prescribed duration.
Continuous infusion: Infuse solution through IV line initially at prescribed rate, then adjust rate to control arrhythmias.

CONTRAINDICATIONS & CAUTIONS
• Contraindicated in hypersensitivity to quinidine or cinchona derivatives and in myasthenia gravis.
• Also contraindicated in cardiac glycoside–induced AV conduction disorders, complete AV block, severe

intraventricular conduction defects associated with a widened QRS complex, or escape junctional or ventricular rhythms.
• Use cautiously in the elderly.
• Administer cautiously to patients with asthma, emphysema, weakness, febrile infection, and hepatic or renal impairment.
• Use cautiously in incomplete AV, heart failure, hypotension, digitalis toxicity, hypokalemia, or history of thrombocytopenia.

SPECIAL CONSIDERATIONS
• Signs of overdose include absence of P waves and widening of QRS complex and PR and QT intervals, anuria, apnea, ataxia, extrasystoles, hallucinations, hypotension, irritability, lethargy, respiratory distress, seizures, thrashing, twitching, and ventricular arrhythmias. If these signs develop, promptly discontinue drug and give oxygen and ventilatory support.
• During infusion, continuously monitor blood pressure and cardiac function (including ECG).
• Monitor serum quinidine and potassium levels; quinidine levels above 8 mcg/ml are toxic.
• Know that GI adverse effects, especially diarrhea, are signs of toxicity.

ranitidine

Zantac

Pregnancy Risk Category: B

INDICATIONS & DOSAGES
Active duodenal or gastric ulcer and pathologic hypersecretory conditions, such as Zollinger-Ellison syndrome and multiple endocrine adenomas, in hospitalized patients who cannot take oral medication—
Adults: 50 mg q 6 to 8 hours. Maximum dosage is 400 mg daily.
Note: Adjust dosage in renal impairment.

R

PREPARATION & STORAGE
Available in 2- and 10-ml vials containing 25 mg/ml. Store at room temperature. Protect from light and freezing. For direct injection, dilute 50 mg dose with compatible IV solution (such as 0.9% NaCl, D_5W or dextrose 10% in water, lactated Ringer's, sodium bicarbonate 5%) to a total volume of 20 ml. For intermittent infusion, dilute 50-mg dose with 100 ml of a compatible IV solution. For continuous infusion, dilute 150 mg in 1,000 ml of a compatible solution. Solutions remain stable for 48 hours at room temperature. Do not use if drug is discolored or if a precipitate is present.

Incompatibility
Incompatible with amphotericin B, chlorpromazine hydrochloride, clindamycin phosphate, methotrimeprazine, midazolam hydrochloride, opium alkaloids hydrochloride, and pentobarbital sodium.

ADMINISTRATION
Direct injection: Inject diluted drug into a patent IV line over at least 5 minutes.
Intermittent infusion: Infuse diluted drug into a patent IV line through a piggyback set over 15 to 20 minutes.
Continuous infusion: Infuse over 24 hours at a rate of 6.25 mg/hour. No loading dose is required.

CONTRAINDICATIONS & CAUTIONS
• Contraindicated in hypersensitivity.
• Use cautiously in breast-feeding women and in renal or hepatic impairment because of possible increased serum levels.

SPECIAL CONSIDERATIONS
• Drug can be removed by hemodialysis.
• Monitor AST levels if patient receives 400 mg daily for 5 days or longer. Begin on day 5 of therapy and check daily until discontinuation.

• Instruct patient to inform doctor if rash, sore throat, fever, or easy bruising or bleeding occurs.

respiratory syncytial virus immune globulin intravenous, human (RSV-IGIV)

RespiGam

Pregnancy Risk Category: C

INDICATIONS & DOSAGE
Prevention of serious lower respiratory tract infections caused by RSV in children under age 24 months with bronchopulmonary dysplasia (BPD) or history of premature birth (35 weeks' gestation or less)—
Premature infants and children under age 2: single infusion monthly. Give 1.5 ml/kg/hour for 15 minutes; then, if clinical condition allows a higher rate, increase to 3 ml/kg/hour for 15 minutes and then to maximum of 6 ml/kg/hour until infusion is complete. Maximum recommended total dosage per monthly infusion, 750 mg/kg.

PREPARATION & STORAGE
Available as a single-use vial containing 2,500 mg RSV. Store between 35.6° F and 46.4° F (2° C and 8° F). Do not freeze. Do not shake vial; avoid foaming. Discard after use. RespiGam is compatible with the following dextrose solutions (with or without NaCl): 2.5%, 5%, 10%, and 20% dextrose in water. Do not dilute drug more than 1:2 with any of the above-named solutions.

Incompatibility
Administer drug separately from other medications.

ADMINISTRATION
Intermittent infusion: Begin infusion within 6 hours and complete within 12 hours after vial has been entered.

R

Administer drug using a constant infusion pump. Do not predilute drug. If possible, administer through a separate IV line, although it may be piggy-backed into a compatible solution. Although filters are not necessary, an in-line filter with a pore size larger than 15 micrometers may be used.

CONTRAINDICATIONS & CAUTIONS
• Contraindicated in history of severe hypersensitivity to drug or other human immunoglobulin and selective immunoglobulin A (IgA) deficiency.
• Do not use in children with fluid overload.
• Safety and efficacy of drug have not been established in children with congenital heart disease.

SPECIAL CONSIDERATIONS
• Give first dose before RSV season begins and subsequent doses monthly during the RSV season to maintain protection. Children with RSV should continue to receive monthly doses for duration of RSV season.
• Adhere to infusion rate guidelines; most adverse reactions may be related to rate used. In especially ill children with BPD, slower rates may be indicated.
• Assess cardiopulmonary status and vital signs before beginning infusion, before each rate increase, and every 30 minutes thereafter until 30 minutes after completion of infusion.
• Monitor closely for signs of fluid overload. Children with BPD may be at higher risk for this condition.
• If patient develops hypotension, anaphylaxis, or severe allergic reaction, stop infusion and administer epinephrine (1:1,000), as ordered.
• Explain to parents the importance of their child receiving drug monthly throughout the RSV season, even if already infected.

reteplase, recombinant

Retavase
Pregnancy Risk Category: C

INDICATIONS & DOSAGES
Management of acute MI—
Adults: double-bolus injection of 10 + 10 U. Give each bolus by infusion over 2 minutes. If complications, such as serious bleeding or an anaphylactoid reaction, do not occur after first bolus, give second bolus 30 minutes after start of first bolus.

PREPARATION & STORAGE
Available as a sterile, preservative-free lyophilized powder in 10.8-U (18.8 mg) vials. Reconstitute only with materials provided by manufacturer. Reteplase should be reconstituted with 10 ml of sterile water for injection. Reconstitution results in solution containing 1 U/ml. Solution may be used within 4 hours of reconstitution when stored at 36° to 86° F (2° to 30° C). Protect from light. Do not use if particulate matter or discoloration occurs.

Incompatibility
No other medication should be added to the injection solution containing drug.

ADMINISTRATION
Direct injection: Give as an IV bolus over 2 minutes.

CONTRAINDICATIONS & CAUTIONS
• Contraindicated in active internal bleeding, known bleeding diathesis, history of CVA, recent intracranial hemorrhage or intraspinal surgery or trauma, severe uncontrolled hypertension, intracranial neoplasm, arteriovenous malformation, or aneurysm.
• Use cautiously in patients with recent (within 10 days) major surgery, obstetric delivery, organ biopsy, or trauma; previous puncture of non-

R

compressible vessels; cerebrovascular disease; recent GI or GU bleeding; hypertension (systolic pressure of 180 mm Hg or more or diastolic pressure of 110 mm Hg or more); conditions that may lead to left-sided heart thrombus including mitral stenosis; acute pericarditis or subacute bacterial endocarditis; hemostatic defects; diabetic hemorrhagic retinopathy; septic thrombophlebitis; other conditions in which bleeding would be difficult to control; and in patients age 75 or older.
• Use cautiously in breast-feeding patients.
• Use in pregnancy only if the benefit justifies potential risk to the fetus.
• Safety and efficacy in children have not been established.

SPECIAL CONSIDERATIONS
• Reconstitute drug according to manufacturer's instructions using items provided in kit. Reconstitute with sterile water for injection, USP (without preservatives). Solution should be colorless. If foaming occurs, allow vial to stand for several minutes. Inspect for precipitation.
• Potency is expressed in terms of units specific for reteplase and not comparable to other thrombolytic agents.

rifampin

Rifadin
Pregnancy Risk Category: C

INDICATIONS & DOSAGES
Neisseria meningitidis *carriers*—
Adults: 600 mg b.i.d. for 2 days.
Children ages 1 month to 12 years: 10 mg/kg q 12 hours for 2 days.
Infants under age 1 month: 5 mg/kg q 12 hours for 2 days.
Primary treatment in pulmonary tuberculosis—
Adults: 10 mg/kg up to 600 mg daily as a single dose.

Children over age 5: 10 to 20 mg/ kg daily as a single dose. Maximum dose, 600 mg daily.

PREPARATION & STORAGE
Available as lyophilized powder in a 600-mg vial. Store at room temperature, protect from light, and avoid excessive heat (above 104° F [40° C]). Reconstitute using 10 ml of sterile water to make solution of 60 mg/ml; reconstituted solution is stable at room temperature for 24 hours. Immediately before use, withdraw the calculated amount of rifampin and add to 500 ml D_5W and infuse over 3 hours; if patient condition permits, add to 100 ml of D_5W and infuse over 30 minutes. Use either solution within 4 hours to avoid precipitation. Use 0.9% NaCl solution when dextrose is contraindicated; stability is reduced slightly.

Incompatibility
Incompatible with minocycline hydrochloride and many solutions. Use only D_5W or sterile saline as infusion solutions.

ADMINISTRATION
Intermittent infusion: Infuse 100 ml over 30 minutes; 500 ml over 3 hours.

CONTRAINDICATIONS & CAUTIONS
• Contraindicated in history of hypersensitivity to rifamycins and clinically active hepatitis.
• Do not use for treatment of meningococcal disease.
• Use cautiously in patients with hepatic disease or in those receiving other hepatotoxic drugs, carefully assessing benefits and risks.

SPECIAL CONSIDERATIONS
• Avoid extravasation.
• Monitor liver function tests, bilirubin, and blood counts. Watch closely for signs of hepatic impairment.
• Inform patient that urine, feces, saliva, sputum, sweat, and tears may be discolored red or orange and soft

R

contact lenses can be permanently stained.
• Instruct patient to inform doctor if sore throat, fever, malaise, or easy bruising or bleeding occurs.

Ringer's injection

Pregnancy Risk Category: C

COMPOSITION
An isotonic multiple electrolyte solution, Ringer's injection contains the principal ionic constituents of normal plasma. Each 100 ml contains 860 mg of NaCl, 30 mg of potassium chloride, and 33 mg of calcium chloride dehydrate. Each liter of Ringer's injection provides 147 mEq of sodium, 4 mEq of potassium, 4 mEq of calcium, and 155 mEq of chloride. The solution's pH is approximately 6.0.

INDICATIONS & DOSAGES
Replacement of extracellular fluid and electrolyte losses—
Adults and children: dosage highly individualized but usually 1.5 to 3 L daily (2% to 6% of body weight).

PREPARATION & STORAGE
Available in 500- and 1,000-ml containers. Store at room temperature. Avoid excessive heat; however, brief exposure to higher temperatures (up to 104° F [40° C]) does not adversely affect solution. Protect from freezing.
　　Before administration, inspect for precipitates and discoloration. Do not use unless solution is clear and container undamaged.

Incompatibility
Incompatible with ampicillin sodium, cefamandole, chlordiazepoxide, diazepam, erythromycin lactobionate, methicillin, potassium phosphate, sodium bicarbonate, and thiopental.

ADMINISTRATION
Continuous infusion: Infuse through central or peripheral IV line over ordered duration.

CONTRAINDICATIONS & CAUTIONS
• Contraindicated in renal failure, except as an emergency volume expander.
• Avoid use as a blood replacement or a substitute for plasma volume expanders, except in emergencies.
• Use cautiously in heart failure, hyperkalemia, hypoproteinemia, severe renal failure, and sodium retention.
• Administer to pregnant women only if clearly indicated.

SPECIAL CONSIDERATIONS
• Solution may be given with dextrose, other carbohydrates, or sodium lactate.
• IV administration of Ringer's injection can cause fluid or solute overload.
• Electrolyte content is insufficient for treating severe electrolyte deficiencies.
• If an adverse reaction occurs, discontinue infusion, institute symptomatic treatment, and save remainder of solution for examination, if necessary.
• Monitor changes in fluid and electrolyte balance during prolonged therapy.
• Instruct patient to promptly report difficulty in breathing.

Ringer's injection, lactated (Hartmann's solution, Ringer's lactate solution)

Pregnancy Risk Category: C

COMPOSITION
Lactated Ringer's injection consists of multiple electrolytes—130 mEq of sodium, 4 mEq of potassium, 3 mEq of calcium, 109 mEq of chloride, and 28 mEq of lactate per L.

R

Each liter of this isotonic solution contains 9 calories (from lactate). Solutions containing dextrose 5% or 10% provide additional calories.

INDICATIONS & DOSAGES
Replacement of extracellular fluid and electrolyte losses—
Adults and children: dosage highly individualized, but usually 1.5 to 3 L (2% to 6% of body weight) daily.

PREPARATION & STORAGE
Available in 250-, 500-, and 1,000-ml containers. Store at room temperature. Avoid excessive heat; however, brief exposure to temperatures up to 104° F (40° C) does not affect solution adversely.

Incompatibility
Incompatible with amphotericin B, ampicillin sodium, cefamandole, chlordiazepoxide, diazepam, erythromycin lactobionate, methicillin, methylprednisolone sodium succinate, phenytoin sodium, potassium phosphate, sodium bicarbonate, thiopental, and whole blood.

ADMINISTRATION
Continuous infusion: Infuse ordered amount through peripheral or central IV line over 18 to 24 hours.

CONTRAINDICATIONS & CAUTIONS
• Contraindicated in hyperkalemia, severe renal failure, and potassium retention.
• Avoid use in lactic acidosis.
• Use with caution in heart failure, edema, severe renal insufficiency, sodium retention, metabolic or respiratory alkalosis, and hepatic insufficiency.
• Use cautiously because excess lactate levels may cause metabolic acidosis.

SPECIAL CONSIDERATIONS
• Be aware of incompatibility of solution with various other medications when preparing infusion.
• During long-term therapy, monitor fluid and electrolyte balance.

• Instruct patient to report pain or swelling at infusion site.

ritodrine hydrochloride

Yutopar✦
Pregnancy Risk Category: B

INDICATIONS & DOSAGES
Management of uncomplicated preterm labor after gestation of 20 or more weeks, but less than 36 weeks—
Adults: initially 50 mcg/minute, gradually increasing q 10 minutes in 50-mcg increments until contractions cease. (Usual effective dosage, 150 to 350 mcg/minute.) Maintenance dosage, 150 to 350 mcg/minute for 12 to 24 hours after contractions stop. Maximum dosage, 350 mcg/minute.

PREPARATION & STORAGE
Available in concentrations of 10 and 15 mg/ml in 5- and 10-ml ampules, vials, and syringes. Store at room temperature.

For infusion, add 150 mg of ritodrine to 500 ml of D₅W to yield 300 mcg/ml. In patients with fluid restrictions, prepare a more concentrated solution, as ordered. Drug may also be diluted with 10% Dextran 40 in NaCl or 10% invert sugar solution. Avoid diluting with Ringer's injection, 0.9% NaCl, or lactated Ringer's. Also avoid diluting in NaCl solutions except in maternal diabetes because of increased risk of pulmonary edema. Use solution within 48 hours. Discard if discoloration or precipitation is present.

Incompatibility
None reported.

ADMINISTRATION
Continuous infusion: Using a pump to control rate, infuse by IV piggyback into a patent primary line at port closest to the infusion needle.

R

Adjust delivery to 50 mcg/minute (10 drops/minute, using microdrip chamber). Increase by 50 mcg/minute every 10 minutes until contractions or dilation stops, adverse maternal or fetal effects occur, or maximum dosage of 350 mcg/minute (70 drops/minute) is reached. At the recommended dilution, maximum fluid volume after 12 hours is about 840 ml.

CONTRAINDICATIONS & CAUTIONS
• Contraindicated before 20th week of pregnancy because of inadequate research; in antepartum hemorrhage, chorioamnionitis, pregnancy-induced hypertension, or pulmonary hypertension because continuation of pregnancy would be hazardous to patient or fetus; and in intrauterine fetal death or any known abnormality that requires immediate delivery.
• Also contraindicated in patients with hypersensitivity to sulfites, ritodrine, and other beta$_2$-adrenergic receptor agonists.
• Avoid use in hyperthyroidism or cardiac disorders.
• Give cautiously to patients with diabetes mellitus or mild to moderate hypertension.
• Effectiveness of drug in advanced labor (cervical dilation of more than 4 cm or effacement of more than 80%) has not been established.

SPECIAL CONSIDERATIONS
• For most effective results, start therapy as soon as preterm labor diagnosis is confirmed.
• Place patient in left lateral position to minimize hypotension.
• If preterm labor recurs, IV infusion may be repeated. If contractions do not recur after 36 to 48 hours, patient may gradually resume ambulation.
• Sinus bradycardia may follow drug withdrawal.
• Closely monitor intake and output. Also check fetal and maternal heart rates as well as maternal blood pressure, breath sounds, respirations, and uterine activity.

rocuronium bromide
Zemuron
Pregnancy Risk Category: B

INDICATIONS & DOSAGES
Adjunct to general anesthesia to facilitate endotracheal intubation or to provide skeletal muscle relaxation during surgery or mechanical ventilation—
Adults and children over age 3 months: dosage depends on anesthetic used, individual needs, and response. Dosages are representative and must be individualized. Initially, 0.6 mg/kg IV bolus. In most patients, tracheal intubation may be performed within 2 minutes; muscle paralysis lasts about 31 minutes. A maintenance dose for adults of 0.1 mg/kg provides an additional 12 minutes of muscle relaxation to duration of effect; 0.15 mg/kg, an additional 17 minutes; and 0.2 mg/kg, an additional 24 minutes. A maintenance dose for children of 0.075 to 0.125 mg/kg provides clinical relaxation for 7 to 10 minutes. Continuous infusion may be used to maintain neuromuscular blockade. Infusion for adults may start after early evidence of spontaneous recovery from intubating dose. Initiate at rate of 0.01 to 0.012 mg/kg/minute. An infusion for children may start at rate of 0.012 mg/kg/minute after one twitch is present in train-of-four. Dosages are adjusted to patient's twitch response.

PREPARATION & STORAGE
Available in vials containing 10 mg/ml. Store refrigerated at 36° to 46° F (2° to 8° C), but do not freeze. Use vial within 30 days after removal to room temperature (77° F [25° C]). If drug is given by continuous infusion, dilute with D$_5$W, 0.9% NaCl injection, dextrose 5% in 0.9% NaCl injection, sterile water for injection, or lactated Ringer's. Store reconstituted solution in refrigerator.

♦Also available in Canada.   ◊Available in Canada only.

Discard after 24 hours. Inspect for precipitates before use.

Incompatibility
Incompatible with alkaline solutions. Do not mix with other drugs.

ADMINISTRATION
Direct injection: Give undiluted drug by rapid injection.
Continuous infusion: Give diluted drug by infusion pump. Infusion rates are highly individualized but have ranged from 0.004 to 0.016 mg/kg/minute.

CONTRAINDICATIONS & CAUTIONS
• Contraindicated in patients hypersensitive to bromides and rocuronium.
• Use cautiously in hepatic disease, severe obesity, bronchogenic cancer, electrolyte disturbances, neuromuscular disease, and in altered circulation time from CV disease, old age, or edema.
• Drug is not recommended for use during rapid sequence induction for cesarean section.

SPECIAL CONSIDERATIONS
• Have emergency respiratory support materials readily available.
• Know that neuromuscular blockers do not alter consciousness or the pain threshold.
• A nerve stimulator and train-of-four monitoring are recommended to confirm antagonism of neuromuscular blockade and recovery of muscle strength.
• Monitor respirations until patient is fully recovered from neuromuscular blockade, as evidenced by tests of muscle strength (hand grip, head lift, and ability to cough).

sargramostim

Leukine

Pregnancy Risk Category: C

INDICATIONS & DOSAGES
Acceleration of myeloid reconstitution after autologous bone marrow transplantation in patients with malignant lymphoma, acute lymphoblastic leukemia, or Hodgkin's disease undergoing autologous bone marrow transplantation (BMT)—
Adults: 250 mcg/m² daily for 21 consecutive days over 2 hours, beginning 2 to 4 hours after BMT. In clinical studies, doses of 60 to 1,000 mcg/m²/day have been used.
BMT failure or engraftment delay—
Adults: 250 mcg/m²/day for 14 days, over 2 hours. May be repeated after 7 days off therapy if engraftment has not occurred; a third course of therapy at 500 mcg/m²/day for 14 days may be tried after 7 days off therapy have passed. If no improvement is shown, further treatment will likely not be beneficial.
Neutrophil recovery following chemotherapy in acute myelogenous leukemia—
Adults: 250 mcg/m²/day over 4 hours starting on approximately day 11 or 4 days after completion of induction chemotherapy, if day 10 bone marrow is hypoplastic with fewer than 5% blasts. If second cycle of induction chemotherapy is necessary, administer approximately 4 days after completion of chemotherapy if bone marrow is hypoplastic with fewer than 5% blasts. Continue until an absolute neutrophil count (ANC) exceeds 1,500/mm³ for 3 consecutive days or a maximum of 42 days.
Mobilization of peripheral blood progenitor cells (PBPC)—
Adults: 250 mcg/m²/day over 24 hours. Dosing should continue at the same dose through the period of PBPC collection.
Post-PBPC—

S

Adults: 250 mcg/m²/day over 24 hours beginning immediately after infusion of progenitor cells and continuing until ANC exceeds 1,500/mm³ on 3 consecutive days.

PREPARATION & STORAGE
Available as a lyophilized powder in 250- and 500-mcg preservative-free single-dose vials. Do not reuse single-dose vial; do not use 6 hours after reconstitution or dilution, and discard unused portion.

Reconstitute with 1 ml sterile water, directing stream against side of vial and swirling contents gently to minimize foaming. Dilute in 0.9% NaCl solution to make a concentration greater than 10 mcg/ml. If final concentration is below 10 mcg/ml, add human albumin at a final concentration of 0.1% to the 0.9% NaCl solution *before* adding sargramostim to prevent adsorption. For a final concentration of 0.1% human albumin, add 1 mg human albumin/1 ml 0.9% NaCl solution.

Incompatibility
Do not add other medications unless specific compatibility data are available. Use only 0.9% NaCl solution for reconstitution and dilution.

ADMINISTRATION
Intermittent infusion: Infuse over 2 to 4 hours by a central line; do not use in-line membrane filter.
Continuous infusion: Administer recommended dose over 24 hours.

CONTRAINDICATIONS & CAUTIONS
• Contraindicated in patients with excessive leukemic myeloid blasts in bone marrow or peripheral blood; and in hypersensitivity to drug or its components or yeast-derived products.
• Use cautiously in patients with pre-existing cardiac disease or fluid retention, hypoxia, pulmonary infiltrates, heart failure, or impaired renal or hepatic function.
• Safety and efficacy in children have not been established.

SPECIAL CONSIDERATIONS
• Do not administer within 24 hours of last dose of chemotherapy or within 12 hours after last dose of radiotherapy in acceleration of myeloid reconstitution.
• Monitor CBC with differential biweekly, including examination for blast cells.
• If blast cells appear or increase to 10% or more of WBC count, or if progression of the underlying disease occurs, discontinue therapy. If ANC is above 20,000 cells/mm³ or if WBC count is above 50,000 cells/mm³, discontinue therapy temporarily or reduce dose by half.
• Transient rash and local injection site reactions may occur.
• Closely monitor respiratory symptoms during and immediately after infusion.

secobarbital sodium

Seconal✦

Controlled Substance Schedule II

Pregnancy Risk Category: D

INDICATIONS & DOSAGES
Acute agitation in psychosis—
Adults: initially, no more than 250 mg; additional doses given cautiously after 5 minutes if initial dose does not produce desired response. Usually a dose of 1.1 to 1.7 mg/kg produces moderate to heavy sedation, 2.2 mg/kg produces hypnosis, and 3.3 to 4.4 mg/kg calms extremely agitated patients. Maximum dose is 500 mg.
Status epilepticus—
Adults: 250 to 350 mg.
Tetanic seizures—
Adults: 5.5 mg/kg, repeated q 3 to 4 hours, p.r.n.
Children: 3 to 5 mg/kg or 12.5 mg/m².
Preoperative anesthesia—
Adults: 50 to 250 mg in divided doses.
Insomnia—

Adults: 100 to 150 mg.

PREPARATION & STORAGE
Available in concentrations of
50 mg/ml in 1- and 2-ml prefilled
syringe cartridges and 20-ml vials.
Store in refrigerator at 36° to 46° F
(2° to 8° C). Protect from light. Do
not use if solution is discolored or
contains a precipitate. Drug may be
administered as supplied or diluted
with sterile water for injection, 0.9%
NaCl injection, or Ringer's injection.

Incompatibility
Incompatible with alkali-labile drugs
(such as penicillin), atracurium, benzquinamide, chlorpromazine, cimetidine, clindamycin phosphate, codeine phosphate, diphenhydramine,
droperidol, ephedrine, glycopyrrolate, hydrocortisone sodium succinate, isoproterenol hydrochloride,
lactated Ringer's injection, levorphanol, metaraminol, methadone
hydrochloride, methyldopate hydrochloride, norepinephrine, pancuronium, pentazocine lactate,
phenytoin sodium, procaine, regular
insulin, sodium bicarbonate, streptomycin, succinylcholine, and vancomycin.

ADMINISTRATION
Direct injection: Inject drug slowly
(not exceeding 50 mg/15 seconds)
through a primary IV line containing
a free-flowing, compatible solution.
Slow administration usually prevents
hypotension in hypertensive patients.

CONTRAINDICATIONS & CAUTIONS
• Contraindicated in hypersensitivity
to barbiturates and in acute intermittent porphyria, variegate porphyria,
bronchial pneumonia, or other severe pulmonary insufficiency.
• Also contraindicated in breast-
feeding women.
• Use cautiously in debilitated or elderly patients and in those with severe anemia, hyperkinesis, hyperthyroidism, and asthma.
• Also, use cautiously in patients
with borderline hypoadrenalism,

acute or chronic pain, hepatic or renal impairment, hepatic coma, cardiac disease, and hypertension.
• Give carefully during pregnancy or
labor and delivery.
• Use extreme caution in giving
drug to patients with history of drug
abuse or dependence and to depressed patients.

SPECIAL CONSIDERATIONS
• Avoid extravasation. Use large
veins to minimize irritation and risk
of thrombosis.
• Maintain airway with ventilation
and oxygen administration as needed. Administer chest physiotherapy.
• Discontinue drug if skin eruptions
occur; these may precede potentially
fatal reactions.
• Risk of barbiturate-induced hypothermia may increase in elderly
patients, especially with high doses
or acute overdose.
• Always keep resuscitation and mechanical ventilation equipment available.
• Monitor vital signs.
• Monitor fluid balance. Avoid sodium or fluid overload, especially in
cardiac disorders.
• After drug discontinuation, be
alert for withdrawal symptoms.
Those that require medical attention
include anxiety or unusual restlessness, dizziness, hallucinations, lightheadedness, muscle twitching, nausea and vomiting, seizures, insomnia,
trembling hands, vision problems,
and unusual weakness.

sodium bicarbonate

Sodium Bicarbonate
Pregnancy Risk Category: C

INDICATIONS & DOSAGES
Dosage reflects severity of acidosis,
test results, and patient's age,
weight, and condition.
Cardiac arrest—
**Adults and children age 2 and
older:** 200 to 300 mEq of bicarbon-

S

ate, with additional doses depending on arterial blood gas (ABG) measurements, if available.
Children under age 2: 1 mEq/kg initially. If ABG and pH levels are available, further doses are given q 10 minutes and calculated in milliequivalents of NaHCO₃. Multiply 0.3 by body weight (kg). Then multiply this figure by base deficit (mEq/L). If ABG and pH levels are unavailable, further doses of 1 mEq/kg are given q 10 minutes during arrest. Maximum dosage is 8 mEq/kg daily.
Metabolic acidosis associated with chronic renal failure—
Adults and older children: initially, 2 to 5 mEq/kg; subsequent doses are determined by response to drug and test results (total carbon dioxide [CO₂], blood pH).
Urinary alkalinization—
Adults and children: 2 to 5 mEq/kg.

PREPARATION & STORAGE
Available in 5-ml (2.4 mEq) flip-top and pin-top vials containing 4% solution (0.48 mEq/ml); 10-ml (5 mEq) disposable syringes containing 4.2% solution (0.5 mEq/ml); 500-ml (297.5 mEq) containers of 5% solution (0.595 mEq/ml); 10-ml (8.9 mEq) ampules and 50-ml (44.6 mEq) ampules and disposable syringes containing 7.5% solution (0.892 mEq/ml); and 10-ml (10 mEq) disposable syringes and 50-ml (50 mEq) vials and disposable syringes containing 8.4% solution (1 mEq/ml).
Store at room temperature, always below 104° F (40° C), and protect from freezing and heat. Stability may be increased by refrigerating sodium bicarbonate injection and syringes before preparation, rinsing syringes twice with refrigerated sterile water for injection, and minimizing contact with air. To do this, expel air from syringes and tape the plungers in place to reduce movement caused by escaping CO₂. The 7.5% solution in polypropylene

syringes is stable up to 100 days if refrigerated or up to 45 days at room temperature. Do not use solution if it is cloudy or contains a precipitate.
To dilute for infusion, follow manufacturer's instructions, using sterile water for injection or other standard electrolyte solutions. In neonates and children under age 2, use 4.2% sodium bicarbonate solution or dilute 7.5% or 8.4% sodium bicarbonate solution 1:1 with D₅W.

Incompatibility
Incompatible with alcohol 5% in dextrose 5%, amino acids, ascorbic acid injection, calcium salts, carmustine, cisplatin, codeine phosphate, corticotropin, dextrose 5% in lactated Ringer's injection, dobutamine, dopamine, epinephrine hydrochloride, fat emulsion 10%, glycopyrrolate, hydromorphone, insulin (regular), Ionosol B, D, or G with invert sugar 10%, isoproterenol hydrochloride, labetalol hydrochloride, levorphanol, magnesium sulfate, meperidine, methadone hydrochloride, methicillin sodium, methylprednisolone sodium succinate, metoclopramide, morphine sulfate, norepinephrine bitartrate, penicillin G potassium, pentazocine lactate, pentobarbital sodium, phenobarbital sodium, procaine hydrochloride, promazine hydrochloride, Ringer's injection and lactated Ringer's injection, secobarbital sodium, sodium lactate (1/6 M), streptomycin sulfate, succinylcholine chloride, thiopental sodium, vancomycin hydrochloride, and vitamin B complex with vitamin C.

ADMINISTRATION
Direct injection: For cardiac arrest, flush IV line before and after use. In adults, inject rapidly into patent primary IV line. In neonates and children under age 2, inject ordered dose into patent primary IV line over 1 to 2 minutes. Overly rapid injection (10 ml/minute) can cause hypernatremia, decreased CSF pres-

sure, intracranial hemorrhage, and severe alkalosis, accompanied by hyperirritability or tetany.
Continuous infusion: Flush IV line before and after use. Infuse ordered amount of diluted drug into patent IV line over 4 to 8 hours, as ordered, for metabolic acidosis.

CONTRAINDICATIONS & CAUTIONS
• Contraindicated in metabolic or respiratory alkalosis.
• Also contraindicated in chloride loss from vomiting or continuous GI suctioning, in hypocalcemia, and in patients at risk for development of diuretic-induced hypochloremic alkalosis.
• Give cautiously in hypertension, renal insufficiency, and edematous sodium-retaining conditions.
• Drug should only be given when clearly needed during pregnancy.

SPECIAL CONSIDERATIONS
• Administer repeated small doses to avoid overdose and resultant metabolic alkalosis.
• Use of drug in cardiac arrest should be preceded by manual or mechanical hyperventilation to lower partial pressure of carbon dioxide levels.
• Do not attempt full correction of bicarbonate deficit during first 24 hours of therapy; this may produce metabolic alkalosis from delayed compensatory mechanisms.
• If alkalosis develops, have patient breathe expired air from a mask or paper bag. If alkalosis is severe, administer calcium gluconate IV, as ordered.
• Throughout therapy, monitor ABG and pH, serum bicarbonate, renal function (especially in long-term therapy), and urine pH (especially when drug is used for alkalinization).

sodium chloride

0.45% Sodium Chloride Injection, 0.9% Sodium Chloride Injection, 3% Sodium Chloride Injection, 5% Sodium Chloride Injection
Pregnancy Risk Category: C

COMPOSITION
These solutions consist of NaCl and sterile water with no bacteriostatic or antimicrobial agents or added buffers. They have a pH of 4.5 to 7.
The 0.45% concentration is hypotonic with 77 mEq/L of sodium and of chloride and an osmolarity of 154 to 155 mOsm/L. The 0.9% concentration is isotonic, contains 154 mEq/L of sodium and of chloride, and has an osmolarity of 308 to 310 mOsm/L. The 3% concentration is hypertonic and contains 513 mEq/L of sodium and of chloride with an osmolarity of 1,026 to 1,030 mOsm/L. Also hypertonic, 5% NaCl contains 855 mEq/L of sodium and of chloride. Its osmolarity is 1,710 to 1,711 mOsm/L.
Concentrations of 0.225% and 0.3% NaCl are not commercially available. These hypotonic solutions contain 38.5 mEq/L of sodium and of chloride for the 0.225% concentration and 51 mEq/L for the 0.3% concentration.

INDICATIONS & CONCENTRATION
Dosage depends on the disorder and patient's age, weight, and fluid, electrolyte, and acid-base balance. For children, concentration and dosage are based on weight or body surface area.
Fluid and electrolyte replacement—
Adults: usually 1 L daily of 0.9% NaCl or 1 to 2 L daily of 0.45% NaCl.
Fluid and electrolyte replacement in ketoacidosis—
Children: 0.225% or 0.3% NaCl.

S

Severe NaCl depletion requiring rapid replacement—
Adults: 100 ml of 3% or 5% NaCl over 1 hour, then additional doses determined by serum electrolyte measurement.
Adjunct to blood transfusions and hemodialysis—
Adults: 0.9% NaCl.
Hyperosmolar diabetes—
Adults: 0.45% NaCl.

PREPARATION & STORAGE
Available in glass or flexible polyvinyl chloride containers. Solutions of 0.45% NaCl come in 500- and 1,000-ml containers; 0.9% NaCl in 50-, 100-, 150-, 250-, 500-, and 1,000-ml containers; and 3% and 5% NaCl in 500-ml containers. Solutions of 0.9% NaCl are also supplied in 25-, 50-, and 100-ml containers as diluents for drug delivery. Store solutions at room temperature.

Incompatibility
Incompatible with amphotericin B, benzquinamide, chlordiazepoxide, diazepam, fat emulsion, methylprednisolone sodium succinate, and phenytoin sodium.

ADMINISTRATION
Direct injection: Used only as drug diluent.
Intermittent infusion: Used only as drug diluent.
Continuous infusion: Infuse through a peripheral or central vein at ordered rate. Infuse 3% or 5% solutions through a large vein, at a rate not exceeding 100 ml/hour. Avoid extravasation. Observe infusion site carefully for signs of phlebitis.

CONTRAINDICATIONS & CAUTIONS
• Contraindicated in conditions in which sodium and chloride administration is hazardous.
• Use hypertonic solutions only in patients with severe sodium and chloride deficits.
• Use with extreme caution in patients with heart failure, other sodi-

um-retaining conditions, and severe renal disease or insufficiency.
• Give carefully in elderly or postoperative patients.

SPECIAL CONSIDERATIONS
• If fluid overload occurs, discontinue infusion and initiate corrective measures.
• Monitor serum electrolytes, especially sodium and potassium. Also check chloride and bicarbonate levels.
• Encourage patient to report pain at IV site immediately.

streptokinase

Kabikinase, Streptase◆

Pregnancy Risk Category: C

INDICATIONS & DOSAGES
Pulmonary embolism, deep vein thrombosis, arterial embolism or thrombosis—
Adults: loading dose 250,000 IU; maintenance dose 100,000 IU/hour.
Acute, obstructing coronary artery thrombi associated with evolving acute MI—
Adults: 1.5 million IU over 60 minutes.
Arteriovenous cannula occlusion—
Adults: 250,000 IU in 2 ml of IV solution.

PREPARATION & STORAGE
Available in powder form in 5-ml vials containing 250,000, 600,000, or 750,000 IU; in 6.5-ml vials containing 250,000, 750,000, or 1.5 million IU; and in 50-ml infusion bottle of 1.5 million IU. Store unopened vials at room temperature.

For arteriovenous cannula clearance, reconstitute using 2 ml of 0.9% NaCl injection or dextrose 5% injection for each 250,000 IU of streptokinase. Add diluent slowly, directed at the side of the vial (rather than onto the powder). Roll and tilt the vial gently; avoid shaking, which may cause foaming and an increase in flocculation. Slight flocculation does not interfere with safe use; however, solutions containing many particles should be discarded.

For infusion, reconstitute with 0.9% NaCl injection or dextrose 5% injection. Further dilute, generally to a volume of 45 ml (loading dose infusion) or to a multiple of 45 ml to a maximum of 500 ml (continuous maintenance infusion), with the same solution used for reconstitution. Infusions should be administered through a 0.22- or 0.45-micron filter. Use volumetric or syringe pumps because reconstituted streptokinase solution may alter drop size, influencing the accuracy of drop-counting infusion devices.

Store reconstituted solutions at 36° to 39° F (2° to 4° C); discard after 24 hours. Do not add any other drugs to the solution.

Incompatibility
Drug is incompatible with dextrans. Do not mix with other medications.

ADMINISTRATION
Direct injection: To clear arteriovenous cannula obstruction, use an infusion pump to slowly deliver 250,000 IU of reconstituted drug into each occluded cannula over 25 to 35 minutes. Then, clamp off the cannulas for 2 hours. Closely observe patient for possible adverse reactions. After 2 hours, aspirate contents of the cannulas and flush with 0.9% NaCl. Reconnect cannula.
Continuous infusion: For loading dose in pulmonary embolism, deep vein thrombosis, or arterial embolism or thrombosis, give diluted drug through a peripheral IV line, using an infusion pump to deliver 250,000 IU over 30 minutes. Set rate at 30 ml/hour (for 750,000 IU vial) or 90 ml/hour (for 250,000 IU vial) with dilution equaling 45 ml.

For maintenance dose, set infusion pump to deliver 100,000 IU/hour. Continue infusion for 24 hours for pulmonary embolism, for 24 to 72 hours for arterial embolism or thrombosis, and for 72 hours for deep vein thrombosis.

For coronary artery thrombi, give diluted drug through a peripheral IV line, using an infusion pump with rate set at 1.5 million IU/hour for 1 hour. No maintenance dose is required.

CONTRAINDICATIONS & CAUTIONS
• Contraindicated in active internal bleeding, intracranial neoplasm, severe uncontrolled hypertension, or recent (within 2 months) CVA or intracranial or intraspinal surgery.
• Also contraindicated in previous severe allergic reaction to drug.
• Use with extreme caution in conditions with associated risk of bleeding, such as dissecting aneurysm, CVA or disease (within 2 months), childbirth, invasive procedures or surgery within past 10 days, uncontrolled coagulation defects or other hemostatic defects, subacute bacterial endocarditis, diabetic hemorrhagic retinopathy, severe GI bleeding within the past 10 days, GI lesion or ulcer, moderate hypertension, recent trauma, and active tuberculosis with cavitation of recent onset.
• Use cautiously in mitral stenosis with atrial fibrillation or other indications of probable left heart thrombus and in conditions with risk of cerebral embolism.
• Give cautiously in sepsis at or near thrombus site, obstructed intravenous catheter, or occluded arteriovenous cannula.
• Administer carefully in patients with recent streptococcal infection (and in patients receiving drug).

SPECIAL CONSIDERATIONS
• Avoid invasive arterial procedures before and during therapy. If necessary, use an upper extremity.
• Perform venipunctures carefully and as infrequently as possible.
• Avoid IM injections and unnecessary handling of patient.

S

• Because exposure to streptococci (source of streptokinase) is common, a loading dose is used to neutralize the antibodies present in many patients. Do not give loading dose exceeding 1 million IU.
• In hemorrhage, discontinue drug immediately. If necessary, administer whole blood (fresh blood preferred), packed RBCs, and cryoprecipitate or fresh frozen plasma. Do not use dextrans. Aminocaproic acid may be administered in an emergency, although its use as an antidote has not been established.
• Before initiating therapy, obtain a blood sample to determine thrombin time, APTT, PT, hematocrit, and platelet count.
• Monitor vital signs and clotting status.

succinylcholine chloride

Anectine✦, Anectine Flo-Pack✦, Quelicin, Sucostrin

Pregnancy Risk Category: C

INDICATIONS & DOSAGES
Dosages below are guidelines.
Skeletal muscle relaxant for short procedures, such as endotracheal intubation, endoscopy, and orthopedic manipulations—
Adults: initially, 0.6 mg/kg (range 0.3 to 1.1 mg/kg). Subsequent doses based on response to drug.
Children: initially, 1 to 2 mg/kg. Subsequent doses based on first dose.
Skeletal muscle relaxant for prolonged surgical procedures—
Adults: 2.5 to 4.3 mg/minute (0.5 to 10 mg/minute) by continuous infusion (preferred method). Or initially, 0.3 to 1.1 mg/kg by intermittent injection; subsequent doses 0.04 to 0.07 mg/kg, p.r.n., to maintain relaxation.
Electroshock therapy—

Adults: 10 to 30 mg given about 1 minute before shock is administered, although dosage must be individualized by patient size and condition.

PREPARATION & STORAGE
Available in 10-ml vials containing 20 or 100 mg/ml and in 10- and 20-ml ampules containing 50 mg/ml. Also available in powder form in strengths of 100 mg, 500 mg, and 1 g in 5-ml unit-dose vials.

Reconstitute powder with compatible diluent, such as dextrose 5% injection or 0.9% NaCl, according to manufacturer's instructions. Store solutions at 36° to 46° F (2° to 8° C). Multidose vials are stable for 14 days at room temperature. Powders do not require refrigeration.

For continuous infusion, dilute to a concentration of 1 to 2 mg/ml. Add 1 g of powder, 10 ml of solution (100 mg/ml), or 20 ml of solution (500 mg/ml) to 1 L or 500 ml of compatible diluent, such as dextrose 5% injection, dextrose 5% in 0.9% NaCl, 0.9% NaCl, or 1/6 M sodium lactate. Alternatively, add 500 mg of powder, 5 ml of solution (100 mg/ml), or 10 ml of solution (50 mg/ml) to 500 or 250 ml of diluent to yield 1 or 2 mg/ml succinylcholine, respectively.

For direct injection, use prepared solution if possible, or dilute with compatible solution to yield concentration, volume, and dosage ordered.

Discard unused solutions within 24 hours.

Incompatibility
Decomposes in a solution with pH above 4.5. Incompatible with barbiturates, nafcillin, and sodium bicarbonate.

ADMINISTRATION
Direct injection: Inject ordered amount of commercially prepared or diluted drug over 10 to 30 seconds

---

✦ Also available in Canada. ◇ Available in Canada only.

S

into a primary IV line containing a free-flowing, compatible solution. *Continuous infusion:* Infuse diluted drug through an IV line containing a free-flowing, compatible solution at 2.5 mg/minute initially; then adjust to 0.5 to 10 mg/minute, depending on patient response.

To avoid overdose and detect development of nondepolarizing neuromuscular blockade, monitor neuromuscular function with a peripheral nerve stimulator when giving drug by infusion.

CONTRAINDICATIONS & CAUTIONS
• Contraindicated in patients with low pseudocholinesterase levels and myopathies associated with elevated serum CK levels.
• Also contraindicated in patients with personal or family history of malignant hyperthermia and in angle-closure glaucoma and penetrating eye injuries.
• Use cautiously in recent digitalis therapy or digitalis toxicity, severe burns, degenerative or dystrophic neuromuscular disease, paraplegia, spinal cord injury, or severe trauma.
• Give carefully in bronchogenic carcinoma, electrolyte or acid-base imbalance, conditions in which histamine release would be hazardous, and hyperkalemia.
• Also give carefully in anemia, dehydration, exposure to neurotoxic insecticides, severe hepatic disease or cirrhosis, malnutrition, pregnancy, recessive hereditary trait, pulmonary impairment, respiratory depression, severe obesity, or neuromuscular disease.
• In open eye injury or chronic open-angle glaucoma or during ocular surgery, use drug cautiously.
• Also use cautiously in fractures, muscle spasm, hyperthermia, hypothermia, and hepatic or renal impairment.
• Continuous IV infusion is considered unsafe in infants and children.

SPECIAL CONSIDERATIONS
• In prolonged administration, if the depolarizing neuromuscular blockade changes to nondepolarizing blockade (determined by nerve stimulator), give small doses of an anticholinesterase drug (antagonist), as ordered. Administer atropine with an anticholinesterase agent to counteract muscarinic adverse effects. Observe patient for at least 1 hour after reversal of nondepolarizing blockade for possible return of muscle relaxation.
• Administer test dose of 10 mg IV to determine patient's sensitivity and recovery time, as ordered.
• Premedicate with atropine, scopolamine, or thiopental sodium, as ordered.
• Give drug after unconsciousness has been induced.
• Use a peripheral nerve stimulator to determine nature and degree of neuromuscular blockade. Overdose may result in prolonged respiratory depression or apnea and CV collapse. If apnea or prolonged paralysis occurs, maintain airway and administer manual or mechanical ventilation until independent respiration resumes. Administer fluids and vasopressors as needed to treat shock or severe hypotension.
• When administering succinylcholine, keep emergency resuscitation equipment available.

sufentanil citrate

Sufenta

Controlled Substance Schedule II

Pregnancy Risk Category: C

INDICATIONS & DOSAGES
Dosage depends on concurrent drug administration (especially anesthetics), type and expected length of surgery, and patient's age, ideal weight, size, physical condition, underlying disorder, and response to drug.

S

Adjunct in anesthesia—
Adults: low initial dose, 1 to 2 mcg/kg, with supplemental doses of 10 to 25 mcg p.r.n. to maintain analgesia or anesthesia; moderate initial dose, 2 to 8 mcg/kg, with supplemental doses of 10 to 50 mcg p.r.n.

If used with nitrous oxide and oxygen for procedures lasting 8 hours or longer, total dosage is 1 mcg/kg/hour or less.

Primary anesthesia—
Adults: initially, 8 to 30 mcg/kg with 100% oxygen, with supplemental doses of 25 to 50 mcg p.r.n. to maintain anesthesia. Loading dose followed by continuous infusion is recommended for prolonged procedures.

Children under age 12 undergoing CV surgery: initially, 10 to 25 mcg/kg with 100% oxygen, with supplemental doses of 25 to 50 mcg p.r.n. (maximum total, 1 to 2 mcg/kg) to maintain anesthesia.

PREPARATION & STORAGE
Available in preservative-free 1-, 2-, and 5-ml ampules containing 50 mcg/ml. Store at room temperature, always below 104° F (40° C). Protect from light and freezing. For continuous infusion, dilute with a compatible solution.

Incompatibility
None reported.

ADMINISTRATION
Direct injection: Inject slowly, especially with large doses, over 1 to 2 minutes. Use a 1-ml syringe for small doses.
Continuous infusion: After loading dose, infuse 1 mcg/kg or less over 1 hour.

CONTRAINDICATIONS & CAUTIONS
• Contraindicated in sensitivity to sufentanil or other fentanyl derivatives.
• Use with extreme caution in patients receiving MAO inhibitors within the previous 14 days and in those with altered respiratory function.
• Use cautiously in patients with head injury and increased intracranial pressure.
• Use cautiously in elderly or debilitated patients and neonates.
• Also administer carefully in patients with bradyarrhythmias or poor cardiac reserve.
• Give lowered doses in hypothyroidism and hepatic or renal impairment.

SPECIAL CONSIDERATIONS
• High doses may produce muscle rigidity, which can be reversed by administering neuromuscular blocking agents.
• During therapy with sufentanil, keep resuscitation equipment available.
• In cases of overdose, maintain airway patency and provide respiratory support. Give naloxone as needed to reverse respiratory depression. Also administer IV fluids and vasopressors, as ordered, to maintain blood pressure and neuromuscular blockers to relieve muscle rigidity.
• Monitor patient's breathing for at least 1 hour after dose.
• Closely monitor for signs of withdrawal when discontinuing sufentanil after prolonged use.

teniposide (VM-26)

Vumon✦

Pregnancy Risk Category: D

INDICATIONS & DOSAGES
Malignant lymphomas—
Adults: as a single agent: 30 mg/m^2/day q 5 days, or 30 mg/m^2/day for 10 days, or 50 to 100 mg/m^2/day once weekly; in combination therapy: 60 to 70 mg/m^2/day once weekly.
Neuroblastomas—
Adults: 130 to 180 mg/m^2/day as a single agent once weekly; or

100 mg/m² daily q 21 days in combination therapy.
Acute lymphocytic leukemia—
Adults: 165 mg/m²/day twice weekly in combination therapy.
Acute lymphocytic leukemia induction therapy in childhood—
Children: optimum dose has not been established. One protocol reported by manufacturer is 165 mg/m² IV teniposide with cytarabine 300 mg/m² IV twice weekly for eight or nine doses.

PREPARATION & STORAGE
Use extreme caution when preparing and administering drug to avoid mutagenic, teratogenic, and carcinogenic risks. Use a biological containment cabinet, wear gloves and mask, and use syringes with luer-lock fittings to prevent drug leakage. Avoid contaminating work surfaces, and dispose of needles, syringes, ampules, and unused drug correctly. Avoid inhaling drug particles or solutions or allowing contact with skin or mucosa. If contact occurs, wash the area immediately with soap and water.

Supplied in ampules of 50 mg/5 ml that must be refrigerated and protected from light. For infusion, dilute to a final concentration of 0.1 mg/ml, 0.2 mg/ml, 0.4 mg/ml or 1 mg/ml with D₅W or 0.9% NaCl. In glass containers, solutions of 100 to 200 mcg/ml are stable for 24 hours using D₅W or sterile water; 100 to 400 mcg/ml solutions are stable for 24 hours using 0.9% NaCl. In plastic containers, 100 mcg/ml solutions are stable for 8 hours using 0.9% NaCl or sterile water. However, drug is unstable in plastic containers at concentrations above 100 mcg/ml, and teniposide concentrate may soften plastic, causing cracking and leaking. Glass bottles and nonpolyvinyl chloride plastic administration sets are recommended. Solution may appear slightly opalescent from surfactants in the formulation.

Incompatibility
Incompatible with heparin sodium.

ADMINISTRATION
Continuous infusion: Using a 23G or 25G winged-tip needle, administer over at least 45 minutes to avoid hypotension. Use distal rather than major veins. Choose a new site for each infusion.

If extravasation occurs, apply ice to the area. Injection of a corticosteroid and irrigation with copious amounts of 0.9% NaCl may decrease swelling.

CONTRAINDICATIONS & CAUTIONS
• Contraindicated in patients who have demonstrated a previous hypersensitivity to teniposide or polyoxyethylated castor oil.
• Use with caution in patients with renal or hepatic dysfunction.

SPECIAL CONSIDERATIONS
• Keep diphenhydramine, epinephrine, hydrocortisone, and an airway available in case of anaphylaxis.
• Stop infusion; notify doctor if systolic pressure falls below 90 mm Hg.
• Be aware that dosages for malignant lymphoma, neuroblastomas, and acute lymphocytic leukemia in adults apply only in Canada.
• Monitor blood pressure before, during, and after infusion.
• Monitor CBC during and after treatment.
• Monitor for phlebitis at injection site.
• Monitor liver function studies.

terbutaline sulfate

Brethine, Bricanyl
Pregnancy Risk Category: B

INDICATIONS & DOSAGES
Treatment of premature labor (after 20 weeks' gestation)—
Adults: initially, 10 mcg/minute, increased by 10 mcg/minute q 20 minutes until contractions stop or

reach maximum rate of 80 mcg/
minute. Once contractions have
ceased for 30 to 60 minutes, reduce
dose by 5 mcg/minute and maintain
at minimum effective rate for 4
hours. Then switch to oral form.

PREPARATION & STORAGE

Available in 2-ml ampules containing
1 mg/ml. Solution is clear and colorless; do not use if discolored. Store
ampules at room temperature and
protect from light. For infusion, add
10 mg of drug to 250 ml of D_5W,
0.9% NaCl, or 0.45% NaCl to yield
40 mcg/ml.

Incompatibility
Incompatible with bleomycin sulfate.

ADMINISTRATION

Continuous infusion: Before administration, start a primary IV infusion.
Hang terbutaline solution as a secondary IV line to allow immediate
discontinuation if adverse effects occur. Use an infusion pump and continuously monitor cardiac status.

CONTRAINDICATIONS & CAUTIONS

• Contraindicated in hypersensitivity
to sympathomimetics.
• Also contraindicated in arrhythmias caused by digitalis toxicity because of enhanced risk of drug-
induced tachycardia.
• Use cautiously in patients with hypothyroidism, diabetes mellitus,
glaucoma, pheochromocytoma, hypertension, vasomotor instability, or
a history of seizures.

SPECIAL CONSIDERATIONS

• To reduce risk of pulmonary edema, avoid using NaCl as a diluent
when possible.
• Monitor serum potassium and glucose levels closely during infusion.
• Monitor fetus continuously for CV
effects.
• After delivery, observe neonate for
hypoglycemia.

thiotepa (TSPA, TESPA)

Thioplex

Pregnancy Risk Category: D

INDICATIONS & DOSAGES

Dosage reflects response to the drug
and appearance or degree of toxicity.
Maintenance doses are based on
hematologic studies.
*Adenocarcinomas of breast and ovary,
lymphomas, bronchogenic carcinoma
(palliative treatment)—*
**Adults and children age 12 and
over:** 0.3 to 0.4 mg/kg q 1 to 4
weeks.

PREPARATION & STORAGE

Use extreme caution in the preparation and administration of drug to
avoid mutagenic, teratogenic, and
carcinogenic risks. Use a biological
containment cabinet, wear gloves
and mask, and use syringes with luer-
lock fittings to prevent drug leakage.
Dispose of needles, vials, and unused
drug correctly, and avoid contaminating work surfaces.

Available as a powder in 15-mg
vials. Reconstitute with 1.5 ml of
sterile water for injection to yield a
concentration of 10 mg/ml. For infusion, further dilute drug in NaCl
injection, dextrose injection, dextrose and NaCl injection, Ringer's
injection, or lactated Ringer's injection.

Refrigerate powder and reconstituted solution at 36° to 46° F (2° to
8° C), and protect from light. Reconstituted solution is stable for 5
days if refrigerated (0.5 mg/ml solution in Ringer's injection is stable
for 15 days refrigerated or at room
temperature). Do not use if solution
is grossly opaque or contains precipitates; microbial contamination is
possible.

Incompatibility
None reported.

T

ADMINISTRATION
Direct injection: Using a 21G or 23G needle, inject rapidly.
Intermittent infusion: Give diluted drug over ordered duration. Start a primary IV line or use the infusion port of an existing primary line.

CONTRAINDICATIONS & CAUTIONS
• Contraindicated in hypersensitivity to drug and during pregnancy.
• Also contraindicated in existing or recent exposure to chickenpox or herpes zoster.
• Use cautiously in patients with infections, bone marrow depression, gout, or history of urate renal calculi.
• Also use cautiously in tumor cell infiltration of bone marrow, previous cytotoxic drug therapy, radiation therapy, or in renal or hepatic impairment.
• Dosage not established for children under age 12.
• In recent cytotoxic drug or radiation therapy, therapy is not recommended until depressed WBC and platelet counts start to recover.

SPECIAL CONSIDERATIONS
• At the first sign of a sudden large drop in WBC (particularly granulocyte) or platelet counts, discontinue drug or reduce dosage, as ordered, to prevent irreversible myelosuppression.
• Provide adequate oral hydration, which may prevent or delay uric acid nephropathy. Allopurinol administration may also be helpful.
• Drug is highly toxic with a low therapeutic index; many adverse effects are unavoidable.
• Before and during therapy, monitor WBC and platelet counts and BUN, hematocrit, AST, ALT, bilirubin, creatinine, LD, and uric acid levels.

ticarcillin disodium
Ticar♦

Pregnancy Risk Category: B

INDICATIONS & DOSAGES
Septicemia; respiratory tract, skin, soft tissue, intra-abdominal, female pelvic, and genital tract infections—
Adults and children weighing over 88 lb (40 kg): 200 to 300 mg/kg/day in divided doses q 4 to 6 hours.
Children weighing up to 88 lb: 200 to 300 mg/kg/day in divided doses q 4 to 6 hours.
Neonates weighing 4.5 lb (2 kg) and over: 75 mg/kg q 8 hours for first week of life; then 100 mg/kg q 8 hours.
Urinary tract infections (complicated)—
Adults and children weighing over 88 lb: 150 to 200 mg/kg/day in divided doses q 4 to 6 hours.
Children weighing up to 88 lb: 150 to 200 mg/kg/day in divided doses q 4 to 6 hours.
Urinary tract infections (uncomplicated)—
Adults and children weighing over 88 lb: 1 g q 6 hours.
Children weighing up to 88 lb: 50 to 100 mg/kg/day in divided doses q 6 to 8 hours.
Note: Dosage in renal failure reflects creatinine clearance.

PREPARATION & STORAGE
Supplied as a white to pale yellow powder or lyophilized cake in 1-, 3-, and 6-g vials and 3-g piggyback bottles. Reconstitute by adding 4 ml of 0.9% NaCl, D_5W, or lactated Ringer's solution for each gram of drug. For continuous infusion, dilute further with 10 to 100 ml of a compatible IV solution. Reconstituted solution is clear and colorless or pale yellow.
  Store powder at room temperature. Refrigerate reconstituted solution or use within 30 minutes. Diluted solutions are stable for 72 hours at room temperature with

T

sterile water for injection, D_5W water, and 0.9% NaCl; and for 48 hours at room temperature with Ringer's injection or lactated Ringer's solution (10 to 100 mg/ml). Solutions with dextrose 5% in 0.225% or 0.45% NaCl or with 5% alcohol are stable at room temperature for 72 hours (10 to 50 mg/ml). All solutions are stable for 14 days when refrigerated at 39° F (4° C) but should not be used for multiple doses if stored longer than 72 hours. Reconstituted solutions may also be frozen at 0° F (−18° C) and are stable for up to 30 days. Use thawed solution within 24 hours.

Incompatibility
Incompatible with aminoglycosides.

ADMINISTRATION
Intermittent infusion: Infuse diluted solution directly into vein via an established IV line. To minimize vein irritation, use solutions containing 50 mg/ml or less and infuse slowly, that is, over 30 minutes to 2 hours in adults or 10 to 20 minutes in neonates.
Continuous infusion: Add the total daily dosage of reconstituted drug to ordered volume of compatible solution. Adjust rate to deliver required 24-hour volume.

CONTRAINDICATIONS & CAUTIONS
• Contraindicated in hypersensitivity to penicillin and other beta-lactam antibiotics.
• Use cautiously in renal impairment and sodium restriction; sodium content of drug is 6.5 mEq/g.
• Give cautiously in patients with hypokalemia, bleeding disorders, and history of allergic disorders, ulcerative colitis, regional enteritis, or antibiotic-associated colitis.

SPECIAL CONSIDERATIONS
• Obtain specimens for culture and sensitivity tests before giving first dose.

• Give drug at least 1 hour before bacteriostatic antibiotics.
• Monitor electrolyte levels (especially potassium) and cardiac status frequently, because high sodium content of drug may cause electrolyte imbalance and arrhythmias.
• Monitor neurologic status.
• If diarrhea persists during treatment, obtain stool culture to rule out pseudomembranous colitis.

ticarcillin disodium/ clavulanate potassium

Timentin

Pregnancy Risk Category: B

INDICATIONS & DOSAGES
Systemic infections and urinary tract infections, particularly those caused by beta-lactamase-producing organisms—
Adults weighing over 132 lb (60 kg): 3.1 g ticarcillin (as 3 g ticarcillin and 100 mg clavulanic acid) q 4 to 6 hours.
Adults weighing under 132 lb and children age 12 and over: 200 to 300 mg/kg/day given in divided doses q 4 to 6 hours.
Note: Dosage in renal failure reflects creatinine clearance.

PREPARATION & STORAGE
Supplied as a white to pale yellow powder in vials containing 3.1 g (3 g ticarcillin and 100 mg clavulanic acid). Reconstitute by adding 13 ml of sterile water or 0.9% NaCl for a ticarcillin concentration of 200 mg/ml and a clavulanate concentration of 6.7 mg/ml. Before infusion, dilute solution in 50 to 100 ml of 0.9% NaCl, D_5W, or lactated Ringer's solution. Drug is also available in pharmacy-mixed reconstituted piggyback infusion bottles.
Store powder at 70° to 75° F (21° to 24° C). After reconstitution, solutions of 200 mg ticarcillin/ml

T

are potent for 6 hours at room temperature and for up to 72 hours if refrigerated. Lactated Ringer's solution and 0.9% NaCl solutions of 10 to 100 mg ticarcillin/ml remain potent for 24 hours at room temperature and for 7 days if refrigerated. D_5W solutions remain potent for 24 hours at room temperature and for 3 days if refrigerated. Solutions of 100 mg ticarcillin/ml or less in 0.9% NaCl or lactated Ringer's solution may be frozen and stored up to 30 days; 7 days for solutions in D_5W. Use thawed solutions within 8 hours.

Incompatibility
Incompatible with aminoglycosides and sodium bicarbonate. Do not use with other anti-infective agents.

ADMINISTRATION
Intermittent infusion: Give diluted dose over 30 minutes by infusion through a Y-tubing, or use the piggyback method. Temporarily discontinue administration of primary solutions during administration.

CONTRAINDICATIONS & CAUTIONS
• Contraindicated in hypersensitivity to penicillin and other beta-lactam antibiotics.
• Use cautiously in renal impairment, sodium restriction, and electrolyte imbalance.
• Give cautiously in ulcerative colitis, regional enteritis, or antibiotic-associated colitis and history of allergic disorders.

SPECIAL CONSIDERATIONS
• Obtain specimens for culture and sensitivity tests before giving first dose.
• Before giving drug, ask patient about allergic reactions to penicillin.
• If patient is receiving dialysis, administer drug after session is complete.
• Monitor serum sodium and potassium levels closely. Drug has a high sodium content, and clavulanic acid

contributes about 0.15 mEq (6 mg) of potassium per 100 mg.
• Monitor CBC, PT, and bleeding times. Watch for bleeding tendencies and discontinue drug if bleeding occurs.
• If diarrhea persists during therapy, obtain stool culture to rule out pseudomembranous colitis.

tobramycin sulfate

Nebcin ◆

Pregnancy Risk Category: D

INDICATIONS & DOSAGES
Serious bacterial infections, including septicemia, lower respiratory tract infections, meningitis, intra-abdominal infections, complicated or recurrent urinary tract infections, and infections of skin, bone, and skin structures—
Dosage based on actual pretreatment body weight.
Adults: 3 mg/kg daily in equal doses q 8 hours. May be increased to 5 mg/kg daily in three or four equal doses for life-threatening infections.
Children: 6 to 7.5 mg/kg daily in three or four equal doses.
Neonates under age 1 week:
4 mg/kg daily or less in equal doses q 12 hours.
Acute pelvic inflammatory disease—
Adults: initially, 2 mg/kg, then 1.5 mg/kg q 8 hours.
   Note: Adjust dosage in renal impairment.

PREPARATION & STORAGE
Available as a clear, colorless solution in rubber-stopped vials containing 80 mg/2 ml or 20 mg/2 ml and as pediatric injection in 2-ml vials containing 10 mg/ml. Also available as a dry powder (1.2 g), which should be reconstituted with 30 ml of sterile water for injection to a 40 mg/ml concentration. For adults, further dilute the calculated dose in 50 to 100 ml of 0.9% NaCl or dextrose 5%

T

injection. For children, dilution depends on patient needs.

Diluted tobramycin is stable for 24 hours at room temperature.

Incompatibility
Incompatible with beta-lactam antibiotics; cefamandole nafate; cefoperazone; cefotaxime sodium; dextrose 5% in Isolyte E, M, or P; heparin sodium; and IV solutions containing alcohol. Because of other potential incompatibilities, manufacturer recommends that other drugs not be mixed with tobramycin.

ADMINISTRATION
Intermittent infusion: Infuse diluted solution over 20 to 60 minutes.

CONTRAINDICATIONS & CAUTIONS
• Contraindicated in hypersensitivity to drug or other aminoglycosides.
• Use cautiously in elderly patients, neonates, premature infants, and patients with renal impairment or dehydration.
• Also use cautiously in cranial nerve VIII damage.
• In infant botulism, myasthenia gravis, and Parkinson's disease, give cautiously.
• Advise women that drug may cause fetal harm when administered during pregnancy.

SPECIAL CONSIDERATIONS
• Usual duration of treatment is 7 to 10 days.
• Obtain specimens for culture and sensitivity tests before giving first dose.
• In cases of overdose, ensure adequate airway, oxygenation, and ventilation. Ensure adequate hydration and urine output. Hemodialysis effectively reduces serum drug levels and may be necessary in those with abnormal renal function.
• Monitor serum drug levels, especially in neonates, elderly patients, and those with renal impairment. Therapeutic concentration is 4 to 10 mcg/ml.

• Monitor renal function by obtaining periodic BUN and serum creatinine levels.

topotecan hydrochloride

Hycamtin

Pregnancy Risk Category: D

INDICATIONS & DOSAGES
Metastatic carcinoma of the ovary after failure of initial or subsequent chemotherapy—
Adults: 1.5 mg/m^2 given over 30 minutes daily for 5 consecutive days, starting on day 1 of a 21-day cycle. Minimum of four cycles should be given.

Note: Reduce dosage in renal impairment and in severe neutropenia.

PREPARATION & STORAGE
Use caution with preparation and prepare under a vertical laminar flow hood while wearing gloves and protective clothing. If solution contacts the skin or mucous membranes, wash thoroughly with soap and water. Available in 4-mg single-dose vials. Store the vials at controlled room temperature (68° to 77° F [20° to 25° C]). Protect from light. Reconstitute each 4-mg vial with 4 ml of sterile water for injection. Further dilute the appropriate volume of the reconstituted solution with either 0.9% NaCl intravenous infusion or 5% dextrose IV infusion before administration. Use reconstituted product immediately. Reconstituted vials diluted for infusion are stable at room temperature and ambient lighting conditions for 24 hours.

Incompatibility
None reported.

ADMINISTRATION
Intermittent infusion: Infuse ordered amount over 30 minutes.

CONTRAINDICATIONS & CAUTIONS
• Contraindicated in hypersensitivity reactions to drug or to its ingredients; in pregnant or breast-feeding patients, and in those with severe bone marrow depression.
• Use with caution in patients with hepatic or renal impairment.
• Advise women of childbearing age to avoid becoming pregnant during treatment.

SPECIAL CONSIDERATIONS
• Administer granulocyte colony-stimulating factor as ordered.
• Bone marrow suppression is the dose-limiting toxicity of topotecan. Nadir occurs in about 11 days.
• Duration of thrombocytopenia is about 5 days, nadir at 15 days. Blood or platelet transfusions may be necessary.
• Inadvertent extravasation of topotecan has been associated with mild local reactions, such as erythema and bruising.
• Frequently monitor CBC.
• Baseline neutrophil count should be above 1,500 cells/mm³ and platelet count above 100,000 cells/mm³ before first dose is administered.

torsemide

Demadex

Pregnancy Risk Category: B

INDICATIONS & DOSAGES
Treatment of edema associated with heart failure—
Adults: 10 or 20 mg once daily. If response is inadequate, double the dose until desired diuretic response is obtained. Single doses of higher than 200 mg have not been adequately studied.
Chronic renal failure—
Adults: 20 mg once daily. Titrate dosage upward by doubling previous dose until desired diuretic response is obtained. Single doses of higher than 200 mg have not been adequately studied.
Hepatic cirrhosis—
Adults: 5 or 10 mg once daily administered with an aldosterone antagonist or a potassium-sparing diuretic. Titrate dosage upward by doubling previous dose until desired diuretic response is obtained. Single doses of higher than 40 mg have not been adequately studied.

PREPARATION & STORAGE
Available in clear ampules containing 2 ml (20 mg) or 5 ml (50 mg) of a 10 mg/ml solution. Store at room temperature. Do not freeze.

Incompatibility
None reported.

ADMINISTRATION
Direct injection: Give slowly over 2 minutes.

CONTRAINDICATIONS & CAUTIONS
• Contraindicated in hypersensitivity to drug or sulfonylureas and in anuric patients.
• Use cautiously in patients with cirrhosis and ascites.
• As with other ototoxic loop diuretics, exercise caution when administering torsemide.

SPECIAL CONSIDERATIONS
• Flush IV line with NaCl injection USP before and after administration.
• In diuretic potency, 10 to 20 mg torsemide is approximately equivalent to 40 mg furosemide or 1 mg bumetanide. It has a longer duration of action than furosemide, allowing once-daily dosing.
• Monitor for clinical evidence of electrolyte imbalance, hypovolemia, or prerenal azotemia.

T

urokinase

Abbokinase, Abbokinase Open-Cath

Pregnancy Risk Category: B

INDICATIONS & DOSAGES
Pulmonary embolism—
Adults: 4,400 IU/kg initially by infusion, then continuous infusion of 4,400 IU/kg/hour for 12 hours.
Venous catheter occlusion—
Adults: 1 ml of 5,000 IU/ml solution for each clearing procedure.

PREPARATION & STORAGE
Supplied as lyophilized white powder in vials containing 250,000 U. Reconstitute with 5 ml of sterile water for injection (without preservatives) for a solution of 50,000 IU/ml. Do not use bacteriostatic water; it contains preservatives. Dilute solution further with 0.9% NaCl or D_5W. Total volume administered should not exceed 200 ml.

Reconstituted solution should be clear, practically colorless, and without precipitates. To avoid filament formation, roll and tilt vial during reconstitution; avoid shaking. Solution may be filtered through a 0.45-micron or smaller cellulose filter.

Refrigerate vials at 35° to 47° F (2° to 8° C). Because urokinase contains no preservatives, reconstitute immediately before use and discard unused portion. Do not use highly colored solutions, and do not add other drugs to the solution.

Incompatibility
None reported; however, manufacturer recommends that urokinase not be mixed with any other drugs.

ADMINISTRATION
Direct injection: To clear a venous catheter occlusion, slowly inject solution into occluded line, wait 5 minutes, then aspirate. Repeat aspiration attempts q 5 minutes for 30 minutes. If not patent after 30 min-utes, cap line and let urokinase work for 30 to 60 minutes before aspirating. Second injection may be required.
Continuous infusion: Administer initial dose of diluted solution over 10 minutes using an infusion pump. Infuse subsequent doses, as ordered, over 12 hours.

CONTRAINDICATIONS & CAUTIONS
• Contraindicated in active internal bleeding; within 2 months of CVA, intracranial neoplasm, or intracranial or intraspinal surgery; within 10 days of major surgery, severe GI bleeding, organ biopsy, obstetric delivery, or puncture of noncompressible vessels; in severe uncontrolled hypertension; and in recent serious trauma.
• Also contraindicated in recent minor trauma (including CPR), high risk of left heart thrombus, pregnancy, infectious endocarditis, cerebrovascular disease, diabetic hemorrhagic retinopathy, and hemostatic defects.
• Use with extreme caution in any condition in which bleeding would be hazardous or especially difficult to manage.
• Use cautiously in atrial fibrillation or other conditions with risk of cerebral embolism.
• Safe use in children has not been established.

SPECIAL CONSIDERATIONS
• Have typed and crossmatched RBCs and whole blood available to treat hemorrhage.
• Maintain alignment of involved extremity to prevent bleeding at infusion site.
• Avoid IM injections, unnecessary handling of patient, and arterial or venous invasive procedures.
• Follow with heparin, usually within 1 hour after discontinuation of urokinase, to prevent recurrent thrombosis.
• In hemorrhage, stop drug immediately. Give plasma volume expanders (other than dextrans) to replace volume deficits. For severe blood loss,

U

give packed RBCs (rather than whole blood). For rapid reversal of hyperfibrinolysis, possibly give aminocaproic acid (efficacy is not established).
• Monitor for bleeding every 15 minutes for first hour, every 30 minutes for the next 7 hours, and then once each shift.
• Monitor vital signs. Also monitor pulses, color, and sensitivity of extremities every hour.
• Know that hematocrit, plasma fibrinogen, and plasminogen levels may decrease for 12 to 24 hours after therapy stops. Fibrin split products increase similarly. Monitor these levels.

vancomycin hydrochloride

Lyphocin, Vancocin, Vancoled

Pregnancy Risk Category: C

INDICATIONS & DOSAGES
Severe systemic infections caused by susceptible organisms when less toxic drugs are ineffective—
Adults: 500 mg q 6 hours or 1 g q 12 hours.
Children over age 1 month: 40 mg/kg daily in divided doses.
Neonates: 15 mg/kg initially, then 10 mg/kg q 8 hours (older than age 8 days) or 10 mg/kg q 12 hours (age 8 days or younger).
Prophylaxis for bacterial endocarditis in penicillin-allergic patients undergoing dental procedures or upper respiratory tract procedures—
Adults: 1 g 30 to 60 minutes before procedure, followed by oral erythromycin.
Children: 20 mg/kg 30 to 60 minutes before procedure, followed by oral erythromycin.
Prophylaxis for bacterial endocarditis in penicillin-allergic patients undergoing GI or GU procedures—
Adults: 1 g 30 to 60 minutes before procedure in combination with gentamicin.

Children: 20 mg/kg 30 to 60 minutes before procedure in combination with gentamicin.
Note: Adjust dosage in patients with renal impairment.
For anephric patients on dialysis, initial dose is 15 mg/kg, followed by maintenance dose determined by serum levels given q 3 to 7 days.

PREPARATION & STORAGE
Available as an off-white to buff powder in 500-mg and 1-g vials. Reconstitute 500-mg vial with 10 ml and 1-g vial with 20 ml of sterile water for injection for an average concentration of 50 mg/ml. Reconstituted solution is clear and light yellow to light brown. Before administration, dilute in 100 to 200 ml (500 mg in at least 100 ml, 1 g in at least 200 ml) of D_5W or 0.9% NaCl. For continuous infusion, dilute 1 to 2 g in the ordered volume for 24 hours. Inspect before administration for precipitates or discoloration.
Before reconstitution, store vials at room temperature. Reconstituted solutions may be refrigerated for 14 days. When diluted, solutions are stable for 24 hours at room temperature.

Incompatibility
Incompatible with alkaline solutions, aminophylline, amobarbital sodium, chloramphenicol, chlorothiazide, corticosteroids, heavy metals, heparin, methicillin sodium, pentobarbital, phenobarbital, secobarbital sodium, and sodium bicarbonate.

ADMINISTRATION
Intermittent infusion: Infuse diluted dose over at least 60 minutes to reduce risk of local reactions and "redneck" syndrome.
Continuous infusion: Use only when intermittent infusion is not feasible. Add ordered dose to compatible solution and give by IV drip over 24 hours.

V-Z

CONTRAINDICATIONS & CAUTIONS
• Contraindicated in vancomycin hypersensitivity.
• Use cautiously in severe renal insufficiency, in elderly patients, in premature neonates and young infants.
• Also use cautiously in hearing loss, intestinal obstruction, and during pregnancy.

SPECIAL CONSIDERATIONS
• When used preoperatively, give 60-minute infusion before anesthetic induction to reduce risk of infusion-related reactions.
• If "red-neck" syndrome occurs, stop infusion and notify doctor.
• When drug is used to treat staphylococcal endocarditis, therapy should continue for at least 4 weeks.
• Monitor vital signs, especially blood pressure.
• Monitor renal function, WBC counts, and auditory function.
• Also monitor serum vancomycin levels for efficacy and toxicity.

vasopressin (antidiuretic hormone [ADH])

Pitressin Synthetic

Pregnancy Risk Category: C

INDICATIONS & DOSAGES
GI hemorrhage—
Adults: 0.2 to 0.4 U/minute, with increases to 0.9 U/minute if needed. Dosage must be individualized based on patient's response and tolerance.

PREPARATION & STORAGE
Available in 0.5-ml and 1-ml ampules with a concentration of 20 U/ml. For IV infusion, dilute to a concentration of 0.1 to 1 U/ml with 0.9% NaCl or 5% dextrose injection. Store at 59° to 86° F (15° to 30° C). Do not freeze.

Incompatibility
None reported.

ADMINISTRATION
Continuous infusion: Infuse diluted solution through a peripheral vein with a controlled infusion device.

CONTRAINDICATIONS & CAUTIONS
• Contraindicated in chronic nephritis complicated by nitrogen retention.
• Use cautiously in patients with seizure disorders, migraine, asthma, heart failure, vascular disease, angina, coronary thrombosis renal disease, goiter with cardiac complications, arteriosclerosis, or other disease in which rapid addition to extracellular fluid may be hazardous.
• Also use cautiously in children and the elderly.

SPECIAL CONSIDERATIONS
• Use extreme caution to avoid extravasation because of risk of necrosis and gangrene.
• Discontinue vasopressin and restrict water intake until polyuria occurs. Severe water intoxication may require osmotic diuresis with mannitol, hypertonic dextrose, or urea, either alone or with furosemide.
• Establish baseline vital signs and intake and output ratio before therapy.
• Monitor blood pressure twice daily, intake and output, and daily weights.
• Observe for signs of early water intoxication, including drowsiness, listlessness, headache, confusion, and weight gain.
• Monitor electrolytes and ECG periodically.

vecuronium bromide

Norcuron

Pregnancy Risk Category: C

INDICATIONS & DOSAGES
Adjunct to general anesthesia, to facilitate endotracheal intubation and to provide skeletal muscle relaxation

V-Z

during surgery or mechanical ventilation—
Dose depends on anesthetic used, individual needs, and response. Doses are representative and must be adjusted.
Adults: 0.08 to 0.1 mg/kg initially. Maintenance dose, 0.01 to 0.015 mg/kg 20 to 40 minutes after initial dose, then q 12 to 15 minutes, p.r.n., or continuous infusion started at 1 mcg/kg/minute (0.001 mg/kg/minute).
Children: dosage individualized.
  Note: Reduce dosage in patients with renal or hepatic impairment.

PREPARATION & STORAGE
Supplied as a sterile, nonpyrogenic, freeze-dried buffered cake composed of fine crystalline particles. Available in 5- and 10-ml vials containing 10 mg drug and diluent. For infusion, dilute further by adding 10 ml of reconstituted drug to 100 ml of D_5W, 0.9% NaCl, dextrose 5% in 0.9% or 0.45% NaCl, or dextrose 5% in lactated Ringer's solution. Vecuronium is compatible with all IV solutions.
  Before reconstitution, store at room temperature and protect from light. After reconstitution with bacteriostatic water, use within 24 hours; with other solutions, use within 8 hours.

Incompatibility
None reported.

ADMINISTRATION
Direct injection: Inject dose directly into tubing of an IV line containing a free-flowing, compatible solution.
Continuous infusion: Begin infusion 20 to 40 minutes after initial dose by direct injection. Determine rates by carefully observing neuromuscular blockade with a peripheral nerve stimulator. Infusion rates range from 0.8 to 1.2 mcg/kg/minute (0.0008 to 0.0012 mg/kg/minute) with a 1:10 dilution.

CONTRAINDICATIONS & CAUTIONS
• Contraindicated in hypersensitivity to drug.
• Use cautiously in neuromuscular disease, bronchogenic carcinoma, CV impairment, edema, electrolyte imbalance, or dehydration.
• Also administer cautiously in elderly or debilitated patients.
• Use with caution in patients with myasthenia gravis, renal failure, hepatic disease, pulmonary impairment, respiratory depression, or severe obesity.

SPECIAL CONSIDERATIONS
• Patients with bromide intolerance may also be sensitive to vecuronium.
• Know that infants are especially sensitive to drug effects.
• Provide mechanical ventilation with endotracheal intubation until reversal of neuromuscular blockade is adequate. As ordered, reverse blockade with acetylcholinesterase inhibitors, such as neostigmine, pyridostigmine, or edrophonium given with atropine or glycopyrrolate.
• Continuously monitor patient throughout infusion.
• A nerve stimulator and train-of-four monitoring are recommended to assess recovery of muscle strength.

verapamil hydrochloride

Calan, Isoptin ◆
Pregnancy Risk Category: C

INDICATIONS & DOSAGES
Supraventricular arrhythmias—
Adults: 0.075 to 0.15 mg/kg (5 to 10 mg) by IV push over 2 minutes, with continuous ECG and blood pressure monitoring. Repeat dose in 30 minutes if no response occurs.
Children ages 1 to 15: 0.1 to 0.3 mg/kg as bolus over 2 minutes, with continuous ECG monitoring.

V-Z

Repeat dose in 30 minutes if no response occurs.
Children under age 1: 0.1 to 0.2 mg/kg as bolus over 2 minutes, with continuous ECG monitoring. Repeat dose in 30 minutes if no response occurs.

PREPARATION & STORAGE
Supplied as a solution of 2.5 mg/ml. Store at room temperature and protect from light and freezing. Drug is stable for 24 hours at 77° F (25° C) in most common infusion solutions when protected from light. It is compatible with D_5W, 0.9% NaCl, and lactated Ringer's solution.

Incompatibility
Incompatible with albumin, aminophylline, amphotericin B, ampicillin sodium, co-trimoxazole, dobutamine, hydralazine, mezlocillin sodium, nafcillin, oxacillin sodium, sodium bicarbonate, and trimethoprim.

ADMINISTRATION
Direct injection: Administer undiluted drug at a rate of 5 to 10 mg over at least 2 minutes. Inject into vein or into an IV line containing a free-flowing, compatible solution. In elderly patients, give over at least 3 minutes to reduce adverse effects.

CONTRAINDICATIONS & CAUTIONS
• Contraindicated in hypersensitivity to drug.
• Also contraindicated in second- or third-degree AV block; in severe hypotension, cardiogenic shock, or pulmonary artery wedge pressure exceeding 20 mm Hg; and in Wolff-Parkinson-White syndrome.
• Use cautiously in children (particularly neonates).
• Also use cautiously in Duchenne-type muscular dystrophy, extreme bradycardia, heart failure, hypertrophic cardiomyopathy, moderate ventricular dysfunction, sick sinus syndrome, and mild to moderate hypotension.
• Give with caution in renal impairment and renal or hepatic failure.

• Caution women against breast-feeding during therapy.

SPECIAL CONSIDERATIONS
• If giving digoxin concomitantly, reduce digoxin dose by half and monitor ECG for possible AV block.
• Notify the doctor if signs of heart failure, such as dependent edema or dyspnea, develop.
• Administer dose over 3 minutes in older patients.
• Monitor ECG.

vinblastine sulfate (VLB)

Velban, Velbe◇, Velsar
Pregnancy Risk Category: D

INDICATIONS & DOSAGES
Vinblastine may be used alone or in combination with other drugs in various schedules and regimens. Dosage reflects response to drug and degree of bone marrow depression.
Hodgkin's disease and malignant lymphomas (including lymphocytic lymphoma and diffuse, poorly differentiated, well-differentiated, or histiocytic lymphomas); breast, testicular, renal cell, or head and neck cancer; Kaposi's sarcoma; advanced mycosis fungoides; choriocarcinoma; Letterer-Siwe disease (histiocytosis); germ-cell ovarian tumors; chronic leukemias; neuroblastoma—
Adults: initially 0.1 mg/kg weekly or 3.7 mg/m² weekly. Successive weekly doses increased by increments of 0.05 mg/kg (or 1.8 to 1.9 mg/m²) until WBC count falls to 3,000/mm³, tumor size decreases, or maximum dose of 0.5 mg/kg (or 18.5 mg/m²) is reached (usual range, 0.15 to 0.2 mg/kg or 5.5 to 7.4 mg/m²). Subsequent maintenance doses (one increment smaller than final initial dose q 7 to 14 days, or 10 mg once or twice monthly) should not be given until WBC

◆ Also available in Canada. ◇ Available in Canada only.

count (after preceding dose) returns to 4,000/mm³.

Children: initially 2.5 mg/m² weekly, then successive weekly doses increased in increments of 1.25 mg/m² until WBC count falls to 3,000/mm³, tumor size decreases, or a maximum dose of 7.5 mg/m² is reached. Subsequent maintenance doses (one increment smaller than final initial dose q 7 to 14 days) are not recommended until WBC count (after preceding dose) returns to 4,000/mm³.

PREPARATION & STORAGE
To avoid mutagenic, teratogenic, and carcinogenic risks when preparing and administering drug, use a biological containment cabinet, wear disposable gloves and mask, and use syringes with luer-lock fittings to prevent drug leakage. Dispose of needles, syringes, vials, and unused drug properly, and avoid contaminating work surfaces.

Avoid drug contact with eyes because severe irritation and possibly corneal ulceration may result. If contact occurs, wash the eye with water immediately.

Supplied in 10-mg vials. Reconstitute by adding 10 ml of 0.9% NaCl injection containing phenol or benzyl alcohol as a preservative to yield 1 mg/ml. Also available in 10-ml aqueous solution of 10 mg/ml. Store powder and reconstituted solution at 36° to 46° F (2° to 8° C). Solution is stable at these temperatures for up to 30 days without significant potency loss.

Incompatibility
Incompatible with furosemide.

ADMINISTRATION
Direct injection: Inject dose rapidly into side port of a free-flowing patent IV line or inject directly into vein over 1 minute. (Avoid injecting drug into extremity veins with compromised circulation because of enhanced risk of thrombosis.)

If extravasation occurs, stop the injection immediately and inject remaining dose into another vein. Treat the affected area immediately.

CONTRAINDICATIONS & CAUTIONS
• Contraindicated in hypersensitivity to drug or if WBC count is below 3,000/mm³.
• Also contraindicated in bacterial, fungal, or viral infection and in existing or recent chickenpox or herpes zoster infection.
• Use cautiously in skin ulcers, bone marrow depression, metastasis to the bone marrow, and with previous cytotoxic drug therapy or radiation therapy.
• Use with caution in hepatic impairment, history of gout or urate renal calculi, and in debilitated or elderly patients.
• Advise women to avoid becoming pregnant during treatment.

SPECIAL CONSIDERATIONS
• Provide adequate oral hydration and, as ordered, also give allopurinol to alkalinize urine.
• Therapy should continue for 4 to 6 weeks or longer.
• Before and during therapy, monitor hematocrit, platelet count, total and differential WBC count, AST, ALT, and serum bilirubin, creatinine, LD, BUN, and uric acid levels.
• Monitor for life-threatening acute bronchospasm and notify doctor immediately if this occurs.
• Advise patient to report fever, sore throat, chills, sore mouth, or unusual bleeding or bruising, especially if receiving myelosuppressant drugs.
• Advise patient to report symptoms of neurotoxicity (such as paresthesia or loss of deep tendon reflexes).

V-Z

vincristine sulfate

Oncovin◆

Pregnancy Risk Category: D

INDICATIONS & DOSAGES

Dosage adjustment (usually reduced) may be necessary. Vincristine may be used in combination with other drugs, altering incidence or severity of adverse effects.

Leukemias (especially acute lymphoblastic leukemia); Hodgkin's disease and malignant lymphomas (mainly diffuse histiocytic or lymphocytic); osteogenic and other sarcomas (including Kaposi's sarcoma and Ewing's sarcoma); Wilms' tumor; rhabdomyosarcoma; multiple myeloma; medulloblastoma; neuroblastoma; mycosis fungoides; lung, breast, and ovarian carcinoma—

Adults: depending on protocol, 0.01 to 0.03 mg/kg weekly as single dose or 0.4 mg to 1.4 mg/m² weekly as single dose.

Children weighing over 22 lb (10 kg): 1.5 to 2 mg/m² weekly as single dose.

Children weighing 22 lb or less: 0.05 mg/kg weekly.

PREPARATION & STORAGE

Use extreme caution when preparing and administering vincristine to avoid mutagenic, teratogenic, and carcinogenic risks. Use a biological containment cabinet, wear disposable gloves and mask, and use syringes with luer-lock fittings to prevent drug leakage. Dispose of needles, syringes, vials, and unused drug properly and avoid contaminating work surfaces.

Avoid drug contact with eyes because severe irritation and possibly corneal ulceration may result. If contact occurs, wash eye immediately with water.

Supplied in 1-, 2-, and 5-ml vials containing 1 mg/ml. For infusion, dilute to ordered concentration and volume with a compatible IV solution, such as D_5W or 0.9% NaCl injection. Undiluted drug is best stored at 36° to 46° F (2° to 8° C); however, it is stable at room temperature for at least 1 month. Protect from light to prevent degradation.

Because vincristine is a vesicant, assemble necessary supplies for managing extravasation before administration. Also ensure a patent IV line.

Incompatibility

Incompatible with furosemide.

ADMINISTRATION

Direct injection: Inject dose over 1 minute directly into vein or into side port of a newly started IV line. Use a 23G or 25G winged-tip infusion set. If possible, use distal rather than major veins, which allows for repeated venipuncture if necessary.

If extravasation occurs, stop the injection immediately and inject the remaining dose into another vein. Give a local injection of hyaluronidase and apply moderate heat or cold compresses to minimize discomfort and cellulitis.

Intermittent infusion: not recommended; however, drug has been diluted and given as a slow infusion over 4 to 8 hours.

Continuous infusion: not recommended.

CONTRAINDICATIONS & CAUTIONS

• Contraindicated in hypersensitivity to drug.

• Also contraindicated in existing or recent exposure to chickenpox or herpes zoster and in patients with the demyelinating form of Charcot-Marie-Tooth syndrome.

• Use cautiously in hepatic impairment, infection, or neuromuscular disease and when large fluid intake is required.

SPECIAL CONSIDERATIONS

• Start a prophylactic bowel regimen before treatment and continue throughout treatment.

• Hematologic toxicity with vincristine is less than that with other antineoplastic agents. Mild leukopenia, anemia, and thrombocytopenia are rare at usual doses. However, drug is highly toxic with a low therapeutic index.
• Provide adequate oral hydration and give allopurinol, as ordered, to alkalinize urine.
• As ordered, administer anticonvulsant doses of phenobarbital and give enemas to prevent ileus. Monitor CV function and hematologic studies.
• Before and during therapy, monitor hematocrit, platelet count, ALT, AST, total and differential WBC counts, and serum bilirubin, creatinine, LD, BUN, and uric acid levels. Leukopenia usually reaches nadir within 4 days.
• Notify patient that sensorimotor dysfunction may become progressively more severe with treatment.

vinorelbine tartrate

Navelbine

Pregnancy Risk Category: D

INDICATIONS & DOSAGES

Alone or as adjunct therapy with cisplatin for first-line treatment of ambulatory patients with nonresectable advanced non-small-cell lung cancer (NSCLC); alone or with cisplatin in stage IV of NSCLC; with cisplatin in stage III of NSCLC—
Adults: 30 mg/m^2 weekly. In combination therapy, 30 mg/m^2 with 120 mg/m^2 of cisplatin, given on days 1 and 29, then q 6 weeks.
Note: Adjust dosage for hematologic toxicity.

PREPARATION & STORAGE

Exercise caution when handling and preparing the solution of Navelbine. The use of gloves is recommended. Skin reactions may occur with accidental exposure. If the solution contacts the skin or mucosa, immediately wash with soap and water. If contact with the eyes occurs, flush eyes with water thoroughly and immediately to prevent severe irritation.

Supplied in 1-ml and 5-ml single-use vials at a concentration of 10 mg/ml. For direct injection, dilute calculated dose to a concentration between 1.5 and 3 mg/ml, with 5% dextrose injection or 0.9% NaCl injection, USP. For infusion, the calculated dose should be diluted to a concentration between 0.5 and 2 mg/ml, with 5% dextrose injection, 0.9% NaCl injection, USP; 0.45% NaCl injection, USP; 5% dextrose and 0.45% NaCl injection, USP; Ringer's injection, USP; or lactated Ringer's injection, USP.

Store the vials under refrigeration at 36° F to 46° F (2° to 8° C). Protect from light. Avoid freezing. Diluted Navelbine may be used for up to 24 hours under normal room light when stored in polypropylene syringes or polyvinyl chloride bags at 41° to 86° F (5° to 30° C).

Incompatibility

None reported.

ADMINISTRATION

Direct injection: administer over 6 to 10 minutes into the side port of a free-flowing IV line closest to the IV bag followed by flushing with at least 75 to 125 ml of one of the solutions.
Intermittent infusion: administer diluted solution over 6 to 10 minutes as above.

CONTRAINDICATIONS & CAUTIONS

• Contraindicated in patients with pretreatment granulocyte counts below 1,000 cells/mm^3.
• Use with extreme caution in patients whose bone marrow reserve may have been compromised by prior or radiation or chemotherapy or whose bone marrow function is recovering from the effects of previous chemotherapy.
• Use with caution in patients with hepatic impairment.

V-Z

SPECIAL CONSIDERATIONS
• Avoid extravasation because of risk
of severe tissue irritation, necrosis,
and thrombophlebitis. If extravasation occurs, discontinue drug immediately and use different vein for remaining infusion.
• Provide supportive therapy, with
antibiotics and blood transfusions as
needed.
• Continue to monitor peripheral
blood count throughout therapy.
• Monitor deep tendon reflexes; loss
may be associated with toxicity.
• Monitor patient for hypersensitivity reactions.
• Advise patient to report fever, sore
throat, chills, bleeding, or bruising
immediately.

V-Z

APPENDICES
AND
INDEX

Electrolyte components of IV solutions

SOLUTION	Sodium (mEq/L)	Potassium (mEq/L)	Osmolarity (mOsm/L)
Aminosyn 3.5% M	47	13	477
Aminosyn 7% with electrolytes	70	66	1,013
Aminosyn 8.5% with electrolytes	70	66	1,160
Ammonium chloride 2.14%	-	-	Additive is hypertonic
Dextrose 2.5% in half-strength lactated Ringer's solution	65	2	265
Dextrose 5% in electrolyte no. 48	25	20	348
Dextrose 5% in electrolyte no. 75	40	35	402
Dextrose 5% in sodium chloride 0.11%	19	-	290
Dextrose 5% in sodium chloride 0.2%	34 or 38.5	-	320-330
Dextrose 5% in sodium chloride 0.33%	51 or 56	-	355-365
Dextrose 50% with electrolyte pattern A	84	40	2,800
Dextrose 50% with electrolyte pattern N	90	80	2,875
Dextrose 50% with electrolytes #1	110	80	2,917
50% Travert and electrolyte no. 2	56	25	449
FreAmine III 3% with electrolytes	35	24.5	405
Ionosol B in dextrose 5% in water	57	25	426
Ionosol MB in dextrose 5% in water	25	20	352
Ionosol T in dextrose 5% in water	40	35	432
Isolyte E	140	10	310
Isolyte G with dextrose 5%	65	17	555
Lactated Ringer's solution	130	4	275
Normosol-M in dextrose 5% in water	40	13	363
Plasma-Lyte A	140	5	294
Plasma-Lyte R	140	10	312
ProcalAmine	35	24	735

*Tonicity key: 1 = hypotonic; 2 = isotonic; 3 = hypertonic.

Tonicity*	Calcium (mEq/L)	Magnesium (mEq/L)	Chloride (mEq/L)	Acetate (mEq/L)	Phosphate (millimoles)	Other (mEq/L)
3	-	3	40	58	3.5	amino acids 3.5%
3	-	10	96	124	30	amino acids 7%
3	-	10	98	142	30	amino acids 8.5%
3	-	-	400	-	-	ammonium 400
2	1.4-1.5	-	54-55	-	-	lactate 14
2	-	3	24	-	3	lactate 23
3	-	-	48	-	15	lactate 20
2	-	-	19	-	-	-
2	-	-	34 or 38.5	-	-	-
2	-	-	51 or 56	-	-	-
3	10	16	115	-	-	gluconate 13 sulfate 16
3	-	16	150	-	28	sulfate 16
3	-	16	140	36	24	-
3	-	6	56	-	12.5	lactate 25
3	-	5	41	44	3.5	amino acids 3%
3	-	5	49	-	7	lactate 25
2	-	3	22	-	3	lactate 23
3	-	-	40	-	15	lactate 20
2	5	3	103	49	-	citrate 8
3	-	-	149	-	-	ammonium 70
2	2.7-3	-	109 or 110	-	-	lactate 28
3	-	3	40	16	-	-
2	-	3	98	27	-	gluconate 23
2	5	3	103	47	-	lactate 8
3	3	5	41	47	3.5	amino acids 3% glycerin 3%

(continued)

Electrolyte components of IV solutions *(continued)*

SOLUTION	Sodium (mEq/L)	Potassium (mEq/L)	Osmolarity (mOsm/L)
Ringer's solution	147 or 147.5	4	310
Sodium bicarbonate	598	-	1,190- 1,203
Sodium chloride 0.45%	77	-	154
Sodium chloride 0.9%	154	-	308
Sodium chloride 3%	513	-	1,030
Sodium chloride 5%	855	-	1,710
Sodium lactate 1/6 M	167	-	330
Travasol M 3.5% with electrolyte no. 45	25	15	450
Travasol 5.5% with electrolytes	70	60	850
Travasol 8.5% with electrolytes	70	60	1,160
Fat emulsion 10%, 20%, 30%	-	-	258- 310

*Tonicity key: 1 = hypotonic; 2 = isotonic; 3 = hypertonic.

Tonicity*	Calcium (mEq/L)	Magnesium (mEq/L)	Chloride (mEq/L)	Acetate (mEq/L)	Phosphate (millimoles)	Other (mEq/L)
2	4 or 4.5	-	155 or 156	-	-	-
3	-	-	-	-	-	-
1	-	-	77	-	-	-
2	-	-	154	-	-	-
3	-	-	513	-	-	-
3	-	-	855	-	-	-
2	-	-	-	-	-	lactate 167
3	-	5	25	52	7.5	-
3	-	10	70	102	30	-
3	-	10	70	141	30	-
2	-	-	-	-	-	-

Estimating body surface area in children

Pediatric drug dosages should be calculated on the basis of body surface area or body weight. If your pediatric patient is of average size, find his weight and corresponding surface area in the box. Otherwise, to use the nomogram, lay a straightedge on the correct height and weight points for your patient, and observe the point where it intersects on the surface area scale. *Note:* Don't use drug dosages based on body surface area in premature or full-term newborns. Instead, use body weight.

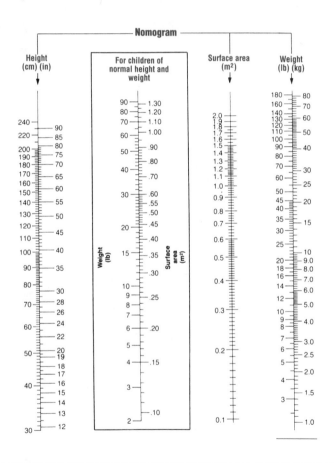

Nelson Textbook of Pediatrics, 15th edition. Courtesy W.B.Saunders Co., Philadelphia.

Estimating body surface area in adults

Lay a straightedge from the patient's height in the left-hand column to his weight in the right-hand column. The intersection of this line with the center scale reveals the body surface area. The adult nomogram is especially useful in calculating dosages for chemotherapy.

Height	Body surface	Mass

Geigy Scientific Tables, vol. 5, 8th ed. (1990). Courtesy Novaritis, Basel, Switzerland.

Infusion therapy manufacturers

This chart shows selected manufacturers of infusion therapy–related products along with their Web site addresses and phone numbers. A key (below) designates general categories of products made by each manufacturer.

Name	1	2	3	4	5
Abbott Laboratories	X	X	X	X	X
Alaris	X				
Arrow International Inc.	X			X	
B. Braun Medical/McGraw Inc.	X		X	X	
Bard Access Systems	X	X	X	X	X
Baxa Corporation	X		X		
Baxter Healthcare Corp.	X	X	X	X	
Becton Dickenson Infusion Therapy Systems		X	X	X	
Block Medical, Inc.	X				
Catheter Innovations				X	X
Centurian Products		X			
Cook Inc.				X	X
Davol Inc.		X	X		
Eli Lilly and Company					
Gesco International Inc.	X			X	
Gish Biomedical Inc.	X		X		
HDC Corporation				X	X
ICU Medical Inc.				X	
Infusion Technology Inc.	X	X	X		
IV House			X		
Johnson and Johnson Medical Inc.		X	X	X	
Kawasumi Laboratories America, Inc.	X				
Luther Medical Products			X	X	
McGaw Incorporated					
3M Health Care		X			
10MED					
Medi-flex Hospital Products		X	X	X	X
Medi-Tech/Boston Scientific Corporation				X	X
Microject	X				
Option Care Inc.	*				
Repro-Med, Inc.	X				
SIMS Deltec	X		X	X	X
Strato Infusaid					X
Tristate Hospital Supply Corporation					
U.S. Medical Instruments, Inc.					
Venetec International		X			
Vygon Corporation		X	X	X	

Key: 1. Delivery devices and infusion pumps. 2. Dressings. 3. Procedure kits/supplies.
4. Midline and PICC catheters. 5. Tunneled catheters and implanted ports.
6. Peripheral IV catheters. 7. Pharmaceuticals. 8. Needleless systems.

* National Home Infusion Provider

6	7	8	Web site address	Phone number
X	X		www.abbott.com	1-800-ABBOTT3
			www.alarismed.com	1-800-458-7854
X	X	X	www.arrowintl.com	1-800-523-8446
		X	www.bbraunusa.com	1-800-523-9676
X		X	www.bardaccess.com	1-800-555-PICC
		X	N/A	1-800-525-9567
	X	X	www.baxter.com	1-800-422-9837
X		X	www.bd.com	1-800-237-4554
			N/A	1-800-944-1501
			www.pasv.com	1-800-418-2828
			N/A	1-800-248-4058
			www.cookgroup.com	1-800-457-4500
			www.davol.com	(401) 463-7000
		X	www.lilly.com	1-800-951-0674
			N/A	1-800-531-5814
X		X	N/A	1-800-938-0531
			N/A	1-800-227-8162
		X	www.icumed.com	1-800-824-7890
		X	N/A	1-800-999-9484
			N/A	1-800-530-0440
X	X	X	www.johnsonandjohnson.com	1-800-465-3141
			N/A	(813) 630-5554
X		X	www.luthermedical.com	1-800-227-2918
		X	N/A	1-800-624-2963
			N/A	1-800-228-3957
		X	www.10med.com	1-800-621-3347
			N/A	1-800-554-0880
			www.bsci.com	1-800-225-3238
			N/A	1-888-642-7646
			www.optioncare.com	1-800-879-6137
			N/A	1-800-624-9600
			www.deltec.com	1-800-426-2448
			N/A	1-800-637-5006
		X	754573663@compuserve.com	1-800-248-4058
		X	N/A	1-800-723-3762
			N/A	1-800-833-3895
		X	N/A	1-800-544-4907

Infusion therapy organizations

Below is a list of selected organizations related to infusion therapy along with their phone numbers and Web site addresses where available.

Organization	Phone number	Web site address
Academy of Medical/Surgical Nurses	(609) 256-2323	N/A
American Association of Critical Care Nurses	1-800-899-2226	www.aacn.org
American Association of Neuro-science Nurses (AANN)	1-800-477-AANN	www.aann.org
American Association of Nurse Anesthetists (AANA)	(847) 692-7050	www.aana.com
American Nephrology Nurses Association (ANNA)	(609) 256-2320	www.inurse.com/~ANNA/
American Pharmaceutical Association (APA)	(202) 628-4410	N/A
American Red Cross Blood and Tissue Services	1-888-545-7800	www.redcross.org
American Society of Health System Pharmacists (ASHP)	(301) 657-3000	www.ashp.org
American Society of Parenteral and Enteral Nutrition (ASPEN)	1-800-727-4567	www.clinnutr.org
American Society of Peri-anesthesia Nurses (ASPAN)	(609) 845-5557	www.aspan.org
Association of Operating Room Nurses (AORN)	1-800-755-2676	www.aorn.org
Association of Pediatric Oncology Nurses	(847) 375-4724	www.apon.org
Canadian Intravenous Nurses Association (CINA)	(416) 292-0687	N/A
Emergency Care Research Institute (ECRI) (independent medical device testing agency)	(610) 825-6000	N/A
Emergency Nurses Association (ENA)	(847) 698-9400	www.ena.org
Intravenous Nurses Society (INS)	(617) 441-3008	www.ins1.org
Intravenous Nurses Certification Corporation	(617) 441-3008	www.ins1.org
League of Intravenous Therapy Education	(412) 678-5025	www.lite.org
National Alliance for Infusion Therapy	(202) 624-7289	N/A
National Association of Orthopedic Nurses (NAON)	(609) 256-2310	www.naon.inurse.com
National Association of Vascular Access Networks (NAVAN)	1-888-57NAVAN	N/A
National Home Infusion Association (NHIA)	(703) 549-3740	N/A
Oncology Nursing Society (ONS)	(412) 921-7373	www.ons.org
US Food and Drug Administration	1-800-741-8138	www.fda.gov

Selected references

American Hospital Formulary Service 1998 Drug Information. Bethesda, Md: American Society of Health-System Pharmacists, Inc., 1998.

Andris, D.A., and Krzywda, E.A. "Catheter Pinch-Off Syndrome: Recognition and Management," *Journal of Intravenous Nursing* 20(5):233-37, September-October 1997.

CDC. "Guideline for Prevention of Intravascular Device-Related Infections," *American Journal of Infection Control* 24(4):262-93, 1996.

Comeau, C. J. "The Nurses's Role in Informed Consent," *Journal of Nursing Law* 1(2):5-15, 1996.

Giving Drugs by Advanced Techniques. Springhouse, Pa.: Springhouse Corporation, 1993.

Hadaway, L. "Vascular Access in Home Care: 1997 Update," *Infusion* 4(1):18-36, 1997.

Intravenous Nurses Society. "Revised Intravenous Nursing Standards of Practice," *Journal of Intravenous Nursing* 21:15, 1998.

Levin, T. "Central Intravenous Lines: Your Role," *Nursing96* 26:48-49, April 1996.

Masoorli, S., et al. "Danger Points: How to Prevent Nerve Injuries from Venipuncture," *Nursing98* 28(9):35-39, September 1998.

NAVAN's Resource Guide to Vascular Access. Drapier, Utah: National Association of Vascular Access Networks, 1997.

Nurse's Handbook of Home Infusion Therapy. Springhouse, Pa.: Springhouse Corporation, 1997.

Renner, C., et al. "Vascular Access in Home Care: Current Trends," *Infusion* 3(10):11-25, 1996.

Ryder, M. A. "Peripheral Access Options," *Surgical Oncology Clinics of North America,* 4(3):407-08, July 1995.

Smith, J. "Thrombotic Complications in Intravenous Access," *Journal of Intravenous Nursing* 21(2):96-99, 1998.

Terry, J., et al., eds. *Intravenous Therapy: Clinical Principles and Practice.* Philadelphia: W. B. Saunders Co., 1995.

Weinstein, S. *Plumer's Principles and Practice of Intravenous Therapy,* 6th ed. Philadelphia: Lippincott-Raven Pubs., 1997.